PRAISE FOR
THE PAIN CURE

"Remarkably comprehensive."

—Paul J. Rosch, M.D., F.A.C.P., president, The American
Institute of Stress, and clinical professor of medicine
and psychiatry, New York Medical College

• • •

"A must-read for anyone interested in conquering chronic
pain!"

—Ronald Klatz, D.O., president, American
Academy of Anti-Aging Medicine

• • •

"A book about fun....Dr. Khalsa teaches you to overcome different kinds of pain in multiple ways, so you can again love,
live, and succeed. I know this from firsthand experience."

—Somers H. White, C.M.C., C.P.A.E., president,
Somers White Company, Inc.

• • •

"THE PAIN CURE works. It provides the keys to life with less
pain, and sometimes, through prayer and meditation, to life
without pain....It can be the first step or a final step toward
wellness and joy."

—Michael Loes, M.D., Maricopa Medical Center,
Arizona Pain Institute

"Unique...Dr. Khalsa's comprehensive and compassionate approach, backed by extensive clinical experience and scientific evidence, will clearly start you on the right path to healing your chronic pain."

—Ray Sahelian, M.D., director, Longevity Research Center, and author of *5-HTP: Nature's Serotonin Solution*

• • •

"THE PAIN CURE is about more than controlling pain. It is about replacing pain with a healing lifestyle."

—Richard S. Weiner, Ph.D., executive director, The American Academy of Pain Management

• • •

"A readable, user-friendly style...a must-read."

—Hyla Cass, M.D., author of *St. John's Wort: Nature's Blues Buster*

• • •

"Dr. Khalsa knows by experience the challenges of treating chronic pain....His book provides a crucial road map for pain relief."

—Martin L. Rossman, M.D., author of *Healing Yourself: A Step-by-Step Program to Better Health Through Imagery*

THE
PAIN
CURE

THE PROVEN MEDICAL PROGRAM THAT HELPS END YOUR CHRONIC PAIN

DHARMA SINGH KHALSA, M.D.
with CAMERON STAUTH

WARNER BOOKS

A Time Warner Company

The program described in this book is not intended to be a substitute for medical care and advice. You are advised to consult with your health care professional with regard to all matters relating to your health, including matters which may require diagnosis or medical attention. In particular, if you have any special condition requiring medical attention, or if you are taking or have been advised to take (or to refrain from taking) any medication, you should consult regularly with your physician regarding possible modification of the program contained in the book.

The identity of some of the patients referred to in this book, and certain details about them, have been modified or are presented in composite form.

The information provided in this book is based upon sources that the authors believe to be reliable. All such information regarding specific products and companies is current as of August 1998.

Copyright © 1999 by Dharma Singh Khalsa, M.D., and Cameron Stauth
All rights reserved.

Warner Books, Inc., 1271 Avenue of the Americas, New York, NY 10020
Visit our Web site at www.twbookmark.com

W A Time Warner Company

Printed in the United States of America
Originally published in hardcover by Warner Books, Inc.
First Trade Printing: May 2000
10 9 8 7 6 5 4 3

The Library of Congress has cataloged the hardcover edition as follows:

Singh Khalsa, Dharma.
The pain cure : the proven medical program that helps end your chronic pain /
Dharma Singh Khalsa, with Cameron Stauth.
p.   cm.
ISBN 0-446-52305-4
1. Chronic pain—Treatment—Popular works.   I. Stauth, Cameron.
II. Title.
RB127.S521999
616'.0472—dc21   98-36540
                                                        CIP

ISBN 0-446-67586-5 (pbk.)

Cover design by Michael Accordino
Book design by H. Roberts Design

For all people in pain everywhere:
May this book set you free

and
For David Stauth

Acknowledgments

Many of the people who were so instrumental in the success of our first book, *Brain Longevity,* were again very helpful and supportive.

I must first thank my spiritual teacher, The Sri Singh Sahib, Yogi Bhajan, for everything he has done for humanity.

Cameron Stauth, my co-author, worked long and hard to bring this book to production. His research initiative and writing ability are par excellence.

Cam and I again salute the vision of our agent, Richard Pine, who got *The Pain Cure* off the ground. Thank you, Richard, for your unwavering support and insight. Artie Pine was also there when we needed him, and his suggestions were, as always, astute.

Appreciation to Maureen Egen, the President and C.O.O. of Warner Books, for her outstanding leadership. We are very happy and blessed to be working under her guidance. Jackie Joiner, Warner's secret weapon and a real friend, was always helpful in getting things done. Besides that, Jackie is a lot of fun to talk to and work with.

Our editors at Warner Books, Colleen Kapklein and Diana Baroni, did a fantastic job with the manuscript, and we know we have a great future together.

My personal thanks to Arielle Ford of the Ford Group in La Jolla, California, for doing an outstanding job as my publicist. I think Deepak's right: Arielle is the best publicist in the world.

I would like to thank and acknowledge all of my friends and colleagues who reviewed the manuscript and wrote comments.

Special thanks to Jerry Calkins, Ph.D., M.D., and Michael Loes, M.D., of the Arizona Pain Institute; Richard Weiner, Ph.D., of the American Academy of Pain Management; and Mark Hahn, D.O., of the Penn State College of Medicine. I also salute Somers and Susan White for the sage advice in all matters and their priceless friendship.

My love and admiration to my beautiful wife, Kirti, for her tireless efforts in coordinating all our activities and still having energy left over to keep a wonderful home. A big kiss to Sat and Hari, my two children, who make it all worthwhile. God bless you and protect you everywhere.

A note of gratitude to my fine staff: two-time Mr. Universe Nordine Zouareg, M.A., Luz Elena Shearer, M.S., and Linda DiCamillo, my personal assistant during this project.

And to reiterate what I said in the dedication: To all people in pain everywhere—may this book set you free.

Dharma Singh Khalsa, M.D.
Tuscon, Arizona

Dr. Dharma Singh Khalsa, one of the few true innovators in modern medicine, spent many years developing and perfecting a treatment program for chronic pain that now stands as a vital monument to his scientific acumen, to his deep caring for others, and to his spiritual strength, which enabled him to continue well past a point that would have exhausted most people. For including me in this tremendous effort, I will always be grateful.

I am also grateful for the important help and constant good cheer of his wonderful wife, Kirti, whose spirit is one with that of Dr. Khalsa and his work.

Like Dr. Khalsa, I am also indebted to my longtime and loyal friend Richard Pine, and to his father, and to Maureen Egen, Colleen Kapklein, and Diana Baroni.

Thanks, too, to Sandra Stahl, who worked with an ethic of excellence on every page of this book.

Through this book and eleven before it, I've had the constant love of my wife, Shari, and it has been the source of my energy. More recently, I've enjoyed the love of my amazing children, Gabriel and Adrienne. My family is a constant reminder that working hard for people who truly appreciate you is the most important work of all.

Cameron Stauth
Portland, Oregon

Contents

THE
PAIN
CURE

PART ONE

How
Pain
Works

1

Why You Hurt

Pain is a more terrible Lord of mankind than even death itself.
—ALBERT SCHWEITZER

Torture Victims

If you are in chronic pain, you probably feel alone and frightened. You may feel helpless. You might even feel as if life's no longer worth living. I understand. I understand *completely*. You have the worst medical problem a person can have.

Chronic pain is the most devastating physical malady that exists. It's even more overwhelming than having a terminal illness, according to patients of mine who have suffered from both conditions.

Being in pain, hour after hour, day after day, rips away your strength, your hope, your personality, and even your love.

Chronic pain is a demonic force that can destroy everything it touches.

But people are *strong*. I'm constantly amazed by their courage. When life knocks them down, they struggle back up. They do it again and again, all their lives.

If you're a pain patient who is reading this page right now, you must *certainly* be strong, because you're still trying to find a way out of your suffering. Despite everything, you still have hope. I salute your bravery. In my eyes, you're a hero.

But you can only stand so much, right? You're human: that's your blessing, but it's also your vulnerability. You probably suffered stoically for months or even years, but after a while your endurance gave out and the pain took over. Finally, you probably began to feel alone and helpless.

By now, you may even feel like a victim of torture. Researchers have found that torture victims and chronic pain patients endure a very similar experience—a horrific experience that can kill the will of even the strongest person.

Right now, you may be hoping that I'll say, "The good news is, I can help you."

It's true. I *can* help you. Your pain can probably be cured.

But I have even better news than that: *You can help yourself.* If you read this book carefully, and put its advice into your life, you'll no longer need me. Your own body has a healing force that will enable you to *rise above your pain,* and feel whole and happy once again.

When I tell this to my patients, some are thrilled—but others are disappointed. They want me to tell them that I'm the hot new medical pioneer with the miraculous new potion for their pain. That attitude is understandable, because modern medicine has packaged itself as a purveyor of technological miracles. Many of today's doctors enjoy being seen as latter-day sorcerers who can fix every ill with a magical pill.

That may be good marketing, but it's not good medicine—because it's just not true.

There *is* "magic" in medicine. But this magic—this almost supernatural force—won't come to you in a bottle. It will come to you when you do the *honest hard work* of tapping into your own inner resources.

When you do this, you will conquer your pain.

The human body performs the greatest miracles of modern medicine all by itself. As physicians, we will never be able to replicate the body's natural healing force. The body's own power lies far beyond the pale mimicry of human engineering.

Your body *can* heal the pain it now feels. When you cut your finger, you fully expect your body to heal the injury, don't you? *You should not expect less of your body in its fight against pain.* Your body's inner healing power is *unimaginably* strong.

Working with my patients—today's true medical pioneers—I have developed a comprehensive, proven program for chronic pain that gives them access to their own inner healing power. I believe that helping patients reach this power is the greatest thing a doctor can do.

About fifteen years ago, when I first began to develop this approach, it was considered very avant-garde. My pain program at the University of Arizona's teaching hospital in Phoenix was the first holistic pain management program in the southwestern United States.

Since then, though, many of the most prominent pain clinics in America have adopted the therapies I employ and have enjoyed superb results.

However, even though my approach has been accepted by many mainstream pain clinics, *most* of the individual physicians in America are still uninformed about this approach to pain, and therefore they often fail to cure pain. One reason they fail is that they do not address the role that the brain plays in pain. That's a big mistake. The brain helps *start* chronic pain—and the brain can help *stop* it.

If you read my first book, *Brain Longevity: The Breakthrough Medical Program that Improves Your Mind and Memory,* you know that I consider the brain one of the most amazing entities in the universe. In that book I showed that if the human brain is properly nurtured and medically supported, it can overcome terrible chronic conditions—even Alzheimer's disease.

In this book I will show you how *your* brain can help you cure your chronic pain.

Your brain, in fact, has virtually no limits, other than those you impose with your own human frailty.

I can show you ways to overcome that frailty. I can show you a path that will lead to your mastery over pain.

But it's up to you to walk that path. It won't be easy. But good things never are.

On this path, you'll have to give up many of the special indulgences that your pain may have granted you: a sedentary lifestyle, a sense of privilege, drugs that temporarily make you feel good, and the pity of others.

But all of your sacrifices will be repaid many times over. You will regain your sense of personal power, and your ability to control your own life. You'll once again have the energy to do the things you love, and to do things for the people you love. You'll even get reacquainted with a very special person: your own true self.

I have seen this happen many, many times. In fact, when patients work hard, it happens *most* of the time. I have helped cure many hundreds of "hopeless" cases of chronic pain.

I have been able to achieve "impossible" victories against pain for one central reason: my pain program has evolved far beyond the old-fashioned, traditional approach to pain. Unlike many doctors who treat pain, I don't rely on just pills, injections, and surgery. That limited approach, which I and many other doctors now consider outdated, often gives temporary relief but rarely stimulates the permanent healing of chronic pain.

My program is different. It battles chronic pain on every level: the biochemical level, the structural level, the psychological level, and the spiritual level. *This thorough approach is absolutely essential—* because if you have chronic pain it has probably invaded *every part* of your life.

To get your life back, to get your true self back, and to overcome the pain that has violated your body, mind, and spirit, you will need to engage in a comprehensive, coordinated program.

My program can be your path to recovery. It will oppose every possible aspect of your pain, and help you reach new heights of mental, physical, and spiritual well-being.

My program, as you will soon see, is unique. It still has components that are not yet commonly used by even the best pain clinics. For example, my program employs many advanced brain-enhancing modalities—some of which were described in *Brain Longevity*—that will give you the extra brain power you'll need to defeat your pain.

In addition, my program draws upon not only the very latest discoveries from modern technological medicine but also employs ancient healing methods that have withstood the test of time.

This combination of modern medicine and ancient healing is still not widely used in America, but it's incredibly potent. It will enable you to marshal your own healing power, and cure your pain.

If you're suffering now, it might be hard for you to imagine feeling whole and happy again. But that feeling—though deeply buried—already exists within you. It's waiting for you.

You can return to a life of feeling great. Others have. Others will.

Now it's your turn.

Let's begin!

Pain Is Not Suffering

Pain and suffering are different things.

Pain is a physical sensation. Suffering is one possible reaction to that sensation. But suffering is not the *only* possible reaction to pain.

It's possible to experience pain without suffering from it.

When you learn to *experience pain without suffering*, you will be set free. You will be able to love your life again, even though your life may still contain some pain, as all lives do.

When you reach this point, your chronic, disabling pain, for all practical purposes, will be cured.

In addition, when you achieve the ability to experience some pain without suffering from it, you will gain much more than just freedom from constant hurt. You will attain a power of mind and spirit that is rare in this world. Generally, this power is achieved only by enlightened yogic masters and by other people who are very

The Modern Epidemic of Chronic Pain

WHY IT'S OCCURRING
- More people than ever before are older than forty-five, the "magic age" for vulnerability to chronic pain.
- More people are surviving accidents.
- More people are surviving degenerative diseases, such as cancer.
- More people than ever before are sedentary and overweight.
- More people than ever before experience high chronic stress levels.

HOW WIDESPREAD IS IT?
- About 13 percent of the American population—more than 20 million people—experience chronic pain on almost *half the days of every year.*
- Chronic pain causes more disability than cancer and heart disease combined.
- More than 25 percent of all Americans experience some form of chronic pain each year: approximately 30 million have arthritis; approximately 20 million have persistent back pain.
- Over 17 percent of all American women suffer from migraine headaches.
- Pain is the second most common reason for a doctor visit, after colds and flu.

spiritually evolved. Why just them? Because, as a rule, only they are *motivated enough* to do the hard work that creates this power.

But you have your *pain* for motivation, and pain is the most powerful motivator of all. Your pain may now be a curse, but when you learn to harness it as a motivator, you will transform your curse into a blessing.

I remember once telling an elderly arthritis patient that his pain need not cause suffering, and he blew up at me. "That's *easy* for you to say," he snapped, waving a gnarled finger in my face, "but if *your* hand hurt like *this* hand hurts, I don't think you'd *say* that. You don't know how this *feels*!"

He was right about one thing: I didn't know how he felt. If you're free of pain, you can never really imagine the dark cruelty of chronic pain. That's one of the reasons chronic pain is so shattering. It separates people. It obliterates understanding and creates isolation. One result of this psychological isolation is that the divorce rate among people with chronic pain is almost 80 percent.

"I don't know how you feel," I told the elderly man, "but I do want to help you, and I think I can. So let's start right now. I'd like you to imagine a hypothetical situation. Let's say you're a kid again, and you're attending a very strict, old-fashioned school. Imagine that you have a mean teacher who constantly singles you out for punishment. One day he asks you a question, and you give the wrong answer. So he stands you in front of the class, makes you hold out your hand, and slaps your palm with a ruler. Smack! It really stings! On this day he dishes out the punishment again and again, and you're powerless to stop it. Pretty soon you're so depressed and angry that when lunchtime comes, you don't even feel like eating your lunch or playing with your buddies. All you can think about is how much your hand is throbbing, and the more you think about it, the more it hurts. You're really suffering.

"Finally, you're saved by the bell—school's out. You go to your Little League baseball game, but you don't even feel like playing. You do play, though, because you're a tough little kid who won't give up.

"You're the catcher. You're a *good* catcher, the only one who can handle your team's best fastball pitcher. The first time he zings one in, though, your poor hand feels like it's going to explode. But the batter is way behind the pitch and he strikes out. Everybody cheers. So you keep calling for fastballs, and you start to dominate the hitters. Three up, three down! Boom, boom, boom! You *could* call for some curves or change-ups—to give your hand a break—but your pitcher's fastball is really hopping, so you stick with the hard stuff. Pretty soon you *own* the batters, and you feel great. Every time the ball slaps into your mitt, you feel like a hero. You're not thinking about your hand anymore, or your teacher, or anything except how good it feels to be in the game. You love the cheers from the crowd, and the smell of the grass, and the friendship of your teammates. Nothing else exists.

"Finally, last out. Game's over. Your coach comes over and pats you on the back. He says, 'Great game! How's your catching hand?' You tell him it's fine, but when you pull off your mitt, your hand looks like a pink balloon. Your coach says, 'Better put some ice on that.' You tell him you will, but then you start playing a pickup game with your buddies. Your hand is hot and sore. But you want to keep playing. You have pain, but you're *not suffering*."

The elderly arthritis patient nodded. He got my point, and looked encouraged. He was a strong man, and that was good, because he was in for the fight of his life.

"My pain program," I told him, "can help you feel good enough to get back in the game, so to speak. Then your own spirit is going to take over. And when that happens, I don't think *anything* is going to stop you."

"What will happen if I don't get back into the swing of things?" he asked.

"If you don't, you'll continue to suffer. It might get worse."

I was understating. In fact, if he didn't get back into a proactive, take-charge lifestyle, he would probably fall victim to the worst nightmare that pain patients face: chronic pain syndrome.

Chronic Pain Syndrome: Your Worst Nightmare

Chronic pain syndrome is the terrible force that turns chronic pain into constant suffering. It is the biggest threat pain patients face.

Chronic pain syndrome is a group of physical and mental characteristics that often accompany chronic pain. It consists of negative behaviors and attitudes that gradually pull pain patients away from their lives, into a ceaseless whirlpool of pain.

Chronic pain syndrome is highly destructive, in and of itself. It also *greatly magnifies the physical sensation of pain.*

To find out if you have chronic pain syndrome, complete the following questionnaire.

DO YOU HAVE CHRONIC PAIN SYNDROME?

T F

1. I've had persistent pain for at least three months, despite my doctor's treatment. ☐ ☐

2. I frequently act as if I'm in pain, by groaning, crying, wincing, or massaging the area that hurts. ☐ ☐

3. I'm not physically able to do as many things as I was before my pain started. ☐ ☐

4. I'm not as interested in my hobbies as I was before my pain began. ☐ ☐

5. I often feel very depressed, or have considerable anxiety. ☐ ☐

6. My nutritional habits have deteriorated. I either have no appetite, or I eat too many "fun foods" to make myself feel better. ☐ ☐

7. People don't seem to enjoy my company as much as they did before my pain began. ☐ ☐

8. It often takes real willpower for me to control my irritability. ☐ ☐

9. My pain interferes with my work at some point during almost every day. ☐ ☐

10. I'm frequently tired. ☐ ☐

11. My medication is my most powerful weapon against pain. ☐ ☐

12. My pain often interferes with my ability to concentrate. ☐ ☐

13. I wish I could take better care of the people in my family, but it's hard enough for me just to take care of myself. ☐ ☐

14. My sleeping patterns are often disrupted by pain. ☐ ☐

15. My nerves are so touchy that I tend to overreact to minor things, such as sudden   ☐ ☐
    loud noises.

16. I've gone from doctor to doctor, looking for someone who can help.   ☐ ☐

17. When I have an important day coming up, I worry that my pain will interfere.   ☐ ☐

18. I've lost the feeling of control over my life.   ☐ ☐

19. I've begun to feel that my life has been ruined by my pain.   ☐ ☐

20. I spend more time thinking about my pain than any other single aspect of my life.   ☐ ☐

If you answered "true" to only questions one, two, and three, you are suffering from chronic pain, but *not* from chronic pain syndrome. If that's the case, you are a person of unusual courage and wisdom.

If you answered "true" to at least ten of the twenty questions, you have moderate chronic pain syndrome. If you answered "true" to fifteen questions, you have advanced chronic pain syndrome. If you answered "true" to eighteen or more questions, you have severe chronic pain syndrome.

If you have *any* degree of chronic pain syndrome, you will almost certainly need help to overcome it. I can provide much of that help with this book.

You probably developed chronic pain syndrome gradually. When you first began to suffer from chronic pain, you may have consciously *chosen* to adopt some of the chronic pain syndrome behaviors, thinking that they would spare you further pain. For example, you might have decided to limit your involvement with your work or hobbies, to save your energy, and to save yourself from extra pain.

But most of the syndrome's characteristics probably invaded your life against your will. You didn't *choose* to become depressed, irritable, or tired. It just happened, because of your pain's biological and psychological impact.

One of the awful things about chronic pain syndrome is that it makes the physical feeling of pain much more intense. It increases the brain's *perception* of pain. Just one example: Arthritis patients who suffer from depression are approximately twice as sensitive to painful stimuli as nondepressed arthritis patients.

Thus, chronic pain syndrome—which is *caused* by pain—also *causes* further pain. It contributes to a physical phenomenon called the "cycle of pain," which haunts the lives of many pain patients.

To break this insidious cycle, you will need to follow a careful, constructive program, such as the one I describe in this book. It's *up to you* to actively implement this program in your own life, and to *defeat* chronic pain syndrome (which is also called "Pain Disorder with Psychological Features").

There are many elements in my pain program that intervene in the cycle of pain, and you can start the program by engaging in almost any of them.

My pain program consists of four fundamental treatment modalities, or levels. Each of them helps break the cycle of pain and eliminate chronic pain syndrome.

The four levels are: (1) *Nutritional Therapy* (including dietary modification, and ingestion of specific nutrients); (2) *Physical Therapies* (including exercise therapy, acupuncture, massage, light therapy, magnetherapy, chiropractic, and advanced yogic mind-body exercises); (3) *Medication* (including use of pain medications, nerve blocks, injections, and brain-enhancement medications); and (4) *Mental and Spiritual Pain Control* (including stress reduction, treatment of anxiety and depression, psychological therapies, and spiritual development).

The vast majority of the pain patients I have treated over the past fifteen years have reported a *dramatic reduction* in the pain that created their chronic pain syndrome. Their pain diminished to the point where it was no longer a significant element in their lives. Many of them still had occasional pain, as all people do, but their debilitating chronic pain, and the suffering it caused, was cured.

In many other patients the pain *disappeared entirely*.

In some cases this disappearance of pain occurred because of the successful treatment of the neurological problems that were perpetuating the cycle of pain.

In other cases, though, the pain disappeared because the underlying problems that caused the pain were eliminated. For example, I have treated arthritis patients whose pain vanished because their arthritis went into remission. This type of occurrence is very rare among patients of conventional "allopathic" (or anti-disease) medicine, because allopathic medicine is generally ineffective at reversing long-standing degenerative diseases, such as arthritis. However, the form of medicine that I practice is not solely anti-disease, but is also strongly *pro-health*. It stimulates the body's own natural healing force. This form of medicine combines conventional Western medicine with Eastern medicine, and is known as "complementary medicine" or, as I now prefer to call it, "integrative medicine."

Integrative medicine can be quite effective against degenerative diseases. A slowly developing degenerative disease is often caused by mistakes in lifestyle; when those mistakes are corrected by integrative medicine, the patient's body is often able to overcome the disease.

One of the simplest examples of this is the elimination of low back pain caused by obesity. When the patient sheds his or her extra pounds through an integrative medicine program that includes nutritional therapy and exercise therapy, the pain often vanishes. However, if the obesity is not corrected, conventional allopathic treatment generally fails.

As you can see, integrative medicine is not always magical or mysterious. Often it's just a good commonsense treatment.

Even if a patient's pain cannot be totally eradicated, though, the patient can still break the cycle of pain, overcome chronic pain syndrome, and begin to feel great. If you doubt that someone who experiences frequent pain can still feel great, consider the lives of professional athletes. Most pro basketball players, for example, feel an assortment of serious pains virtually every day, owing to the extreme rigor of their sport. As a matter of fact, when Michael Jordan first retired from basketball to play baseball, he cited pain as a major factor in his decision, noting that he was "tired of hurting all the time." And yet, Michael Jordan—*despite his pain*—had remarked throughout his career that he felt great on most of the days of his life. He was almost always able to rise above his pain and do what he loved to do. He loved it so much that he quickly ended his retirement, even though he knew he was returning to a life of daily pain. Like many people, including many of my own patients, he was *master* of his pain instead of its *victim*.

I recall clearly one patient of mine who was never able to totally eradicate his pain, but who still managed to reduce it dramatically, turn his life around, and feel great. The first time I saw him, though, I didn't feel very hopeful. The poor guy was really suffering. He was so overcome by chronic pain syndrome that I hardly knew where to begin.

Scott's Story

His name was Scott, and as he began to tell me his story, there was venom in his voice. Pure hatred. He said he hated his doctor. But I could see he hated life itself. Considering the life he was living, I could hardly blame him.

Every day he was being tortured. It lasted for hours and left him sick, weak, afraid, and hateful.

The source of his torture was a chronic disease called polymyositis, a widespread inflammation of the muscles that causes excruciating pain. Scott's doctor had told him that he would escape his torture only through death.

Scott hunched uncomfortably in a chair in my office, leaning slightly forward, his fingers clenched white, as he told me his story.

"Last time I saw my doctor, this doc said to me, 'You're dying, you know.' I said, 'Oh, thanks for *telling* me.' " Scott's face flushed with anger. He felt betrayed—by his own body, by the doctors he'd once trusted, and even by God. "So this doctor looks down his nose at me and says, 'What do you want me to do?'

"I said, 'That's what *I'm* supposed to ask *you.*'" Scott sighed and slumped. "I'm in bad shape," he said simply. "Look at my face." It was red, fat with water, and pitted with acne caused by the anti-inflammatory steroids he was taking. "My back is so thick with acne that I can't even lean back in this chair," he said. Scott was in his mid-forties, but he looked much older. He was withered, frail, and weak. His eyes were hollow with depression.

"The last thing this . . . esteemed physician . . . said to me was, 'Scott! Look at everything you've got in your life that's *good.* Your wife. Your kids. Your friends. Your work. The *only* bad thing you've got is your pain. Focus on the *good.*' I almost laughed out loud. But laughing hurts, too.

"So I said, 'The only bad thing, huh? The *only* thing? Okay, how about this? My wife can't stand me anymore, because all I do is bitch and moan. My kids are scared to death of me. My friends? What friends? To them, I'm the Elephant Man. My work, now that's funny. I've *got* no career left. I can't even think straight. The only job I've got now is fighting with my insurance company. I'm always tired, but I can't sleep. Food makes me sick, because of all the pills I'm taking. Forget about sex. Forget about fun. Oh yeah, I almost forgot—I'm also in *agony* all the time.'"

He looked for a moment as if he would cry, then his face went cold. He hunched further forward, and his eyes froze into a thousand-yard stare.

To begin my intake procedure on Scott, I asked him a number of questions, and he filled out the following chart. Here's how it looked when he finished:

PAIN INTAKE CHART

1. Location of pain:
   All over; in some muscles more than others.

2. Severity of pain, according to patient:

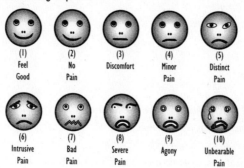

(1)	(2)	(3)	(4)	(5)
Feel Good	No Pain	Discomfort	Minor Pain	Distinct Pain

(6)	(7)	(8)	(9)	(10)
Intrusive Pain	Bad Pain	Severe Pain	Agony	Unbearable Pain

3. Type of pain, in patient's words (throbbing, stinging, burning, etc.):
   Searing; hot; comes in waves

4. Most frequent reactions to pain:
   Take pills; try to hang on

5. Pain medications:
   Xanax, lithium, Ambien, prednisone, aspirin

6. Various triggers of pain:
   Movement; touch

7. Daily patterns of pain:
   Worse at night; worse during physical activity

8. Chronic pain syndrome indices, rated by severity, on a 1–10 scale:
   - Decrease in activities — 9
   - Fatigue — 9
   - Reliance upon medication — 9
   - Decreased socialization — 10
   - Sleep disruption — 9

• Nervousness	8
• Improper nutritional habits	7
• Dissatisfaction with treatment	10
• Worry about pain impact	9
• Loss of sense of control	9
• Sexual dysfunction	10
• Limitation of movement	10
• Cognitive impairment	8
• Anxiety	8
• Depression	9

Scott's responses clearly indicated that he suffered from intense chronic pain and severe chronic pain syndrome.

I looked him straight in the eye.

"I can help stop your suffering," I told him, "but you're going to have to work like an athlete training for the Olympics. Can you afford to make that commitment?"

"I can't afford *not* to," he said.

"Good!" I liked this guy. He was a fighter. "Then let's begin where I always begin. With a goal. What do you *most* hope to achieve?"

Scott had apparently given this a great deal of thought, and he answered quickly. "My doctor told me that pretty soon I'm going to be in a wheelchair, and that then I'll contract pneumonia and die, because the muscles that support my breathing will fail.

"If I die," he said, "I want to die on *my terms*. Which means *no more drugs*. I *hate* this damn stuff they're giving me. It makes my skin crawl. Can you get me *off* all these drugs? Even the pain medications?"

"You're not *taking* any pain medications."

"What about the tranquilizers? My doctor said they killed pain."

"They really don't."

Scott looked exasperated. "Then why would he *tell* me that?"

"Most people," I said, "don't really understand how pain works. Unfortunately, that includes many doctors."

I began to explain the physiology of pain to Scott. He listened intently—like an athlete listening to his coach.

Possible Side Effects of Pain Drugs

(including sedatives, analgesics, nonsteroidal anti-inflammatories, beta-blockers, antidepressants, and muscle relaxers)

- memory loss
- kidney damage
- liver damage
- death
- lethargy
- vomiting and nausea
- heart disease
- ulcers
- osteoporosis

- anxiety
- depression
- high blood pressure
- decreased immunity
- stroke
- insomnia
- rashes
- intestinal bleeding
- convulsions

How Pain Works

I had some wonderful news for Scott. The crux of it was this: Pain travels along a complex pathway in the nervous system, and all along that pathway—in the nerves and in the brain—*there are biological "gates" that can be closed, to shut off pain.*

When these biological gates are closed, the pain is reduced or eliminated.

This concept is called the "gate theory," and it has revolutionized the field of pain management. I am proud to say that I was among the first doctors to clinically incorporate holistic modalities utilizing this theory into my treatment of pain patients.

This theory is now becoming increasingly accepted by pain specialists, but it's still relatively new. Therefore, many doctors who do not specialize in pain management don't really understand it, and don't incorporate it into their treatments of pain. Because of this, their treatments often fail.

In fact, many doctors don't even fully understand what chronic pain *is*. Some of them think that chronic pain is basically the same thing as short-term "acute" pain. They believe that chronic pain is just acute pain that lasts longer.

That's not true.

Chronic pain and acute pain are vastly different. Short-term acute pain is almost always a symptom. It's a warning that something is wrong. When you fix whatever is wrong, the pain usually goes away.

But chronic pain is generally *not* a symptom. Most often it is *not* a warning that something is wrong. For the most part, *chronic pain is a disease.*

Most chronic pain is caused by a malfunction of the nervous system—the nerves and the brain. To a large extent, *chronic pain is in the brain.*

I explained this to Scott but assured him that it did *not* mean his pain was "all in his mind." Much of his pain was in his *brain,* but his brain was much more than just his mind. His brain didn't just think—it also governed every function of his body, including the processing of all his pain signals.

Processing pain signals is a very complicated task, and sometimes our brains make mistakes in this process, just as they do when we add numbers or play the piano.

But those mistakes can usually be corrected.

In Scott's case, I believed that only part of his pain was caused by the ongoing damage from his illness. The rest of it—probably *most* of his pain—was being caused by malfunctions of his nervous system.

Therefore, I believed that if I could correct those malfunctions, and close his pain gates, I could relieve his suffering.

During his previous treatment, his doctor had ignored these pain gates, and the results had been disastrous.

When all of the gates in the nervous system's pain pathway are allowed to remain wide open, pain can begin to "circulate" in a ceaseless cycle.

This cycle begins at the original site of the pain, generally because of an injury or illness. Then pain travels up the spinal cord to the brain. The brain processes the pain signals, then sends nerve impulses back *down* the spinal cord, to the original site of the pain, sensitizing that area, and causing inflammation. This sensitization and inflammation help protect the damaged area, by forcing us to favor it, and it also rushes healing chemicals to the area. But it *magnifies* the pain, and even creates *more* pain. This new pain then travels back to the brain—and the cycle begins again.

The pain impulses can literally begin to have "a life of their own," as pain itself continues to cause *more* pain.

As I've mentioned, this cycle of pain can be reinforced by many of the elements of chronic pain syndrome. Some of these elements tend to *jam open* the gates of the pain pathway and to magnify the sensations of pain.

Also, chronic pain syndrome often makes pain patients feel passive and defeated, and discourages them from doing the many things they must do to make their pain go away.

Now let's take a trip along the pain pathway, and I'll point out

Why Many Doctors Fail

- They do not address the *neurological* aspects of chronic pain, even though *chronic pain is in the brain.*
- They prescribe tranquilizers for chronic pain more often than any other form of medication—even though tranquilizers do not directly decrease pain.
- The primary conventional treatment for chronic pain is administration of drugs. But the top priority at the most successful pain clinics is to get patients off drugs as quickly as possible.
- The most common orthodox medical treatment for back pain is surgery, but surgery is appallingly ineffective for many cases of back pain.
- Drugs often cause "rebound pain" that is worse than the original pain.
- Many doctors ignore the underlying *causes* of pain.

all the various gates where pain can be reduced, blocked, and eliminated.

Then, later in this chapter, I'll tell you about my pain program and show you *how to close those gates.*

A Journey down the Pain Pathway

A pain impulse usually starts its trip along the pain pathway when you suffer an injury or illness. Let's say you cut your finger.

Have you ever noticed that when you cut yourself, you usually feel the sensation of the cut *before* you feel the pain from it? That happens because you have *separate* nerves for touch and for pain—and the "touch" nerves send signals more quickly than the pain nerves. That's why you feel the cut before the pain.

Your fast "touch" nerves shoot signals toward your brain at about 200 miles per hour, while your pain nerves send signals to your brain at a relatively slow speed. Acute pain travels at only about 40 miles per hour, and chronic pain can travel as slowly as 3 miles per hour. This difference in speed occurs mostly because "touch" nerves are generally better insulated.

Whenever you injure your finger, you tend to grab it and squeeze it or rub it, don't you? That's a natural instinct. You do that because it decreases your pain. The reason it decreases your pain is that it shoots fast "touch" signals toward your pain gates, and those fast touch signals *outrun* the slow pain signals. By the time the pain signals arrive, your pain gates are already crowded with touch impulses, and the pain signals have a hard time squeezing through.

So already you know an excellent anti-pain strategy: Give your nervous system a *competing source of input*—especially one that can "outrun" pain signals.

There are many ways to provide a competing source of input, other than just rubbing a painful area. This can also be done bio-chemically, mechanically, electrically—and even with thoughts! Soon you'll know every strategy that exists.

One obvious lesson from this is: Don't be macho by trying to just *ignore* the pain when you first get hurt. Go after it! Beat it! It bothers me when I'm watching a baseball game and the batter gets hit by a pitch and just stands there, not rubbing the injured area, because that would "give the other team satisfaction." That appeals to the athlete in me—but *not* the pain specialist. As you'll soon see, once pain gets started, it can be hard to stop. However, if you take care of your short-term, acute pain right away, you can reduce the chance that it will become a long-standing chronic pain.

Now let's keep traveling along your pain pathway and discover more ways to stop pain.

When pain signals squeeze onto the "elevator" of your spinal cord, headed for your brain, they automatically trigger the release of several chemicals that help them travel to the brain. These chemicals, called neurotransmitters, are the biochemical messengers that carry pain signals from one nerve cell to the next. Your brain, as you probably know, also uses neurotransmitters to carry all of your thoughts and feelings.

The three primary neurotransmitters that "ship" pain signals to the brain are substance P, NMDA (n-methyl-d-aspartate), and glutamate. Of these, substance P seems to be the most active, and most important. Without these three substances—especially substance P—pain signals have a much harder time reaching the brain. However, if there is an *excess* of any of these three substances, pain signals have a much *easier* time reaching the brain.

So, again, we have another way to stop pain: by manipulating the levels of one or more of these neurotransmitters. This can be done in several ways. One way is with pharmaceutical and over-the-counter drugs, and another is with acupuncture. When you learn the details of my pain program, you'll learn *all* the ways.

Here's more good news: The body, in its natural, innate wisdom, has its own way of keeping these pain neurotransmitters from flooding the brain, and overwhelming us with pain. The body forces these pain chemicals to travel through a pain gate that sits near the back of the spinal cord. This pain gate is composed of a substance that has the consistency of jelly; it's called the substantia gelatinosa of the dorsal horn.

Thus we have yet another method of controlling pain: *supporting the function* of this gate. This is achieved by supporting the overall health of the nervous system. If the nervous system is exhausted, stressed, or nutritionally malnourished, this gate will lose its efficiency.

Thus, the better your nervous system functions, the higher your "pain threshold" will be. That's one reason, for example, why you feel more pain when you don't get enough sleep: your lack of sleep hampers the ability of your nervous system to close its pain gates.

However, no matter how well your pain gates are working, some pain signals are certain to reach your brain. This is natural and desirable, of course, because without pain we would constantly be in grave danger of injury.

When pain hits the brain, that's when your body and mind *really* go to war against it—*if* your body and mind are working efficiently, and in proper coordination with each other.

So far, you've just been "playing defense" against pain. But when your brain receives the first pain signals, and realizes that your body is fighting its most vicious enemy, your brain starts to "play offense." It launches a counterattack!

In the next few pages I'll tell you how to make that counterattack *fierce*.

Pain Myth

"Your chronic pain is all in your mind."
(Reality: Chronic pain is in the *brain*—not in the mind.)

Counterattack!

Pain signals enter your brain in an area called the thalamus. The thalamus is where your brain "sorts out" most of its incoming physical signals. For example, besides dealing with pain, your thalamus also handles things like hunger and thirst.

Instantly, your thalamus sends the pain signal to the two most important parts of your brain—your cortex, which does your thinking, and your limbic system, which governs your emotions.

When this happens, your thinking brain and your emotional brain have a dialogue, in which they "compare notes" on the pain signal. They try to decide how serious the pain is, where it's located, what it means, and how to deal with it. They analyze how strong the pain signals are, how frequently they're being sent to the brain, and how long the signals have lasted.

If, during this dialogue, your cortex and limbic system decide the pain signals aren't very serious, they tell your body to relax and tell your neurotransmitter system to pump out a calming brain chemical called serotonin. This causes the nerves that first picked up the pain signal to "quiet down," and it causes the muscles around the injured area to relax. Also, your blood vessels— which had been constricted by alarm—begin to loosen up. Your body soon returns to its normal state. The acute pain soon subsides, and you feel fine again.

However, let's say that when you cut your finger, it *really* hurts, the cut looks deep, and blood is gushing out. Your cortex and limbic system scan your memory, and they don't like what they find. Your memory says, "This is the worst cut you've had in years. It's bound to hurt, and if you're not careful, the finger will get infected." When your cortex and limbic system hear this, they start yelling, "Red alert! Red alert! We've got a *problem!*"

The all-out counterattack begins!

Instead of telling your neurotransmitter system to pump out calming neurotransmitters, your cortex and limbic system put in an order for the stimulating neurotransmitter norepinephrine, which is a form of adrenaline. This always happens when your body is under assault. Suddenly you begin to experience the classic symptoms of the "fight-or-flight response," which is also called the "stress response." Your blood vessels constrict, your heart pounds, your muscles tighten, and your nerves go "on edge," as they wait for further problems.

This is when things can go very wrong. *This is when chronic pain can begin.* If your counterattack doesn't work properly, you can end up with chronic pain. Your counterattack has to be strong, but not *too* strong. If it's not strong enough, or if it's too strong, it can contribute to the neurological malfunctions that create chronic pain.

One thing your counterattack must accomplish is the creation of a reasonable balance between the production of calming serotonin and stimulating norepinephrine. When you're alarmed, your body badly needs serotonin to help calm down, and to begin to close some of the pain gates. Unfortunately, the more alarmed you become, the more those gates are likely to open up, and to even "jam open" indefinitely.

Soon, though, I'll show you how to create abundant supplies of serotonin, so that when you need it, you'll have it.

Another problem that can arise at this point, as mentioned before, is sensitization of the injured area. When pain registers in the brain, the brain begins to closely monitor the injured area, via the nervous system, as part of its counterattack. The nerves around the injured area become more sensitive. They can even start carrying pain signals from stimuli that normally wouldn't cause pain. For example, the skin around your cut finger might hurt when you touch it, even though it's not injured.

Sometimes pain signals can even "jump" bioelectrically from one pain-carrying nerve to a neighboring pain nerve that had previously been free of stimulation. When this happens, it increases the amount of pain headed toward the brain. And when the brain receives these new signals, it sensitizes the injured area even more, contributing to the cycle of pain.

However, the more you nurture your nervous system, with a comprehensive program that builds neurological strength, the less likely this will be to occur. One simple reason why: As your nervous system becomes healthier, the sheaths that insulate your nerves will grow thicker, and help prevent these neurological "leaks."

Another "big gun" in your counterattack against pain is the production of your body's own natural, morphinelike opiates—endorphins, dynorphins, and enkephalins. These substances are ten times stronger than morphine. However, you never build up tolerance to them as you do to drugs.

These natural opioids not only flood the brain—giving physical and psychological relief—but also travel to one of the pain gates in your spine. There they directly "battle" pain-carrying substance P, trying to keep substance P from entering the nerves that go to the brain.

Sometimes you have enough endorphins to overpower your substance P, and stop the pain signals that are trying to get to your brain. But sometimes you don't have enough. When that happens, pain has one less obstacle to overcome.

As you might imagine, though, there are ways to increase your output of endorphins. For example, you can do it with exercise. However, exercise is often avoided by people with chronic pain syndrome. That's a mistake—one you will need to correct to end your chronic pain.

If you don't produce enough endorphins, or enough serotonin, your pain signals begin to increase in intensity, frequency, and duration. When this happens, the signals themselves often "jam open" the pain gates.

Then pain travels freely from the injured area to the brain, and *back* again.

As this happens repeatedly—millions of times per hour—pain signals become "engraved" upon the nervous system. Pain signals literally become a *physical part* of the anatomy of your nervous system, just like the memories that are engraved in your brain.

As your injury heals, *this engraved pain can remain.* It no longer requires the stimuli of the injury. Tragically, it now has a life of its own.

When this happens, the *pain is not a symptom, it's a disease.*

The Biological "Gates of Pain"

What *opens* them (and increases pain)	**What *closes* them** (and decreases pain)
• Lack of sleep	• Relaxation
• Stressful lifestyle	• Exercise
• Fear and anxiety about pain	• Good neurological nutrition
• Repeated trauma to the distressed area	• Medications
	• Acupuncture
• Depression	• Serotonin
• Mentally focusing on pain	• Adequate sleep
• Physical inactivity	• Distraction from pain
• Lack of specific neurological nutrients	• Competing neurological input (e.g., touch)
• Hypoglycemia	• Positive thoughts
• Serotonin deficit	• Endorphins
• Endorphin deficit	• Avoiding nutrients that increase inflammation
• Consumption of nutrients that increase inflammation	• Meditation
	• Mental training

How Healing Can Hurt

Now let me tell you about another problem you face.

As the brain carries out its counterattack against pain, it also launches a counterattack against the injury itself. This counterattack is commonly referred to as the healing process. Unfortunately, the healing process can also contribute to the disease of chronic pain.

One way that healing contributes to pain is through the process of *inflammation*.

Inflammation is a natural part of your body's response to injury. However, inflammation can get out of control. When it does, it can cause great pain.

Inflammation starts when the brain sends "alarm signals" back down to the injured area. Those signals cause increased blood flow to the area, as your body tries to fight infection and repair damage. But some of this extra blood leaks out of its vessels and causes swelling, soreness, stiffness, and warmth. This blood also releases potent chemicals that make the area even more sensitive.

Normally, inflammation goes away when the injury heals. But when pain becomes engraved upon the nervous system, inflammation can remain. At this point it serves no purpose—it just hurts. It's no longer a symptom—it's a disease.

Inflammation is the major culprit in many kinds of pain.

However, there are many effective ways to fight inflammation. You can use anti-inflammatory drugs, such as ibuprofen, or certain nutrients. You can even stop inflammation before it starts, with nutritional therapy. I'll tell you how to do that in the next chapter.

Another way that the healing process causes pain is by creating muscle spasms. A muscle spasm starts out as a natural protective mechanism; it shields a distressed area by immobilizing it. In a way, it's like a plaster cast, or a splint.

Muscle spasms begin when your body experiences pain. When this happens, the body often *contracts* the muscles near the painful area. Frequently, though, those muscles *remain* tight, or in spasm. Part of the reason a muscle stays tight is that the spasm *itself* often hurts. Therefore, it's very easy to create a cycle of pain-spasm-pain-spasm.

If these spasms are ignored, they can become virtually permanent. Muscle tissues can even become, in effect, "glued" together.

Sometimes, ongoing muscle spasms are quite noticeable, and cause great pain. This often occurs in chronic musculoskeletal pain, including back pain and neck pain. At other times, however, the muscle spasms are subtle, and are confined to a very small area. These less noticeable muscle spasms can be insidious, though. One problem they often cause is "referred pain"—pain that exists in a location other than the immediate area of the spasm. For example, a small muscle spasm in the neck can cause a severe headache.

Fortunately, though, there are a number of ways to get rid of these spasms. One of the best ways is with massage, which I'll describe in chapter 3.

A third way that the healing process causes pain is when damaged pain nerves heal *improperly*.

When damaged pain nerves heal and regrow, they often do so imperfectly, and begin to fire *spontaneously*, sending pain signals to the brain for no reason at all.

Frequently the victims of imperfect nerve regrowth get blamed for "making up" their pain, because they no longer have an obvious injury. Often, even their own doctors tell them that their pain is all in their minds. The victims get treated as if they were just neurotic, or cowardly. How unfair! And how stupid!

In fact, there is one very obvious example of this kind of pain: phantom limb pain. Up to 85 percent of all amputees feel pain that seems to come from their missing limbs. In some types of amputations, more than one-third of all patients feel *severe* pain. This pain results, in part, from the improper healing of severed nerves.

However, poor healing of severed nerves isn't the only cause of phantom limb pain. Phantom limb pain is also often caused by the pain that often *preceded* the surgery—the pain from the injury or illness that necessitated the surgery. This pain, if it becomes engraved upon the nervous system, can continue to exist even after the original source of the pain has been surgically removed, with no significant damage to nerves.

Here's another interesting illustration of the fact that pain can become engraved upon the nervous system, including the brain itself. Sometimes paralyzed people feel pain in the parts of their bodies that can no longer move, and that no longer respond to external stimuli. When this happens, doctors sometimes partly sever the patients' spinal cords, to relieve their pain. Occasionally, though, even this does not stop the pain. Unfortunately for the paralyzed people, their pain is no longer in their bodies. It's in their brains.

I'll give you one more really fascinating example that indicates that chronic pain can become "centralized" in the brain. As
you may have heard, it's possible to make people have vivid memories of past events just by stimulating different areas of people's
brains with electrodes. When this happens, memories often come
flooding back with crystal clarity. Knowing about this phenomenon, pain researchers tried to evoke pain in test subjects by electrically stimulating the area of their brains that first receives pain
signals—the thalamus. However, researchers found that subjects
with no history of chronic pain were not affected by stimulation
of the thalamus. But when researchers stimulated this area of the
brain in chronic pain patients, the patients felt intense pain. For
example, one patient who had formerly experienced the chest
pain of angina pectoris reported terrible pain in her chest when
her thalamus was stimulated.

Thus, this angina patient discovered that, for her—as with
other chronic pain patients—*pain is in the brain.*

The Brain Can Stop Pain

As I've indicated, one of the best ways to stop pain is simply to increase the power of the brain. This simple principle was portrayed
dramatically to me shortly after the publication of my first book,
Brain Longevity. In that book, I told readers how to optimize their
brain power—but I said almost nothing in it about using the brain
to defeat pain. Nonetheless, please note the following exchange
of letters.

August 20, 1998
Hartford, CT

Dear Dr. Khalsa,
    I have recently finished reading your book *Brain Longevity.*
It has given me some hope. Recently I was diagnosed as having

a form of dystonia called spasmodic torticollis, a condition that causes severe twisting of the neck, and great pain.

I was given two injections of botulinum toxin, which failed to make a difference. My neurologist has now put me on Tetrabenazine, which also does not seem to be helping. I am 38 years old, very active, and have two daughters.

My neurologist has given me these medications—the only ones available to help me. A cure is not known.

I have started your brain longevity program. It seems to my unscientific mind that it makes sense to try to improve the working order of my brain. The nutritional side is something I can easily handle, but exercise is difficult, since I can't hold my head straight.

Anyway, I am forging ahead, and would love to hear if you think I have any real chance of helping my condition.

Sincerely,
J.M.

I wrote back to this woman—who had a severe neurological disease that is generally unresponsive to treatment—encouraging her to persevere with her brain longevity program. I recommended that she do mind/body exercises and see an acupuncturist, in addition to following a comprehensive program that boosts the power of the brain.

A few months later I received another letter from her.

October 19, 1998
Hartford, CT

Dear Dr. Khalsa,

All of my symptoms are gone! My neurologist had given up on me when the drugs didn't have any effect. I then decided to work on my own, in a holistic mode. I have been successful, and my inspiration came from you. Thank you very much. I continue to take all of the vitamins and supplements you suggested. I also continue with my mind/body exercises, meditation, yoga, good nutrition, and exercise.

Thank you again.

Sincerely,

J.M.

This case clearly illustrates that the brain can have a profound effect upon a supposedly intractable pain condition—even in the absence of a full-fledged pain program.

Furthermore, when the power of the brain is allied with the power of the body, and the power of the spirit—in a comprehensive pain program—almost *anything* is possible!

Now you have a basic understanding of how pain works, and how chronic pain can begin.

Therefore, you already understand—probably better than some doctors do—why the traits of chronic pain syndrome are so devastating to people with chronic pain.

As you'll recall, chronic pain syndrome is characterized by physical inactivity, inadequate sleep, depression, poor nutrition, fear, anxiety, reliance on medications, and mental lethargy. As you now know, these traits are almost certain to lock in—and amplify—pain signals that have become engraved upon the nervous system.

If you are now suffering from chronic pain, I can certainly see why you might have fallen victim to these traits. After all, pain wears you down, and eats away at your strength and your zest for life.

But now that you have a better grasp of how chronic pain gets started, and keeps going, you can probably see that these characteristics of chronic pain syndrome are literally poison for the nervous system. They reduce the natural ability of the nervous system to resist pain. And they allow the brain to focus on pain, and thereby increase the intensity and frequency of pain signals.

Besides being "poisonous" to the nervous system, these characteristics also rob life of its most basic sources of joy: the pleasure of play, the satisfaction of work, and the love of other people.

This loss of joy is not only horrible in itself, but it, too, contributes to the cycle of pain. The less joy, satisfaction, and love you feel, the more you will indulge in harmful habits, and the more you'll focus on the only thing that's left in your life: pain.

The end result is suffering.

If you have been suffering for a long time, you may have come to believe that your only escape from suffering will be through death.

That's what my patient Scott thought. But he was wrong.

> Short-term acute pain is a symptom.
> Long-term chronic pain is a *disease*.

Scott Fights Back

As I described the physiology of chronic pain to Scott, we talked about the particular cause of his own pain.

His immune system, for unknown reasons, had turned against his own body, in an "autoimmune" disorder; it was destroying his muscles, and causing him terrible pain. Shortly after his disease had begun, the pain from his muscle deterioration had become engraved upon his nervous system. It had caused him to suffer almost constant, knifelike jabs of pain. His muscles were disintegrating. He was very thin.

Scott was adamant, though, about discontinuing the use of his medications, including prednisone, a steroid that depresses the immune system and slows the autoimmune attack. He loathed prednisone's side effects of acne, bloating, insomnia, and emotional agitation. He hated these side effects as much as he hated his pain.

But if he *did* stop taking prednisone, a specialist had told him, the disease might intensify, and cause even more agony.

It might also kill him sooner than expected. I asked him how he felt about that, during our first meeting.

"I'll take that chance," he said. His eyes looked watery and regretful. His skin was the color of skim milk, and his body seemed to be a shriveled version of what it once had been. He looked physically and emotionally exhausted.

"How is your doctor monitoring the progress of your disease?" I asked.

"A nurse comes to my house and checks my CPK levels," he said. He was talking about his levels of a chemical called creatine phosphokinase, an enzyme that breaks down muscle tissue. The higher the levels got, the closer he would be to death. "My nurse is part of the hospice program," he said sadly. The hospice program was an in-home service for terminal patients who had only weeks or months to live.

"You'll need to taper off on the prednisone gradually," I said, "because you can die from sudden withdrawal.

"And when you start tapering off on the prednisone, you're going to need an aggressive anti-pain program, because your pain may increase dramatically."

He nodded calmly.

I scanned his medical records. "You're also taking some tranquilizers?"

"Xanax, lithium, and Ambien," he said.

Xanax is a minor tranquilizer, much like Valium, and Ambien is a sleeping pill. Lithium is generally used only for bipolar disorder, or manic depression, which Scott did not have. Xanax and lithium did not seem appropriate for a patient with chronic pain. With Scott's concurrence, I discontinued those two medications and placed him on a full pain program immediately. He began to institute major changes in his life. Even though he had been told he was dying, he participated in his program enthusiastically. I really admired that. In some people the human spirit is just unbeatable.

Here's a brief outline of the four levels of Scott's program:

NUTRITIONAL THERAPY. Scott began to force himself to eat regularly, and carefully. His diet—which I changed to one composed primarily of grains, vegetables, high-protein soy products, and fish—was designed not only to give his nervous system abundant nutritional support, but also to improve his general health. He ate foods that stimulated production of nerve-calming serotonin, and he took the supplements that his brain and nerves needed to achieve regeneration. In addition, he regularly ate nutrients that have anti-inflammatory properties. I'll tell you about those special foods in chapter 2.

Physical therapies. Scott engaged primarily in massage therapy, and yogic mind/body exercises. He also did light work around his house, and a bit of walking, which helped him begin his cardiovascular rehabilitation.

The mild cardiovascular exercise he did stimulated his production of endorphins, and also provided his beleaguered muscles with a much-needed infusion of blood-borne oxygen and nutrients.

The stretching and massage soothed his muscle pain, and helped his nervous system to "unlearn" its patterns of circulating, engraved pain.

The mind/body exercises stimulated his brain, and brought energy to the areas of his nervous system that help control pain.

Medication. This was probably the most important component of Scott's program, since his primary goal had been to stop taking pharmaceutical drugs. Scott's desire to overcome his reliance upon powerful pharmaceutical drugs, though, was not at all uncommon. In fact, at the most prominent pain clinics in America, the first goal of the attending physicians is usually to eliminate their patients' reliance upon drugs. As you'll see in chapter 4, pharmaceutical drugs can play a very positive role in pain management. But they are not panaceas—even though many general practitioners seem to believe they are.

Over the next eighteen months, Scott gradually stopped taking prednisone, and eliminated his use of tranquilizers.

He replaced those pharmaceutical medications with milder

natural medications, including homeopathic remedies and anal-gesic herbs.

I'd feared that his pain might become unmanageable after he discontinued prednisone, but this didn't happen. The natural medications—combined with the other elements of his pain pro-gram—more than compensated.

MENTAL AND SPIRITUAL PAIN CONTROL. To heighten his ability to cognitively reduce his pain signals, Scott began to confront his feelings of anger and worthlessness. These negative emotions in-creased his perception of pain, and reduced his brain's ability to "dampen" pain signals.

Scott had been reared by a difficult father who had convinced him that he didn't deserve to be happy, and never would be. Scott had internalized this neurotic outlook, but was seething with anger toward his dad. To overcome his self-hatred and anger, he used several of the methods of "cognitive therapy," a rationality-based form of psychotherapy that's often quite beneficial for pain patients. As Scott began to shed his sense of self-loathing and his anger, he became much more relaxed, physically as well as emo-tionally. This reduced his perception of pain, increased his ability to accept pain, and heightened his ability to cognitively distract himself from pain.

Having a more positive outlook also helped Scott implement the other self-help measures in his program. It made it much eas-ier for him to rise above his chronic pain syndrome, and to do good things for himself.

I also taught Scott an advanced meditation technique, which I'll soon describe, and his meditation helped him to achieve deep personal insights, and to release much of the negative emotional energy that was heightening his pain.

In addition to his psychological therapy, Scott also began an earnest search for spiritual peace. He started his search the same way many patients do—by asking himself, "Why me?"

This is one of the most fundamental of all spiritual questions about suffering, because spirituality is, essentially, *the search for meaning.*

When patients first ask this question, they usually assume the answer to it will be negative; they assume that they must have been doing something wrong, or that there is something intrinsically wrong with them.

Often this is true, and whatever it is that's wrong must be corrected. But the negative answer is almost never the *complete* answer. Usually there is also a *positive* element to pain. For example, for many people, pain is the only force strong enough to make them back away from the "rat race" and really *live.*

When patients find a positive meaning for their pain, it invariably helps them recover. It reduces their stress response, and heightens the pain-fighting power of their minds. Often it enables them to perceive their pain as less threatening, and helps them forget about it.

Scott found a positive meaning for his pain. He found he could *use* his pain as a path to universal truths, and to greater understanding. From intense study of spiritual literature, he learned that many great holy men had experienced terrible suffering— but had *needed* this suffering to reach enlightenment. Those spiritually advanced people became Scott's role models.

After Scott found a positive meaning for his pain, he never again suffered from it quite so much. When he realized that some good was coming from his pain, he began to see it more as a challenge than as a curse.

Scott, who was a practical man, did not just sit down one day and contrive the meaning of his pain. Instead, he did a lot of hard work. Each day he meditated for a long time, and it helped him to make contact with his inner self. He told me that meditation also helped him to make contact with the realm of the divine spirit.

In addition, each day Scott read extensively in spiritual literature—everything from Buddhism to the Bible. He prayed with conviction and fervor.

He also began a powerful practice called naad yoga, which

employs the chanting of particular mantras. These ancient mantras were devised centuries ago, not only for their literal meaning, but also for the particular vibrations they create in the head, chest, and throat. My own spiritual teacher, Yogi Bhajan, has said that these vibrations stimulate optimal function of the brain and the endocrine glands, which produce hormones. Scott's favorite mantra was *Ra Ma Da Sa Sa Se So Hung*, which means "The healing power of God is in every cell of my body."

For Scott, the turning point in his spiritual exploration was when he finally "gave up" and surrendered to the inescapable fact that sooner or later he would die. When this happened, he remarked to me, "Now that I've given up, I feel like I've *received* everything." By this, he did *not* mean that he had received some sort of "free pass" to immortality. He meant that each day, for at least several blissful moments, he had begun to *experience* his own infinity.

The net effect of Scott's spiritual growth was that he developed an unshakable inner peace. This inner condition was so profound that it had various physical manifestations. One of them was the raising of his pain threshold.

Another manifestation was Scott's physical appearance. After several months he began to look different. His skim-milk skin tone began to be replaced by the luminous, incandescent glow that you sometimes see surrounding holy men. Even the look in his eyes changed. They no longer looked tormented; instead they reflected great compassion, and a deep sense of self-knowledge.

The change in Scott's appearance was very dramatic.

As you can see, there was nothing terribly exotic about his pain program; it was just a combination of good medicine, common sense, and Scott's own hard work.

After he had been on the program for about six months, I got a call from him. "My cardiologist just phoned me," he said. "It was about my CPK levels. We need to talk."

I felt a sick jolt in my stomach. If Scott's CPK levels were becoming dangerously high, his heart muscles might be in danger of immediate failure.

"What did your cardiologist say?" I asked.

"I'd rather talk in person."

Acute Pain/Chronic Pain
There *Is* a Difference

Acute pain
- Short-term.
- Cause is known.
- Hampers physical abilities *temporarily*.
- Causes anxiety.
- Usually responds to treatment.
- Is generally not perpetuated by the brain.

Chronic pain
- Long-term.
- Cause is often unknown.
- Hampers physical abilities *indefinitely*.
- Causes anxiety, fear, depression, and anger.
- Often does not respond to treatment.
- Is generally perpetuated by the brain.

Scott's Story: The Final Chapter

As soon as I saw Scott arrive, I blurted out, "What did he *say*?" I was nervous. I know that some doctors can remain detached and don't become emotionally involved in their patients' lives, but I've never really understood that.

"He said my CPK levels are going *down*," Scott said, flashing a smile as bright as lightning. "*Way* down. As in *normal*."

"Yes!" I jabbed my fist into the air.

"My cardiologist goes, 'I don't know what you're *doing*, but keep *doing* it!'" Scott said, beaming. "The cardiologist said, 'I've read some of that Deepak Chopra stuff, but frankly I just don't get it.' I told him, 'There's nothing to *get*. It's not an intellectual thing, it's an experiential thing. You've just got to *do* it.'"

"How's your pain?" I asked.

"Fine. I don't think about it all that much. Actually, now that

I *do* think about it, it's not fine. My muscles still hurt some. But pain just isn't the be-all and end-all now. I'm working again. Did I tell you that?" Then he was off on a story about work, and I had to steer him back to his medical condition.

"So you still have some residual pain?" I asked.

"I do," he said, "but I know a bunch of ways to rise above it. I know every trick in the book."

"Has it been hard?" I asked.

"You bet. Sometimes it was even harder than being sick. I had to change so *much*—my habits, my diet, my psyche. I had to accept the fact that for forty-two years, most of what I'd been doing was wrong—because look where it got me.

"But having to make so many changes was a *blessing*," he said. "The greater the changes in your life, the greater your healing."

That was three years ago.

Scott's disease is still in remission, as of publication.

Of course, it would be ludicrous of me to purport that my pain program is a miracle cure for polymyositis.

The fact is, Scott transformed his *own* life—body and soul. And when he did, his immune system stopped trying to destroy him, for reasons that are as mysterious as why the disease began in the first place.

As I have said, the body has an almost magical power for self-healing. But no one can control that power. It's a power that can only be served—not commanded.

When I saw Scott again recently, I told him, "I'm so proud of you."

He replied simply, "Thanks, Dharma."

He is very proud, too—that's quite obvious. But he is proud in a way that does not involve his ego. His pride is deeper than that, and more profound.

He loves life now, and his pride—like that of someone who is proud to be in a wonderful family—is the pride of a person who is proud to be a part of life.

PART TWO

The
Pain Cure
Program

2

Level One: Nutritional Therapy

The great art of life is sensation, to feel that we exist, even in pain.
— GEORGE GORDON, LORD BYRON

"You made it!" I said to Marie as she hobbled into my office.

"Barely," she replied.

Her husband, following her in, said, "She usually gets where she really wants to go."

What did that mean? Was it an insult? Or support? I would soon find out.

Marie had called my receptionist an hour earlier and had said she might need to cancel her appointment at my hospital pain clinic. She'd said she had a migraine that felt like "somebody sticking a paring knife in my ear."

As Marie crumpled into a chair, her husband looked at his watch. "When should I come back?" he asked. "About an hour?"

"Or longer," I answered.

"Just to write up a *diet*?"

"It's more complicated than that."

Her husband looked impatient. "Marie's friend said you do *diet* stuff," he said, "instead of medicine."

"Diet *is* medicine," I replied. I smiled, but he didn't respond.

Marie suddenly moaned. She was shielding her eyes from the light.

"You've really been through the mill, haven't you?" I asked.

"Yeah," Marie said softly, without looking up.

"Actually," I said, "I meant your husband."

Her husband looked surprised, as if he wasn't accustomed to attention.

He looked me straight in the eye. "You want the truth?" he said. "The last few years have been a *bitch*."

Marie winced at the profanity. It was possible that she had heard that word too often.

I was starting to fear that Marie's husband was part of the problem—and I needed him to be part of the solution. If he wasn't, there might not *be* a solution.

"You know," her husband said, "we already got a diet from another specialist. He told us all the foods that cause migraines. But it didn't help much, so now I'm sorta dubious."

"I don't blame you," I said. "Everybody hates making sacrifices that don't pay off. But I can tell you a *lot* more than just what foods to avoid. There have been some exciting new discoveries about chronic pain recently, and I know they'll help. I *really* think you ought to stick around," I said to him, "because it's going to take *all* of us to beat this thing."

Again he glanced at his watch. "I'll give it a shot," he said, sighing. His voice was hollow and muffled, as if it were coming from a frightened part of him that was deep in his stomach.

For the first time, Marie looked at her husband. "Thanks, hon." She smiled weakly.

He smiled back, but it was an automatic smile. He had the exhausted look of somebody who had offered too many things that had never helped.

"We're going to *start* with nutrition," I said, "but nutrition is just the first level of my four-level pain program. The other three levels are bodywork, medication, and mental control. That may sound complicated, but let's face facts: *People* are complicated.

They're multifaceted, and it takes a multifaceted program to solve their problems. If we try to take the easy way out, we're not going to *get* out."

Marie's husband nodded.

I caught Marie's eyes and looked into them. "I *know* I can find a way to stop your pain, Marie, because I've helped hundreds of patients with pain that was even worse than yours. What worked for them will work for you.

"The medical community used to think that different kinds of chronic pain functioned differently, and needed different treatments. But I don't believe that anymore, and neither do a lot of other pain specialists. I now think we all experience pain in basically the same way, regardless of its cause. So I'm going to show you not just how to prevent migraines, but how to stop *any* kind of chronic pain. If you happen to develop arthritis in the future, or back pain, or chronic muscle pain, you'll be able to control the pain from those problems with the same basic program. After all, *pain is pain.*

"To beat your pain, though, we're going to have to fight it on every level at once. No level can be ignored, and none is more important than the others. They all work together.

"We've got to start somewhere, so let's start with nutritional therapy. But I'm not just talking about avoiding foods that trigger migraines. That's kindergarten stuff. I'm talking about eating specific nutrients that stop pain."

Marie's husband seemed to perk up as he listened. He pulled a notebook and a pen out of his briefcase. "*What* nutrients?" he asked.

For the first time I saw that he was very much on her side. We were going to win.

"I've got four main nutritional strategies against pain," I said. "Let me tell you about them."

Marie reached out, and took her husband's hand.

Severity of Pain

Most *painful*	10	Migraine headache, or severe burn
	9	Infant colic
	8	Giving birth
	7	Invasive tumor pain
	6	Severe arthritis, or fibromyalgia
	5	Back pain
	4	Phantom limb pain, or broken bone
	3	Mild arthritis, or moderate tension headache
	2	Sprain
Least *painful*	1	Moderate sunburn

Four Nutritional Strategies Against Pain

In just the past few years, as the study of pain management has progressed dramatically, researchers have found that certain nutrients have a profound effect upon how much pain people feel. As a clinician, I have enthusiastically applied these new findings.

I have also applied ancient nutritional measures that have been used in Eastern medicine for thousands of years. Because many of these measures have not undergone extensive testing by governmental agencies, most Western doctors have never even heard about them.

This combination of ancient and modern nutritional remedies has worked extremely well. With it, I have achieved far better results than most other pain specialists, or pain clinics.

My nutritional anti-pain strategies can help virtually *anyone*, because these strategies address the most fundamental functions of the nervous system, which are *similar among all people*. In effect, these are "generic" anti-pain strategies, which are just as effective against arthritis pain as they are against headache pain or back pain. These strategies oppose any cycle of pain that has been engraved upon the nervous system.

The other three levels of my pain program also work on *all forms* of centralized, engraved pain, regardless of the source of that pain. Therefore, the next four chapters—which describe my general pain program—apply to *all people with chronic pain.*

For all people, pain is pain—and *pain is in the brain.* That's why this general program is effective against back pain, headache pain, joint pain, and every other type of chronic pain.

Of course, there are also some specific therapies in my program that are uniquely appropriate for specific problems. In the final section of this book, I'll address a number of specific conditions—including back pain, migraine, arthritis, and fibromyalgia—and help you fine-tune your general program to fit your own special condition.

To get started on the general program, let's look at the four "generic" nutritional strategies against pain:

I. EAT NUTRIENTS THAT RELIEVE INFLAMMATION. As I've mentioned, inflammation is a major cause of pain. It's present in everything from migraines to back pain to muscle pain to arthritis. Certain nutrients have a powerful anti-inflammatory action. Other common nutrients, though, badly aggravate inflammation, and should be strictly avoided.

2. EAT NUTRIENTS THAT BUILD PAIN-BLOCKING SEROTONIN. You may recall that the neurotransmitter serotonin is one of your body's most powerful weapons in its counterattack against pain. Serotonin helps close your pain gates. If you have a shortage of serotonin, you'll be far more vulnerable to pain. A serotonin shortage has been linked to a variety of chronic pain conditions, including migraine, back pain, muscle pain, and many other maladies.

In addition, a shortage of serotonin has also been closely linked to many of the characteristics of chronic pain syndrome, which "locks in" pain. These characteristics include depression, dependence upon drugs and alcohol, overeating, and insomnia.

One reason that a serotonin deficit is common among pain patients is that pain causes the body to "burn up" its supply of serotonin. When this happens, the pain gets worse. Then the body's supply of serotonin becomes even *more* depleted. Thus, a destructive cycle is created. But you can stop this cycle by nutritionally replenishing your body's supply of serotonin.

3. EAT NUTRIENTS THAT BOOST THE HEALTH OF YOUR BRAIN AND NERVES. As I indicated in the first chapter, the healthier your nervous system is, the higher your pain threshold will be. A well-functioning brain can suppress pain. But your brain will not be able to do this unless it is receiving powerful nutritional support.

If your brain is functioning well enough, you'll be able to help banish pain with just your *thoughts.* As you may remember, one proven method of defeating pain is to provide the brain with a competing source of input. Thoughts can be an extremely strong competing source. Some people can literally "think" pain away.

But this is only possible when cognitive powers are razor-sharp. That's one of the reasons why pain hurts more when you're tired—you just don't have the mental energy to distract your brain from pain.

4. AVOID THE CLASSIC DIETARY PAIN PITFALLS. There are a few common dietary mistakes that many pain patients make. Any one of them can markedly increase pain, and can contribute to chronic pain syndrome. These mistakes can have disastrous results.

The most frequent mistakes are allowing yourself to overeat; allowing yourself to undereat; allowing yourself to eat foods that cause allergies or food sensitivities; and allowing yourself to eat foods that destabilize hormonal balance.

Often, in the early stages of chronic pain, these seductive dietary pitfalls are used as a temporary refuge from pain. However, they then often become part of chronic pain syndrome, and begin to perpetuate the cycle of pain.

Avoiding these mistakes is relatively easy.

Now let's take a close look at each of the four basic nutritional strategies.

These strategies are virtually certain to help you. By the end of this chapter, you're going to be able to marshal a *powerful force* against your pain.

This will be your first step on your journey toward curing your chronic pain.

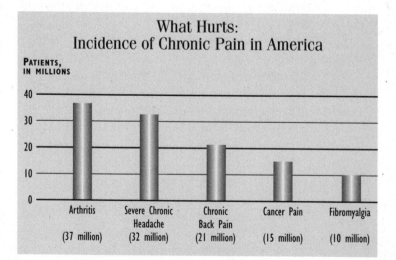

What Hurts:
Incidence of Chronic Pain in America

Nutrients that Start—and Stop—Inflammation

Remember how the process of inflammation works? The inflammation process—which is meant to heal, but can also cause great harm—is part of your body's counterattack against injury or illness. When an area of your body is under attack from injury or illness, your body floods the area with blood. This provides the distressed area with extra white blood cells, which kill infection, and it also gives the area the nutrients it needs for healing.

But some of this extra blood leaks out. This causes swelling, pressure on pain nerves, stiffness, and warmth. Also, this leaking blood releases potent chemicals that sensitize the area. This sensitization is a great survival mechanism, because it makes you favor the distressed area.

Obviously, inflammation helps you heal. However, inflammation can get *out of control.*

If your injury or illness creates engraved "central" pain, your inflammation can remain indefinitely, even after your injury or illness has healed.

Furthermore, because inflammation is *itself* a source of pain, it, too, can contribute to your cycle of perpetual pain.

Here's even more bad news. One of the chemicals that your body rushes to an injured area is serotonin—the "feel good" neurotransmitter that your brain uses to help close pain gates. When serotonin is diverted to an injury, though, it robs your brain and spinal cord of the serotonin they need to close these gates. The shortage of serotonin in your brain and spinal cord then *increases* your pain. This, in turn, causes release of more serotonin at the site of the injury.

At the site of the injury, serotonin isn't even used to block pain. Instead, it's used by the body to activate other chemicals that are part of the inflammation process. The most important of these chemicals are called prostaglandins. When you learn how to control prostaglandins, you'll have a powerful method of controlling pain.

Some prostaglandins have a very positive effect. They help injuries to heal, without increasing inflammation. They even help reduce inflammation.

However, there are also "bad" prostaglandins. "Bad" prostaglandins are also part of the healing process, but they are the *main cause* of inflammation. In fact, without these "bad" prostaglandins, there wouldn't be any inflammation.

But now here's some good news: Both your "good" and your "bad" prostaglandins are made out of specific nutrients. Therefore, you can control prostaglandins by eating certain foods. When you control prostaglandins nutritionally, you exert great power over inflammation. You can relieve existing inflammation, and stop future inflammation before it even starts.

Here's how to do it. The dosages set forth are merely suggested guidelines; you should consult your doctor to tailor this program to your specific needs.

The first step is to *eat the right types of fat in the right amounts.* Fat is used by the body in the production of prostaglandins, so if you alter your fat consumption, you can alter your prostaglandin production.

If you eat the right kinds of fat, you'll help your body to produce mostly "good" prostaglandins. "Good" prostaglandins cause your blood's clot-forming platelets to flow easily, and not stick together. When blood is flowing easily, it quickly exits the inflamed area, and doesn't collect in painful pockets of swollen tissue.

However, if you eat the *wrong* types of fats, you'll produce mostly "bad" prostaglandins. "Bad" prostaglandins cause your blood platelets to clump together, reducing blood flow and *increasing* inflammation.

Here are the fats you *should* eat:

EPA (EICOSAPENTAENOIC ACID). You get this type of fat from eating fish.

EPA is a fatty acid that originates in various types of seaweed and algae. The seaweed and algae are then eaten by fish. When these fish are consumed by people, the people metabolize the

EPA. The best sources of EPA are not white fish, but darker, cold-water fish, such as salmon, tuna, herring, mackerel, and sardines.

Pain patients who are not vegetarians should try to eat two to five servings of fish per week. This should supply enough EPA to help reduce inflammation.

EPA, which is an *omega-3 acid,* can also be taken as a supplement. To improve severe, long-standing inflammatory conditions, such as arthritis, you may need to take up to fifteen one-gram pills of EPA daily.

EPA supplements are easy to find. They're sold in health-food stores, pharmacies, and supermarkets.

Many migraine sufferers have reported relief just from using EPA alone.

Some patients, however, choose not to use EPA, because of concerns about the pollution of the oceans. As a substitute for EPA, patients occasionally use flaxseed oil, which has properties similar to those of EPA. Flaxseed oil can be purchased in health-food stores. Whole flaxseeds, ground in a coffee grinder, are also a rich source of flaxseed oil, and can be used as a garnish.

GLA (GAMMA-LINOLENIC ACID). This type of fat is similar to EPA, but does not appear to have as strong a therapeutic effect. It is most often sold in the form of evening primrose oil, which is available in health-food stores. An appropriate dosage would be approximately 500 mg daily. This oil may be used in combination with other helpful fatty acids, such as EPA.

ALA (ALPHA-LINOLENIC ACID). This fatty acid is found primarily in green vegetables. It is not generally sold as a supplement, so no daily dosage level has been established.

One very rich source of ALA, as well as GLA, is chlorophyll-based "green foods," such as spirulina, blue-green algae, wheat grass, alfalfa, and chlorella. These foods, which contain a wide spectrum of micronutrients, can have a strong anti-inflammatory effect. Patients of mine who have used these products have reported improvements in inflammatory conditions ranging from gingivitis to skin inflammations to arthritis. Green foods are also a general tonic for cognitive function, and can help the brain defeat pain by increasing the brain's level of energy. For sources of the best "green foods," see Appendix III, "Resources and Referrals."

Although all of the oils I've mentioned are safe in reasonable dosages, you should not take excessive amounts of them. In very high amounts, they may interfere with blood clotting. Also, the fish oils contain high levels of vitamin A, which can be toxic in extremely high dosages. Pregnant women, in particular, should avoid high levels of vitamin A, because it can cause birth defects.

Furthermore, a small percentage of patients report that these oils actually aggravate their inflammation, instead of reducing it, so you should be cautious. Some people think that nutritional therapy is invariably safe just because it's natural. But that's not true. Concentrated nutrients can have powerful, far-reaching effects, and should be used prudently, under the care of a pain specialist trained in nutrition.

Now let's talk about the types of fat to *avoid*.

Unfortunately, these are the types of fat you probably now often eat.

The chief culprit is animal fat. Common cooking oils are also bad for inflammation, including corn oil, safflower oil, sunflower oil, sesame oil, and canola oil.

These types of fat contain enzymes that create a substance called arachidonic acid, which is used by the body to produce prostaglandins. For most people this substance is harmless, but for pain patients it's poison.

Therefore, if you have any chronic inflammation, you should significantly reduce—or, preferably, eliminate—your consumption of meat, and substitute olive oil for the other, more common vegetable oils. You should also eat nonfat dairy products, such as fat-free milk, yogurt, ice cream, cheese, and sour cream. In addition, you should avoid processed and prepared foods that contain fats and oils. This could include anything from crackers to cake. Check the labels on the processed foods you eat.

If you are now eating the typical modern diet, this reduction

of fat may be difficult—because the average diet in many industrialized countries, including America, consists of about *33 percent fat.*

However, there are now many delicious fat-free products available, and these should help you to satisfy your desire for rich-
tasting foods.

When you reduce your fat intake, you will not only decrease
your inflammation, but you will also fight pain in two other ways:

(1) You will improve the function of your liver—which is hurt
by excessive fat consumption. This will help stabilize your hormonal levels. As I've mentioned, disruption of hormonal balance
is one of the classic dietary pain pitfalls.

(2) Eating less fat will help you fight pain by improving your
blood circulation. Good circulation boosts the function of the
brain, which uses *20 percent of all blood pumped by the heart.* Good
circulation also brings extra healing power to distressed areas. In
addition, improved circulation has direct benefits for some forms
of pain. For example, some types of muscle pain are relieved by
increased blood flow.

Reducing fat consumption is also one of the single most important things you can do to spare yourself future pain caused by
degenerative disease. Many of the most common forms of cancer,
including cancers of the prostate, the colon, and the breast, are
linked to overconsumption of fat. Eating too much fat is also the
biggest single risk factor in cardiovascular disease, which can
cause many types of pain. Furthermore, recent research indicates
that overconsumption of fat is a significant risk factor for developing Alzheimer's disease and rheumatoid arthritis. Also, both di-
abetes and osteoarthritis are associated with obesity, which is
often caused by eating too much fat.

Here's a newly discovered fact, though, that's very encouraging. In one of the most recent large-scale studies of fat consumption, it was found that when people began eating mostly low-fat
foods, their blood pressure dropped significantly within just *two
weeks.* This indicates how quickly your body can begin to rid itself
of dietary fat.

In my clinical practice, I've seen inflammation respond to reduced fat consumption within just a matter of days.

So start today! There's no reason to wait.

Other Nutrients that "Put Out the Fire" of Inflammation

In addition to the fatty acids that reduce inflammation, several other foodstuffs also have a demonstrated ability to decrease inflammation.

TURMERIC. This common yellow spice may be the single most powerful natural anti-inflammatory substance; it has long been recognized for this property in the Eastern pharmacopeia. It can be taken in commercially prepared capsules, or used as a spice in a wide variety of recipes—particularly curry dishes.

Western studies have shown that the active anti-inflammatory ingredient in turmeric is curcumin, which has been shown in controlled studies to be as effective as the powerful anti-inflammatory drugs cortisone, ibuprofen, and phenylbutazone. But, unlike these drugs, curcumin can be safe when taken in higher dosages.

Turmeric is about 95 percent pure curcumin.

In one study that compared turmeric to anti-inflammatory drugs, patients with rheumatoid arthritis responded to turmeric with improvements in morning stiffness and joint swelling that were equal to those achieved by phenylbutazone (a drug that can cause gastrointestinal ulcers and immune suppression).

Laboratory tests indicate that the most potent form of turmeric, sodium curcuminate, is a more powerful anti-inflammatory agent than the drug cortisone.

Western herbalists recommend oral ingestion of the herb, but in the Eastern medical tradition it is sometimes applied topically to inflamed areas, as part of a poultice. When taken orally, absorption can be improved by also taking protein-digesting enzymes, such as bromelain.

Turmeric is thought to reduce inflammation by increasing the activity of the natural steroid hormone cortisol, which has strong anti-inflammatory properties.

If you have read my book *Brain Longevity*, you know that I consider cortisol to be neurotoxic when it is present in the system at very high levels over a long period. It is unlikely, though, that the use of turmeric could contribute to this extreme chronic elevation of cortisol. The primary cause of chronic cortisol elevation is chronic stress.

There is no established dosage for turmeric. I generally advise patients to begin using the drug in small dosages, such as 100–200 mg daily, and to then increase the dosage, if necessary. It is generally sold in capsules of 100 mg. Significant side effects have not been reported by my patients, but mild stomach upset may occasionally occur if you take very high dosages. If this happens, reduce the dosage.

Turmeric is available as a spice in almost all supermarkets, but turmeric capsules are somewhat harder to find. Many health-food stores do not carry them, so you may need to order them from one of the sources in Appendix III, "Resources and Referrals."

Turmeric is also often available as a major component of natural anti-pain formulations. Sources for some of the better formulations are also listed in Appendix III.

BOSWELLIN. This is another ancient Asian remedy—long a staple of Indian Ayurvedic medicine—that has recently been proven effective in laboratory experiments and controlled clinical trials. Boswellin comes from the gum of the *Boswellia serrata* tree, which is also the source of the aromatic herb frankincense. In one recent animal experiment, a derivative of Boswellin, boswellic acid, reduced inflammation in arthritic animals by 28 to 55 percent.

In a study of 175 rheumatoid arthritis patients, 67 percent of the patients reported a good-to-excellent response to Boswellin. Results included reduction of stiffness, pain, and swelling.

Boswellin is believed to relieve inflammation by reducing the number of white blood cells that "migrate" to an inflamed area.

A reasonable beginning dosage of Boswellin is 300 mg daily. When taken in such moderate dosages, my patients have generally not reported significant side effects.

Boswellin may be relatively difficult to find. You may need to order it through the mail from a reputable supplier of specialty supplements.

GINGER. For thousands of years, Asian healers have used ginger as an anti-inflammatory agent. It is believed that ginger relieves inflammation by decreasing the number of "bad" prostaglandins.

The noted medical author Andrew Weil, M.D., an ardent advocate of botanical medicine, has stated that ginger might be as effective as some of the nonsteroidal anti-inflammatory drugs. However, as he points out, ginger *protects* the lining of the stomach, while the nonsteroidal anti-inflammatories *irritate* the stomach lining.

Ginger can be eaten fresh, and is commonly served this way in many Chinese dishes. However, it has a more powerful anti-inflammatory effect when it is dried. Dried ginger, sold in capsules, is available in many health-food stores. It generally comes in capsules of 500 mg.

A reasonable beginning dosage is two 500 mg capsules, taken two to four times daily.

PROTEIN-DIGESTING ENZYMES. These enzymes—including protease, bromelain, trypsin, lipase, pancreatin, amylase, and papain—have a significant anti-inflammatory effect. They help the immune system distinguish between harmless foreign substances and invasive substances that trigger the inflammatory response.

In several controlled clinical studies, protein-digesting enzymes (also known as proteolytic enzymes) were found to provide significant relief from arthritis. In one study of one thousand patients with various inflammatory rheumatic diseases, almost 70 percent showed a good-to-excellent response, with minimal side effects.

An added benefit of these enzymes is that they will almost certainly aid your digestion of foods, and thereby help heal your gastrointestinal system.

ANTIOXIDANTS. Several antioxidant vitamins, including a form of vitamin E called gamma-tocopherol, do not directly prevent inflammation, but do protect the body from the damage done by inflammation.

Gamma-tocopherol is the only known substance that can rid the body of a highly destructive chemical called peroxynitrite, which is produced by inflammation. This chemical can start processes that lead to cancer and heart disease. In addition, the gamma-tocopherol in vitamin E traps and removes nitrogen oxide, a chemical commonly found in polluted air. A reasonable daily dosage of vitamin E is 400–800 mg.

There is also evidence that other antioxidative nutrients—including vitamin C, vitamin A, and selenium—help protect tissues that are invaded by inflammation. These nutrients help keep muscles, tendons, and ligaments from being permanently damaged by chronic inflammation.

A reasonable dosage of vitamin C is 1000 mg, three times daily. In some people this causes mild gastrointestinal upset. If this occurs, reduce the dosage until the problem goes away. Other people, however, thrive on a dosage of up to two grams of vitamin C, taken three times daily.

A prudent daily dosage of vitamin A is 10,000 IU (international units). Pregnant women, however, should take vitamin A only under the care of a physician, because, as mentioned before, high dosages during pregnancy can cause birth defects.

Selenium, the most powerful mineral antioxidant, should be consumed in dosages of 50–100 mcg daily. At this dosage, it may also have a mild anti-anxiety effect.

Those are the most powerful anti-inflammatory nutrients. If you regularly take some of them—or all of them—you will almost certainly reduce your inflammation.

When you combine anti-inflammatory nutritional therapy with the other three elements of nutritional therapy—and with the other levels of my anti-pain program—your inflammatory pain will no longer be in control of you; you will be in control of *it*.

Anti-inflammatory Nutrients

Helpful

- EPA (oil)
- GLA (oil)
- ALA (oil)
- Turmeric
- Boswellin
- Ginger
- Protein-digesting enzymes
- Gamma-tocopherol, and other antioxidants (vitamins C and A, and selenium).

Harmful

- Animal fat
- Common cooking oils (including corn oil, safflower oil, sesame oil, canola oil). Instead, *use olive oil.*

After I finished telling Marie and her husband about the nutrients that reduce inflammation, I gave them a list like the one in the sidebar above.

Marie's husband, Paul, who was in his forties, folded the list carefully and put it in his notebook. He was an engineer, and liked things to be well organized.

"Quick question," he said. "Why does Marie always seem to get a migraine just before her period starts?"

"I've noticed that, too," said Marie.

"About 60 percent of all migraines," I told them, "are directly related to menstrual cycles. There's a new theory about why this happens. To me, the theory makes a lot of sense.

"You may not have realized it," I said, "but lots of the most common forms of chronic pain—including migraines, back pain, and chronic muscle pain—strike women far more often than men. Chronic muscle pain is ten times more common among women, and migraines and back pain are three times more common. Two-thirds of all patients at pain clinics are women.

"Do you remember my saying that there is a neurotransmitter that helps close the pain gates?"

Paul glanced at his notes. "Serotonin," he said. I slapped his knee and grinned. I love it when patients and their families listen carefully to what I'm saying, and take responsibility for solving their own problems. You'd be amazed at how many people expect me to do everything.

"Good answer!" I said. "Serotonin is probably the body's single best pain-fighter. It's even more important than endorphins.

"Now here's the theory. It looks as if fluctuation of the female hormone estrogen *destabilizes* levels of serotonin. But the male hormone testosterone *stabilizes* serotonin. Therefore, women may be more vulnerable to pain than men. Women are *particularly* vulnerable when menstruation disrupts their estrogen levels."

"But I always heard women had a higher pain threshold than men," said Paul.

"It's possible that because women experience more pain, they learn to tolerate it better," I said. "But they do not appear to have a higher pain threshold. In fact they seem to have a *lower* pain threshold."

I asked Marie if she tended to have severe premenstrual symptoms. She said she did. "Including depression?" I asked.

Marie and Paul both said, "Yes!"

I told them that elevated premenstrual symptoms and depression both indicate a possible serotonin deficit.

"However," I said, "serotonin levels can be increased nutritionally. It's not at all hard."

"Tell us how," said Paul. He opened his notebook to a new page.

Before I started, though, I had Marie complete the patient intake forms. While Paul got a cold drink, I scanned the forms. What I saw was sad. Marie wasn't just "in pain"—she was *suffering*. Her headaches caused true agony that seemed endless. On the pictograph indicating degree of pain, Marie had sketched over the teardrops falling down the patient's face, making them dark and huge. I'd never seen anyone do that. In addition, she clearly had many of the characteristics of chronic pain syndrome.

One notation she made was, "My pain makes it hard for me to feel love. And it makes it hard for my husband to love me."

Still—here they were. Still hoping. Still trying. Still together. People are strong, and their incredible strength touches me deeply.

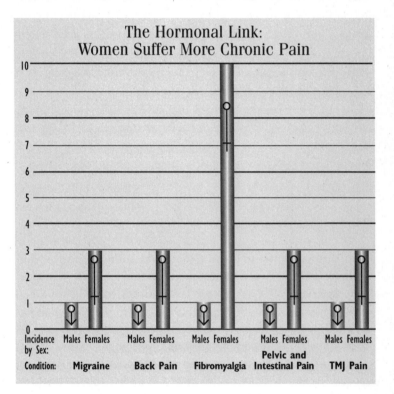

The Hormonal Link: Women Suffer More Chronic Pain

Increasing Serotonin to Raise Your Pain Threshold

Serotonin is your pain's worst enemy. Look at all the ways that serotonin fights pain:

SEROTONIN REDUCES PAIN-CARRYING "SUBSTANCE P." Remember substance P? It's one of the main chemical carriers of pain. Think of it as "substance Pain." Secreted in your spinal column in response to pain signals from nerves, it carries those pain signals to the brain. If pain signals don't reach the brain, you feel no pain—because, ultimately, *pain is in the brain.* Serotonin can decrease the release of substance P. When it does this, it slams shut some of your pain gates.

SEROTONIN FIGHTS PAIN IN THE BRAIN. Even after some pain signals reach the brain, serotonin *still* fights them. The brain's thalamus—its "pain receiving center"—is full of serotonin-system nerve cells. When the thalamus receives pain signals, these cells help launch the counterattack against pain.

In the brain, serotonin actually blocks the *perception* of pain, modulating the intensity of pain signals. In addition, it helps your brain control its counterattack against pain by keeping your brain from overreacting to pain, and "centralizing" pain in your nervous system.

SEROTONIN IMPROVES YOUR MOOD. As you now know, if you react to pain with fear and depression, the pain hurts more. You not only *perceive* it more acutely, but you're less able to launch a controlled, effective counterattack.

Serotonin, though, improves your mood, and helps quiet your fears and relieve your depression. This enables you to fight pain with your peak brain power.

SEROTONIN HELPS REGULATE YOUR SLEEP CYCLES. As I've mentioned, if your brain has been weakened by lack of sleep, you will be far less able to effectively fight pain. Serotonin, though, helps you to sleep. Along with another important "sleep hormone," melatonin, serotonin helps you fall asleep and stay asleep, even when you are experiencing pain.

SEROTONIN AIDS THE FLEXIBILITY OF BLOOD VESSELS. This helps people with chronic inflammatory conditions. When blood vessels are more flexible, they're not as likely to "leak" blood, and cause painful irritation. Serotonin increases blood vessel elasticity, and helps prevent "leakage." One condition this helps is migraine headaches, which are caused primarily by blood vessel leakage in the brain. As you'll see in chapter 7, one of the best ways to prevent and treat migraines is to increase serotonin levels.

As you can see, serotonin powerfully opposes pain in a number of ways.

However, as I've stated, pain itself lowers levels of serotonin. Serotonin gets "used up" at the site of inflammation, and when that happens, you have even more vulnerability to pain. You are also more prone to depression, and more apt to have insomnia. It's a vicious cycle.

But there's a solution: *Create more serotonin.*

This can be done with medication, with light therapy, and with mind/body exercises. However, one of the more effective ways to increase serotonin levels is with nutritional therapy. I'll tell you how.

Serotonin is manufactured by the body from a partial protein (or "amino acid") called tryptophan. Tryptophan is in most of the foods we eat.

However, millions of people either don't get enough tryptophan, or don't convert enough of it into serotonin. One indication that a serotonin shortage is a very common problem is the popularity of a drug that increases serotonin levels: Prozac. In recent years, Prozac has become one of the most widely used drugs in the world.

Foods Rich in L-Tryptophan

Food	Milligrams of L-tryptophan
Chicken (3 oz.)	285
Cheddar cheese (3 oz.)	270
Halibut (3 oz.)	211
Egg	210
Peanuts (1/2 cup)	184
Peanut butter (2 tablespoons)	112

Other sources include milk, soybeans, and other forms of cheese.

Please note that many of these foods are very high in fat, and must be eaten in strict moderation.

Prozac and drugs like it (such as Zoloft) can be very helpful for some people, including some pain patients; I will discuss these drugs in chapter 4. However, Prozac frequently has side effects. Also, it's not appropriate for people who have only a mild deficit of serotonin. Therefore, I prefer to help my patients increase their serotonin levels in more natural ways. The simplest and most effective way is to do mind/body exercises, which I will describe later. However, some patients are able to increase their serotonin levels by increasing their nutritional intake of tryptophan.

Tryptophan is available as a supplement, but it is more difficult to acquire than it used to be. Several years ago, a tainted batch of tryptophan tablets, contaminated during the manufacturing process, resulted in a number of illnesses and deaths. Because of this tragedy, the U.S. Food and Drug Administration prohibited the sale of tryptophan as an over-the-counter supplement. Now, in America, tryptophan requires a doctor's prescription, and must be purchased through a "compounding pharmacy," one that mixes its own formulations.

Tryptophan is also available as a supplement in a number of countries outside the United States, including several countries in Europe. A U.S. citizen may legally purchase it from an overseas company, through a buyer's club, such as those listed in Appendix III.

Another source of tryptophan that is currently available in America as a supplement is 5-HTP (or 5-hydroxy L-tryptophan). A modified form of tryptophan, 5-HTP, obtained from plant sources, tends to have an even more powerful positive effect than tryptophan. A reasonable daily dosage is 50 mg. People with severe pain may, however, require a higher dosage. To obtain 5-HTP, please see Appendix III.

If you take tryptophan supplements, an appropriate daily dosage would be 250–500 mg for a healthy person. However, a person with chronic pain may require up to 3,000 mg daily. This relatively high dosage should be taken in several administrations during the day, under the direction of a health care professional.

Many people prefer to take their largest dosage of tryptophan in the evening, because it may cause drowsiness, due to its immediate stimulation of serotonin output. Also, tryptophan triggers release of melatonin, the "sleep hormone." For many years, tryptophan has been popular as a mild and safe sleep aid.

It is possible that if you take too much tryptophan you will not feel calmed, but will instead feel agitated, because serotonin can cause nervous tension if its levels get too high. Like the levels of all other neurotransmitters, serotonin levels should be kept within the optimal range. It's possible to get "too much of a good thing." If you feel agitated after taking tryptophan, reduce your intake.

If you choose not to take tryptophan in supplement form, you can still increase your dietary intake by eating complex carbohydrates in abundance, and eating carbohydrates (starch and sugar) *before* you eat protein. If you eat protein first, your digestive processes will block the absorption of tryptophan.

Many of my patients who suffer from depression have told me that they often crave carbohydrates. I think this is because they need the serotonin boost that carbohydrates often provide.

As you can see, increasing your tryptophan levels by altering your diet is safe and simple. However, to get the high level of tryptophan required to inhibit chronic pain, you may need to ingest tryptophan in supplement form, rather than as part of your diet.

To Build Serotonin Levels
Eat starch or sugar *first*—*then* eat protein.

Now I'll tell you about the third component of my nutritional strategy against pain: beating pain by "building up" the brain.

As I wrote in *Brain Longevity*, "The brain is just flesh and blood." Therefore, the power of your brain can be increased—just like the power of your muscles—with a health-boosting program that includes nutritional therapy. The stronger your brain gets, the better it will fight your pain.

Fighting Pain with the Brain

Your brain does more than just *think*. It also governs every process in your body—directly or indirectly, consciously or unconsciously. One of these processes is the perception, *and the control*, of pain.

We've already discussed *how* your brain helps stop pain. So now let's look at how you can empower your brain.

There are four primary ways to increase the physical health of your brain: (1) with physical and mental exercise; (2) with natural and pharmaceutical medicines; (3) by decreasing stress, especially through meditation; and (4) with nutritional therapy. Because this chapter is about nutrition, we'll now cover nutritional therapy for the brain. In later chapters we'll look at the other methods that increase brain power.

To nourish your brain optimally, you will need to do two things: Eat a good diet, and take a few brain-building supplements.

First, let's discuss diet.

One of the most frequently expressed ideas in *Brain Longevity* is that "what's good for the heart is good for the head." I first heard this from Dr. Candace Pert, the legendary neuroscientist who was one of the discoverers of the endorphin system. What it means is that the heart and the brain *both* thrive on the same general type of diet: low in fat, nutrient-dense, and balanced. I have prescribed this type of diet to many brain longevity patients, and it has helped them overcome brain disorders ranging from mild memory impairment to brain injuries to full-blown Alzheimer's. This type of diet has helped even healthy people to have more mental energy and brain power. I have also prescribed this type of diet to pain patients, and it's helped them tremendously, by giving them the brain power they needed to defeat their pain.

You already know that a diet high in animal fat and common cooking oils increases inflammation. But did you know that a high-fat diet also literally "rots your brain"? Sad but true. Here's why. The brain itself is largely composed of fat; indeed, each brain cell is 60 percent fat. If you bombard this fatty brain tissue with dietary fat—which is loaded with harmful "free radical" molecules that speed up oxidation—you can cause your brain tissues to die from excessive oxidation. In effect, dietary fat turns your brain cells "rancid."

And each time you lose brain cells, you lose part of your ability to fight pain.

Besides "rotting your brain," dietary fat also hurts blood circulation in the brain. This is a disaster because, as I've mentioned, the brain requires 20 percent of all blood pumped by the heart. Anything that starves the brain of blood stops oxygen and nutrients from getting to the brain. It also keeps the brain from flushing away toxins and dead tissue. Eventually, impaired circulation kills brain cells by the billions.

Consequently, a high-fat diet is worse for your brain than any other nutritional mistake.

However, if you stop eating high-fat foods, start exercising, and take a few circulation-enhancing nutrients, in just a matter of days you will begin to clear the fat out of the blood vessels that serve your brain. I've had patients tell me that they've begun to feel more mental energy after just one week on a low-fat diet. Some of these patients were brain longevity patients, who used their new mental vigor for faster thinking, and some were pain patients, who used their new-found brain power to fight their pain.

Your anti-pain diet should also be *dense in nutrients.* You shouldn't eat "empty calories" of sugar and highly refined starches. Instead, eat the wholesome, nutrient-packed foods that supply your brain and nerves with the nutrients they need. Your diet should be composed primarily of whole grains, vegetables, fruits, high-protein soy products, nonfat dairy products, and various kinds of beans (which are very rich in protein).

If you are not a vegetarian, you should eat only occasional small portions of meat—about the size of a chicken breast—and should have several servings of cold-water fish (e.g., salmon or tuna) each week. However, if you avoid meat completely, you will still be able to ingest enough protein, and will avoid the non-fish animal fats that aggravate inflammation.

Your diet should consist of about 15–20 percent fat, 40 percent protein, and 40 percent complex carbohydrates.

The relatively high proportion of protein in this diet will promote muscle growth and regeneration, which will aid recovery from many common types of pain, including back pain, arthritis, and fibromyalgia.

As you can see, it is not a rigid diet; it's extremely flexible, and allows you to eat healthy foods in abundance. A good anti-pain diet is similar to other healthy eating plans, and is also similar to the diets of athletes.

Eating like an athlete may sound somewhat challenging, but

as I once told Scott, my polymyositis patient, people with chronic pain have to be as dedicated as athletes. If they're not, they will find it much more difficult to cure their pain.

Now let's look at the individual nutrients that will make your brain strong enough to defeat pain. You'll get some of these nutrients through your diet, but you'll need to take others as supplements.

VITAMIN A. This powerful antioxidant protects brain cells by fortifying the membranes that surround the cells. Take 10,000–25,000 IU daily. (Pregnant women should take vitamin A only under a doctor's supervision; high dosages can cause birth defects.)

VITAMIN B COMPLEX. Of all vitamins, the B complex is the most important for your nerves. B vitamins are also vital to the brain. A deficit of B vitamins can make you feel irritable, lethargic, nervous, and more sensitive to pain. A severe deficiency, particularly of the B vitamin inositol, can cause inflammation of the nerves. Take a supplement with at least 50–100 mg of the entire complex every day.

VITAMIN C. This nutrient is needed to manufacture several neurotransmitters, and it also protects your brain from free radical molecules. Take 1,000–2,000 mg, three times daily. If this causes mild gastrointestinal upset, reduce the dosage.

VITAMIN E. Besides fighting inflammation, vitamin E slows the aging of the brain, and helps protect the brain from damage by dietary fat. Take 400–800 IU daily.

MAGNESIUM. This "calming" mineral is important for proper function of the nerves, because it helps nerve cells to absorb the nutrients they need. Most people don't get enough magnesium from their diets. Take 200–300 mg daily.

SELENIUM. This mineral is a powerful antioxidant that helps some people to feel more relaxed. However, selenium levels in the body tend to decrease as we age. A prudent daily dosage is 50–100 mcg.

Besides these vitamins and minerals, there are several other important nutritional substances that powerfully enhance the function of the brain. I commonly recommend all of these natural nutritional substances to my brain longevity patients. However, these substances can be just as helpful to patients with chronic pain, because they help to defeat your pain by building your cognitive strength and raising your intellectual acumen, your mood, and your energy. In short, they'll help you to feel great.

LECITHIN (OR PHOSPHATIDYL CHOLINE). This is the primary nutritional "building block" for the main chemical carrier of thought and memory (acetylcholine). It can boost memory dramatically and heighten the ability to concentrate; this makes it of great benefit to pain patients who use mental focus techniques to block pain. Take up to 1,500 mg daily.

PHOSPHATIDYL SERINE. This substance is similar to lecithin's phosphatidyl choline, but is even more powerful. It helps nerve cells to conduct impulses, helps the brain to manufacture neurotransmitters, and blocks the stress hormone cortisol, which can contribute to an increased perception of pain. Because phosphatidyl serine helps produce neurotransmitters, it has been shown in a number of studies to improve short-term memory and concentration. When phosphatidyl serine boosts brain power, it helps the brain launch its counterattack against pain. Take 100–300 mg daily.

ACETYL L-CARNITINE. This nutrient "revs up" energy production in brain cells, and actually helps the two hemispheres of the brain to work together. It may also improve your mood. Most of my patients take 500 mg daily. Patients with severe cognitive decline, though, take up to 1,500 mg daily.

GINSENG. This ancient Eastern herb is an "adaptogen"—so called because it helps the body and brain adapt to biochemical changes. It's a superb buffer against stress, which provokes a cascade of biochemical alterations. Ginseng is a "balanced stimulant" that will give you energy without nervous tension.

Ginseng will improve your energy level by increasing your production of adrenaline without causing the *release* of adrenaline. This can be helpful for pain patients, because a gross deficit of adrenaline can heighten the vulnerability of the nervous system to pain. A therapeutic daily dosage of ginseng is 750–1,500 mg. Most of the commercially available types of ginseng can be of value.

GINKGO BILOBA. This natural herb dramatically improves blood circulation to the brain. In one study, almost 80 percent of patients with poor cerebral circulation benefited significantly from ingestion of ginkgo. Ginkgo has been shown to elicit improvements in cognitive function and psychomotor performance even in Alzheimer's patients. Ginkgo works very quickly. You may notice its effects in as little as one hour. Patients of mine with minimal cognitive decline take 120 mg daily, while patients with severe cognitive decline take up to 320 mg daily.

PHENYLALANINE. This amino acid is vitally important in helping the brain defeat pain. Phenylalanine helps stop the breakdown of endorphins. It is especially beneficial when it is used with other modalities that boost endorphins, such as acupuncture and exercise. A reasonable dosage of phenylalanine, which is also called DLPA, is two to three grams daily.

I do not recommend that all my patients take each supplement, but if you follow these dietary guidelines and take these supplements as recommended by your doctor, I believe that you will increase your brain power. This increase in the functional ability of your brain and nerves will, in turn, help you to overcome your pain. I've seen it happen hundreds of times—and there's no reason it won't happen for you.

Now let's look at the final component of nutritional therapy for pain management: avoiding the classic dietary pain pitfalls.

The Most Important Nutrients for Your Brain and Nerves

Common Nutrients
(daily dosage)

Vitamin A (10,000–25,000 IU)
Vitamin B Complex
 (50–100 mg)
Vitamin C
 (3,000–6,000 mg)
Vitamin E (400–800 IU)
Magnesium (200–300 mg)
Selenium (50–100 mcg)

Special Nutrients
(daily dosage)

Lecithin (1,000–1,500 mg)
Phosphatidyl serine
 (100–300 mg)
Acetyl L–carnitine
 (250–1,500 mg)
Ginseng (750–1,500 mg)
Ginkgo biloba (90–320 mg)
Phenylalanine (2,000–3,000 mg)

The Classic Dietary Pain Pitfalls

If you follow the diet I have recommended, you will already be well on your way to avoiding the four most common dietary mistakes that pain patients make. Even so, you should be well aware of these pitfalls, so that you'll never be tempted to indulge in them.

PAIN PITFALL NO. 1. ALLOWING YOURSELF TO OVEREAT

Many pain patients gradually begin to eat too much. They find that eating is one pleasure they can still enjoy, and it temporarily takes their minds off their pain. It's good to enjoy eating. In fact, it is *important* to enjoy it. But if you give in to gluttony, you will undermine your pain program. Your pain program will require *discipline* and *energy*—both of which can be subverted by overeating.

If you do overeat, you'll find that it will become increasingly difficult to stick to the healthy foods that fight pain. People rarely go on "carrot binges." Also, overeating will probably disturb your hormonal balance and disrupt your blood sugar levels.

In addition, overeating will almost certainly cause you to gain weight, and for some chronic pain conditions—chiefly back pain and arthritis—being overweight drastically increases pain by increasing strain on muscles and joints. Being overweight will probably hurt your self-esteem, too. And you *need* your self-esteem. It's the "fuel" that runs your willpower.

If you find yourself overeating, cut back gradually. *Don't* go on a crash diet. If you do, you'll fall into Pain Pitfall #2: Undereating.

PAIN PITFALL NO. 2. ALLOWING YOURSELF TO UNDEREAT

I know that pain often ruins your appetite, but for a pain patient, undereating can be just as dangerous as not taking necessary medications. Don't forget: nutrition *is* medicine.

If you undereat, you will gradually starve your brain and nerves of the nutrients they need to fight pain. Pain patients need *abundant* intake of many specific nutrients.

Undereating also often triggers low blood sugar (hypoglycemia). Low blood sugar makes pain patients terribly sensitive to pain. It temporarily stops the brain's counterattack against pain.

Certain nutritional deficiencies can *cause* pain all by themselves. These deficiencies include the following:

VITAMIN C DEFICIENCY. This causes a form of subclinical scurvy that creates pain in muscles, joints, and bones. The pain comes from a lack of "connective tissue," which vitamin C helps to manufacture.

VITAMIN D DEFICIENCY. This can cause a condition called *osteomalacia*—a bone-weakening disease that causes pain in bones. The two most common sites of this pain are the legs and back. This condition is often mistaken for osteoporosis.

VITAMIN B COMPLEX DEFICIENCY. If this is severe, it can cause spontaneous "firing" of pain nerves, creating pain throughout the body. A severe deficit of vitamin B_1 can cause pain in the extremities (particularly the feet), as peripheral nerves begin to die.

MAGNESIUM DEFICIENCY. This can contribute to pain in muscles. One particularly disabling form of muscle pain—the heart ailment angina pectoris, which is pain in the muscle of the heart caused by decreased blood flow—is exacerbated by a magnesium deficiency.

A magnesium deficiency also contributes to onset of migraines, because magnesium helps to control the blood vessel contractions and dilations that create migraines. Furthermore, some researchers believe that a magnesium deficiency contributes to fibromyalgia.

CALCIUM DEFICIENCY. This causes leg cramps, particularly at night. Older people often suffer from these cramps because of a lack of calcium.

PAIN PITFALL No. 3. ALLOWING YOURSELF TO EAT FOODS THAT CAUSE ALLERGIES AND FOOD SENSITIVITIES

This pitfall can often be hard to identify, because it may occur in a mild form. Classic, frank food allergies are easy to spot, because they cause overt symptoms, such as hives, dizziness, and wheezing. But mild allergies—and even milder sensitivities—can be quite subtle.

Even when negative reactions to certain foods are muted, though, these reactions can still cause misery for pain patients. Allergic reactions to foods often affect the brain, impairing cognitive function. When this happens, it's called a "cerebral allergy." Even a mild cerebral allergy can heighten sensitivity to pain.

In addition, food allergies mimic the inflammatory response, and can increase inflammation. Both food allergies and inflammation result from the immune system trying to repel a "foreign invader."

One patient, Elizabeth, had suffered from a painful condition, much like chronic fatigue syndrome, for almost twenty years. Although she had bravely endured symptoms that included chronic infections, a foggy memory, severe insomnia, and "migrating" pains, her condition was destroying the quality of her life. She finally discovered—by means of an "elimination diet"— that she was allergic to wheat gluten. When she restricted gluten from her diet, she made a dramatic recovery. Almost all of her symptoms disappeared in a matter of weeks.

If you suspect you may be allergic or sensitive to certain foods, you should try an elimination diet. To do this, try a water fast for one day, and then begin carefully adding foods, one at a time. When you have a reaction, you will know that you are sensitive to the last food you added.

PAIN PITFALL NO. 4. ALLOWING YOURSELF TO EAT FOODS THAT DESTABILIZE HORMONAL BALANCE

Hormones are one of the primary links between your brain and your body. They are secreted into your blood by the eight glands of your endocrine system, and by your liver and kidneys. Hormones have a powerful effect upon your thoughts, feelings, moods, energy level, and perception of pain.

The endocrine glands that have the greatest effect upon your brain are your adrenal glands, your gonads, your pineal gland, and your pituitary. These glands secrete adrenaline, cortisol, testosterone, estrogen, DHEA, and melatonin, all of which profoundly affect your mind and mood. When you are healthy, these hormones tend to achieve a natural balance.

When you experience the constant stress of chronic pain,

however, your hormones generally lose this condition of balance. The results are terribly negative: depression, anxiety, confusion, lethargy, diminished sex drive, and increased sensitivity to pain and stress.

Even when you suffer from chronic pain, though, you can still rebalance your hormones. One of the best ways to do this is with nutritional therapy. The best single nutritional therapy for achieving hormonal balance is to limit dietary fat. Digesting fat taxes your liver, which is an important organ for maintaining hormonal balance. Your liver helps to orchestrate your "hormonal symphony." Any nutrients that stress your liver hurt your hormonal balance. Sugar can be very harmful, and so can chocolate and alcohol.

One of the best nutritional ways to help rebuild your liver is to take abundant amounts of B vitamins, or to eat beets, which help to stimulate proper liver function. Another nutrient that has a powerful healing effect on the liver is milk thistle (or silymarin), an herb that is available at all health-food stores. An appropriate dosage of silymarin is one to two 500-mg capsules daily.

That concludes Level One of my pain program.

As you can now fully appreciate, nutritional therapy is a powerful weapon against pain. It helps stop inflammation, builds your levels of pain-killing serotonin, increases endorphin production, and helps your brain launch a vigorous counterattack against pain.

When you add nutritional therapy to the other three levels of my pain program, you will be able to oppose your pain with a power you never dreamed possible.

So let's move on. But first you probably want to know what happened to Marie.

Marie

Marie and Paul came in together for her last appointment. Since I'd first met her, eight months earlier, she had come to her subsequent appointments alone. She had begun to feel better very early in her program, and had become less dependent upon Paul.

Marie had participated in her program on all four levels—nutritional therapy, physical therapies, medication, and mental control—and it had had a profound impact on her life. She had quickly progressed from the reduction of symptoms to the elimination of symptoms. Then, as her general health and well-being continued to improve, she had begun to feel great.

She still had occasional, relatively mild headaches, but they no longer controlled her life. Now totally free of chronic pain syndrome, she was no longer depressed, her sleeping patterns were normal, she exercised daily, and she was much more involved with her hobbies and work.

As Paul and Marie sat together on a couch in my office, they were smiling and happy. Later that week they were going on a cruise. It was something they had always wanted to do, but Marie had previously been afraid that her migraines would ruin the trip.

"I told Marie if she could go two months without a migraine, I'd take her to the Caribbean," Paul said. "So we're calling this our Victory Tour."

"Two months!" I exclaimed. Before her treatment, Marie had suffered from a migraine almost every week, and it had lasted at least two days.

"Actually," Marie said, "I had one last week."

Paul looked surprised. "The trip's *off*," he said—but he was smiling. "Why didn't you tell me?"

"Oh, my headaches just aren't the *same* anymore," Marie said. "They're just . . . headaches. It doesn't feel like my brain is on fire."

Paul looked at me. "She's my hero," he said proudly.

"Even more than when she was suffering?" I asked.

Paul thought about it. "The truth?" he said. "Yeah. More. Know why? Because I think it takes more courage to *end* suffering than it does to endure it."

Paul was absolutely right.

It takes more courage to end suffering than it does to endure it.

Now let's forge ahead, to the next level of my program, so that we can soon end *your* suffering.

3

Level Two:
Physical Therapies

The process of self-healing is the privilege of every human being.
—YOGI BHAJAN

Tiffany looked at me from her wheelchair with pleading eyes. "Help me to walk again," she implored. *"Please."*

My heart went out to her. She was suffering so much. But I had to be honest.

"All I can do," I said, "is help you make the most of what you still have. And I think that should be your goal—not walking, or even becoming totally pain-free. Those things might happen if you reach your highest possible level of function. But they might not. I can only guarantee you one thing," I said. "If you can find a way to do the absolute *best* with what you have, you'll find peace."

She looked disappointed, as if I'd urged her to settle for a lesser goal. "Tiffany," I said forcefully, "doing your best will be *harder* than walking. I'm talking about healing your whole life—not just your legs."

"My life isn't paralyzed," she said sadly. "Just my legs."

I nodded sympathetically—but she was wrong. Her life *was* paralyzed. She was "stuck"—in her grief, in her anger, and in her chronic pain syndrome. She was also stuck in her wheelchair.

Whether she could accept it or not, her wheelchair was now part of her life.

She wanted me to restore her life by healing her legs, but I didn't think that was possible. The only practical medical approach was to try to heal her legs by healing her life.

If you are trying to heal your own chronic pain, that's also the approach you should take. You should forget about achieving a perfect, pain-free life, and instead put all your energy into becoming the best possible "you." If you can reach that goal, you will find peace, even if you still have some pain.

In this chapter I'm going to tell you how to find relief from pain through various physical therapies, including acupuncture, exercise therapy, chiropractic and osteopathic manipulation, heat and cold therapy, mind/body exercises, aromatherapy, light therapy, magnetherapy, and massage. These therapies will address the physical structure of your body, and make it more resistant to pain. For the most part, these are "mechanical" therapies, but they can ultimately exert far-reaching effects upon the body's biochemistry, including the chemistry of mood and pain. In the case of the mind/body exercises, they can even influence the spirit.

For Tiffany, this aspect of my pain program was vitally important. It will be for you, too.

To begin my consultation with Tiffany, I administered a standard medical workup. I also assessed her degree of chronic pain syndrome.

By the end of both procedures, I knew that Tiffany faced some terrible obstacles.

Tiffany, who was twenty-three, had been on a sharp career ascent until she was horribly injured. Beautiful and sophisticated, she'd been a gifted photographer, but had gotten hurt while she was taking a photo near a railroad track. She had been sucked into the vortex of a speeding train and dragged.

She'd survived, but when she'd been found lying on the railroad tracks, she was little more than a bloodied sack of broken bones. Her spinal cord had been badly stretched, and this had left her paralyzed from the waist down.

During multiple surgeries, she'd had rods inserted along her spinal column, and her vertebrae had been fused. This had helped her to sit upright, but it had not relieved her severe chronic pain.

She still had a modest degree of feeling in her legs, but that only contributed to her pain. She suffered from hyperesthesia, a condition in which even a light touch can hurt badly. Whenever something brushed against her legs, she felt like screaming. She also had a burning pain in her lower back, and suffered frequent, wrenching back spasms. In addition, she had severe centralized pain that felt to her as if it were coming from her legs. This pain, which she described as her "weird pain," often caused goosebumps on her legs.

Also, it appeared as if Tiffany's nervous system had shifted to a state of almost constant excitation. She showed signs of a significant imbalance in the part of her nervous system that governs automatic actions, such as digestion, or breathing. This part of the nervous system consists of two branches—the excitatory sympathetic branch, and the calming parasympathetic branch. In Tiffany, the sympathetic branch appeared to have become markedly dominant. This is not uncommon among pain patients, because frequently their nervous systems interpret their pain as a threat, and stay locked in a state of constant alert. Unfortunately, though, this nervous excitation just magnifies pain.

Partly because of her continual nervous stimulation, Tiffany was on the verge of adrenal exhaustion, and was very depleted in energy.

Psychologically, she suffered from moderate clinical depression. Part of her depression stemmed from her feelings of sadness about the accident. But part of it was biochemical. Chronic pain often causes biochemical depression, primarily because it upsets the balance of the brain's neurotransmitters.

Unfortunately, though, this depression heightens the perception of pain, and lowers the pain threshold. The added pain then causes even more depression. This is a common vicious cycle—and Tiffany was definitely caught in it.

Depression, as you probably recall, is a major component of chronic pain syndrome. However, depression was not the *only* element of chronic pain syndrome that afflicted Tiffany. She also felt isolated and helpless, had trouble sleeping, and was physically inactive. All of these aspects of chronic pain syndrome were robbing Tiffany of her life, and increasing the intensity of her pain.

Based on my workup, I devised a treatment program for Tiffany that consisted of (1) balancing her nervous system; (2) reducing her pain; (3) treating her depression; (4) restoring her depleted physical and mental energy; (5) stimulating the physical regeneration of her lower body; and (6) controlling her chronic pain syndrome.

After my medical workup, I also examined Tiffany with the diagnostic techniques of Traditional Chinese Medicine, or TCM. These techniques include taking "pulses" of life-energy, or *ch'i*, and examining the body for subtle signs of distress and imbalance.

As often happens, the TCM diagnosis yielded results that were similar to those obtained by the Western diagnostic procedures.

However, because the Asian healing tradition is over five thousand years old, the TCM diagnosis was framed in a vastly different form of expression than the Western diagnosis. Five thousand years ago, TCM doctors had no anatomical knowledge about the parasympathetic and sympathetic branches of the nervous system. But they did see that there was a stimulating, aggressive element in the physical energies of all people, and also a calming, passive element. They named these two elements *yin* and *yang*—instead of parasympathetic and sympathetic. Then, as Western doctors often do, they tried to promote healing by balancing these two forces.

However, the practitioners of TCM ascribed the qualities of yin and yang to more than just physical, human energy. TCM doctors believe that there is a natural balance of equal, opposing forces in *all* things—inside the body and out. They believe that the key to healing is to provide the body with the proper balance of yin and yang in *every* aspect of life.

For example, they believe that work should be balanced with play, that acidic foods should be balanced with alkaline foods, that cold should be balanced with heat, that action should be balanced with contemplation, and so on.

This concept is as profound as it is practical. Achieving balance in all aspects of life is a superb way to prevent disease and to activate the body's own natural healing force.

As a healing method, though, promoting balance does not always yield *immediate* results. Therefore, it's not always helpful in a medical crisis. But for long-term, chronic conditions—such as chronic pain—the TCM approach frequently works even better than the Western approach. It activates the body's own natural power with stunning efficiency.

Moreover, if you *combine* the Eastern approach and the Western approach—as integrative medicine—you can achieve the highest *possible* potential for healing. For many years I have practiced integrative, or complementary, medicine, and I have consistently achieved results that have been superior to those commonly attained by practitioners of just Western medicine, or just Eastern medicine.

Tiffany, according to my TCM diagnosis, was grossly imbalanced in many aspects of her life, and this imbalance had badly depleted her life-energy, or ch'i. Her depleted ch'i deprived her of the power that she needed to launch a strong biological counterattack against her pain. It also contributed to her depression, and to her physical inability to regain at least partial use of her legs.

To help Tiffany revitalize her ch'i, I needed to help her rebalance her mind, body, and spirit.

To revitalize ch'i, there must be not only a balance of yin and yang, but also a balance of the metaphorical qualities known as the Five Elements. TCM doctors believe that balancing the Five Elements fine-tunes the overall balance of the entire system. The Five Elements, which symbolically describe the quality of everything in life, are earth, water, metal, fire, and wood. According to TCM, everything that exists—from objects to emotions—is related to one of the Five Elements. For example, a hard "metal emotion" is grief, while a warming "fire emotion" is joy. By the same token, "metal weather" is dry, while "fire weather" is hot.

TCM doctors believe that achieving balance among the Elements—which is to say, achieving balance in *everything*—is the best possible way to rebuild ch'i, and overcome disease.

In the metaphorical language of TCM, Tiffany's grief about the accident had depleted her "metal energy," which she badly needed to nourish her ch'i. Tiffany's depleted metal energy also rendered her unable to "dampen" the "wood energy" of her anger. Without this "dampening," her anger simmered, and fed her degenerative spiral of grief/pain/anger. This spiral kept her depressed and weak, and left her in almost constant pain.

Even though the metaphorical language of TCM may seem strange to you, the fact is, the TCM diagnosis called for basically the same treatments as the Western diagnosis: balancing Tiffany's flow of life-energy, helping her resolve her grief, and nurturing her physical and mental condition.

To achieve all this, I knew that I would need to apply a full-spectrum program of integrative medicine. Part of this program would consist strictly of Western modalities (nutritional therapy, medication, physical rehabilitation, and psychological counseling). But I knew that if I employed *only* these therapies, I would probably fail.

I would also need to apply two of the most powerful modalities of TCM: acupuncture and advanced yogic mind/body exercises.

I thought that if I combined *all* of these Eastern and Western modalities, in a comprehensive, coordinated program of integrative medicine, I just might—with the grace of God—be able to work some "magic."

Tiffany was already familiar with the modalities of integrative medicine, because she had previously consulted with two of the world's most gifted artisans of healing, Deepak Chopra and Andrew Weil. In fact, Dr. Weil—a fellow resident of Tucson, Arizona—had referred Tiffany to me because he respects my work with pain patients.

After I explained my program to Tiffany, she looked encouraged. "Let's get started," she said. "I'm *ready*."

She was very brave. As the husband of my patient Marie had

once noted, "It takes even more courage to *end* suffering than it does to endure it."

Tiffany, I believed, had the courage it would take to end her suffering.

Acupuncture: A Path to Power

The news of acupuncture's power was brought to the West thanks to President Richard M. Nixon. The Lord works in mysterious ways, as they say.

Prior to the Nixon administration, Western medicine had for centuries been largely oblivious to the healing force of acupuncture. In 1971, however, President Nixon "opened" China to the West and exposed Western physicians to acupuncture. During Nixon's first visit to China, a prominent *New York Times* journalist, James Reston, suffered severe pain after undergoing an emergency appendectomy. But Reston's pain was relieved instantly when Chinese doctors treated him with acupuncture. The astonished American delegation spread the word of Reston's "magical" recovery, and acupuncture began its gradual entry into mainstream medicine in the United States.

These days, acupuncture is accepted by most American pain specialists as one of the most effective methods of controlling pain. Nonetheless, many doctors who do not specialize in pain are poorly informed about acupuncture. They consider it to be arcane, ineffective, and unscientific.

That attitude is terribly unfortunate for the patients of those ill-informed doctors.

Despite what these doctors may think, there is abundant evidence, gained from careful scientific testing, that acupuncture can stop pain.

Consider, for example, the following chart, which portrays the success of acupuncture in four large studies. In each of these studies, acupuncture was more successful than conventional Western therapies.

The Success of Acupuncture
Compared with Conventional Treatments

Response to Acupuncture:				
Condition:	Back Pain	Sciatica	Sciatica	Postoperative Pain
Number of Patients:	56	90	188	100
Length of Symptoms:	3 mos. to 2 yrs.	1 year +	1 year +	Not Available
Treatments that Failed:	Medication Rest	Surgery Medication Rest	Manipulation Surgery Exercise	Medication
Country and Year:	Canada, 1980	U.S., 1973	Australia, 1979	U.S., 1973

LEGEND: ■ CURED ▨ MARKED IMPROVEMENT ▧ MODERATE IMPROVEMENT □ NO EFFECT

As with many other medical modalities, it's easier to prove that acupuncture *does* work than to prove *how* it works. However, there are several theories, and it's possible that any or all of them may be true.

Following are the major theories. All except the last are Western theories; the last one is the ancient TCM theory.

• Acupuncture causes the release of endorphins into cerebrospinal fluid.

• Acupuncture stimulates "peripheral" nerves, which travel to the body's extremities and wage the counterattack against pain.

• Acupuncture releases anti-inflammatory agents into the bloodstream.

• Acupuncture reduces tension in the muscles.

• Acupuncture regulates the flow of ch'i through "energy

meridians" that travel, somewhat like nerves, throughout the body.

There are several different forms of acupuncture, but all are based upon the original, ancient approach. The most common forms are standard TCM acupuncture; European acupuncture (which was adapted from TCM); medical acupuncture (a form of European acupuncture now practiced by American medical doctors); and electroacupuncture, which employs mild electrical stimulation.

I practice medical acupuncture, which I learned at the University of California, Los Angeles. The UCLA School of Medicine program is the world's most prominent training venue for medical acupuncture. To find a physician in your area who attended that program, see Appendix III.

I do not believe, however, that medical acupuncture is the only valid form of the modality. Any of the most common forms of acupuncture will probably help you, if administered by a licensed professional.

Some people worry that acupuncture might hurt, since needles are used. It rarely causes significant pain. The needles are so thin that they part the skin without puncturing it. Having an acupuncture needle inserted is nothing like getting jabbed with a thick, hollow hypodermic needle. In most instances people do not even know when the acupuncture needle is inserted. Many people enjoy acupuncture sessions, because acupuncture often creates a sense of inner calm, as energies become balanced.

Often, health insurance covers the cost of acupuncture. Even if your insurance doesn't cover acupuncture, though, it's usually not very expensive. Rates generally run about forty-five dollars to sixty-five dollars per session.

If you have a serious chronic problem, you may require five to ten sessions annually. You may, however, need far fewer sessions.

Acupressure and Shiatsu

There is even a form of acupuncture therapy that you can practice by yourself, in your own home: acupressure. As you may know, acupressure consists of kneading, manipulating, and massaging acupuncture points. The results gained by acupressure are often not as dramatic and gratifying as those achieved by acupuncture, but acupressure does have certain advantages. It's free, and you can do it yourself at any time, for as long as you like.

Before you try to perform your own acupressure, though, it would be wise to attend at least one session with a therapist trained in acupressure. As the therapist performs acupressure, you can ask him or her questions about the technique. One popular form of acupressure is called *shiatsu*, in which the therapist applies pressure to acupuncture points to balance ch'i.

To perform acupressure, you apply pressure on a known acupuncture point with the tip of your finger. If you have accurately located the point, you will probably feel some tenderness or soreness. This soreness, according to the Western interpretation of acupuncture, indicates a blockage in the flow of nerve energy. According to the Asian theory of acupuncture, this soreness indicates a blockage in the flow of ch'i.

After you have located the point, press firmly on it while rotating your fingertip. You may need to press for as little as thirty seconds, or for as long as ten to twenty minutes. You can stop pressing when you feel relief from your problem, or when the soreness begins to fade.

The chart on the following page shows the classic acupuncture points for specific types of pain and discomfort. You'll note that most of the points are named after bodily organs. Treating those points should not only help stop your pain, but may also help improve the function of the organ.

I do believe that acupressure can help, but I do not believe that it is as powerful as acupuncture. If you have a serious chronic pain disorder, I strongly advise you to consider the help of a professional acupuncturist.

Acupressure for Pain Relief

Pain Conditions

Earache:	TH-17	Stomach pain:	CV-12
Headache:	LI-4	Bladder or urethral pain:	CV-8
Chest pain:	CV-17	PMS pain and anxiety:	Ht-7
Sinus pain:	BL-2	Breast pain and swelling:	CV-17
Eye pain:	GB-14	Uterine pain:	CV-4
Neck pain:	GV-14	Irritability and tension:	LI-4 + Li-3 + GB-21
TMJ pain:	SI-3 + SI-19 + St-44	Anxiety and insomnia:	Ht-7 + Sp-6
Nausea:	MH-6	Leg cramps:	Li-3, BL-58 + GB-34

POINTS

1. TH-17
2. GB-39
3. LI-4
4. UB-58
5. CV-17
6. BL-2
7. GB-14
8. GV-14
9. SI-3
10. SI-19
11. St-44
12. MH-6
13. CV-12
14. CV-8
15. Ht-7
16. CV-4
17. Li-3
18. GB-21
19. Sp-6
20. GB-34

ABBREVIATIONS

LI = large intestine
St = stomach
Sp = spleen
Ht = heart
SI = small intestine
BL = urinary bladder
MH = pericardium
TH = "triple heater"
GB = gallbladder
Li = liver
GV = "governing vessel"
CV = "conception vessel"

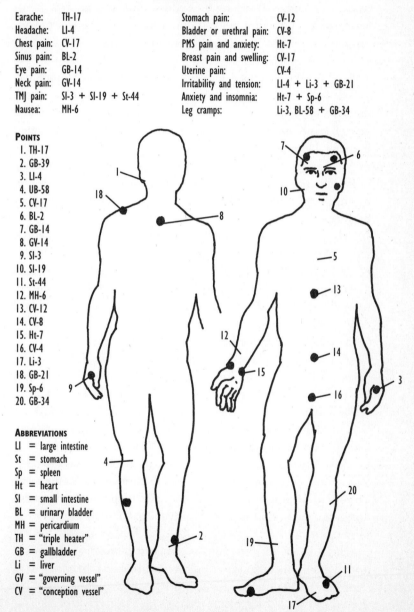

Like virtually every other aspect of my pain cure program, acupuncture works best when it is used in combination with other proven modalities. Don't let the sudden, dramatic improvements caused by acupuncture lull you into abandoning the rest of your program. If you do, you'll risk an eventual relapse.

As I administered a series of acupuncture treatments to Tiffany, her nervous system began to become much more balanced. It shifted away from its condition of sympathetic dominance, and as it did so, she became calmer, less prone to mood swings, less bothered by insomnia, and significantly less depleted in general energy.

As her nervous system regained its balance, her musculoskeletal system also became somewhat more symmetrical. Her posture improved, and it became easier for her to maintain her balance.

The acupuncture also significantly relieved her clinical depression. Acupuncture, along with exercise therapy, can be extraordinarily effective at quickly correcting the chemical imbalances that create "endogenous" biological depression. In fact, in a recent study done for the National Institutes of Health, a group of severely depressed patients who were treated only with acupuncture averaged a 43 percent reduction in depression symptoms.

As Tiffany's depression began to lift, so did her pain. As you know, biological depression opens the "pain gates," and makes the brain much more vulnerable to the recurring cycle of pain. When Tiffany corrected the chemical imbalances that caused her biological depression, her pain gates started to function more efficiently, and began to better protect her brain from pain.

This new freedom from pain, in turn, eased Tiffany's psychological suffering, and this, too, helped control her depression. Thus a positive upward spiral gradually replaced the negative downward spiral that had previously locked Tiffany into her suffering.

Her acupuncture treatments also had a *direct* healing effect upon her chronic pain. After just one treatment, Tiffany began to experience a significant reduction in pain. This may have occurred because of acupuncture's effects upon endorphins, or because of its effects upon nerves, or because of its effects upon "energy meridians." Quite possibly, *all* of these factors helped. The bottom line was that Tiffany's pain became far more manageable. It no longer dominated her life, reminding her constantly of what she had lost.

When Tiffany's life began to improve, she became less obsessed with walking again. As she reintroduced the elements of her life that she'd previously given up—school, work, and socializing—she became more emotionally objective about walking. Walking no longer symbolized life itself. *Life* was life—and walking was just walking.

That was good. As I'd told her the first day we met, the only way she could hope to heal her legs was by healing her life.

One morning, before an acupuncture treatment, she told me she had a surprise. "Look," she said, pointing to her right leg.

With great strain, she lifted her foot slightly off the floor.

I felt so happy I got tears in my eyes.

"Tiffany," I said, "it's time for you to start exercising!"

Exercise Therapy

Exercise is indispensable for *all pain patients*. It has a host of systemic effects that directly block pain.

If you're in chronic pain, exercise may sound repugnant. If so, you've got to find the courage to overcome your aversion. I'm *sure* you can do it. If you weren't a courageous person, you wouldn't be reading this book; you could tell from page one that this isn't a program for weaklings.

To get enough exercise to help block pain, you don't need to run a marathon. The important thing is to do what you can, even if it's only deep breathing exercises. As you persevere, you'll progress.

Here's what exercise does:

EXERCISE BOOSTS OUTPUT OF ENDORPHINS. The endorphin system evolved, in part, as a protective mechanism that enabled people to do hard physical work for long hours. The "second wind" that you sometimes get when you're physically exhausted is, in part, a massive release of endorphins.

EXERCISE INCREASES THE BRAIN'S SUPPLY OF SEROTONIN. As you'll recall, the neurotransmitter serotonin is your pain's worst enemy. In fact, "runner's high"—the mental exhilaration that is usually ascribed to increased endorphin release—is probably more a result of increased *serotonin* release. Researchers believe this because they know that serotonin has a far greater effect on the mind than do endorphins, which mainly just affect the body. One of the great things about the serotonin boost caused by exercise is that it remains long after your last session of exercise.

EXERCISE INCREASES LEVELS OF NOREPINEPHRINE. Norepinephrine is the adrenal neurotransmitter that boosts mood and energy. As you may remember, a gross excess of stimulating norepinephrine can make pain worse. However, the amount of norepinephrine created by exercise won't do that. Instead, it will help activate your counterattack against pain.

EXERCISE HELPS STABILIZE LEVELS OF ESTROGEN. Estrogen is the sex hormone that can interfere with serotonin. Unstable levels of this hormone, as I've mentioned, may partly account for the fact that chronic pain is far more common in women than in men.

EXERCISE IMPROVES THE OVERALL FUNCTION OF THE BRAIN. As I wrote in *Brain Longevity,* "The brain is just flesh and blood." Like everything else that is made of flesh and blood, the brain derives profound benefit from physical exercise. Advanced imaging techniques, such as MRI scans, clearly show that exercise literally "lights up" the brain with increased physical energy.

One way that exercise increases the brain's energy is by providing it with better blood circulation. Because the brain uses 20 percent of all blood pumped by the heart, any improvement in circulation powerfully enhances brain function by providing the brain with extra oxygen, nutrients, and glucose "fuel."

Exercise also increases output of an important brain hormone called *nerve growth factor.* This hormone helps brain cells to function at peak efficiency.

In addition, exercise improves the *metabolism* of the brain. Exercise not only encourages nutrients to enter the brain, but also speeds the removal of toxins and necrotic debris.

Your brain, as you know, can be your best weapon against pain. Therefore you should exercise your *body* to help boost the fitness of your *brain.*

Exercise programs vary greatly among my pain patients. Some patients do intense aerobic exercise and weight work, while others do mostly nonstrenuous activities, such as gardening or walking.

Here are the four most important guidelines for your anti-pain exercise regime:

1. YOUR WORKOUT SHOULD BE INTENSE ENOUGH TO RAISE YOUR HEARTBEAT BY 50 PERCENT. If your resting heartbeat is eighty beats per minute, your heartbeat during exercise should be 120.

This level of intensity will evoke the "training effect," which will speed up your metabolism; cause the secretion of extra endorphins, serotonin, and norepinephrine; burn your stored fat; and place a healthy degree of stress on your cardiovascular system.

If you don't achieve the training effect, your neurological response to exercise will be much more limited.

People who are not very fit can achieve the training effect from doing mild exercise, but people who are in good shape may need to exercise vigorously to achieve it.

An easy way to tell if you're achieving the training effect is to pay attention to your breathing. If you feel like you're slightly out of breath, but can still converse normally, you're in the range of the training effect.

2. YOU SHOULD EXERCISE ALMOST EVERY DAY. If you're sick or injured, you can take some time off. However, the popular concept of "three times a week" is nonsense. This non-challenging approach may enable TV advertisers to sell more exercise equipment, but it won't enable you to wage a serious attack on chronic pain.

If you exercise strenuously, though, you should vary your workouts, and allow yourself at least a day or two of mild workouts each week.

3. YOU SHOULD EXERCISE AT YOUR TRAINING-EFFECT LEVEL FOR AT LEAST HALF AN HOUR. Anything less than this will not have a significant effect upon your metabolism, or upon your brain biochemistry.

If you're trying to lose weight—which can be crucially important for people with arthritis and back pain—you should stay at the training-effect level for at least forty minutes. During approximately the first thirty minutes of exercise, you will not burn stored fat.

In addition to doing at least thirty minutes of brisk exercise every day, you should also do as much *mild* exercise as you can. Any gentle exercise—such as gardening, strolling, or light housework—will be immensely beneficial. It will stretch and tone your muscles, help keep your metabolism elevated, and help to dispel stress.

Over thousands of years, our bodies developed a biological need to be moderately active almost all day long. Thus our current sedentary lifestyles contradict the demands of evolution. The human body was not built to spend half its day sitting at a desk and the other half sitting in front of a TV. That's the kind of lifestyle that helps create chronic pain conditions, and helps perpetuate them.

Above all, avoid being totally sedentary. Researchers discovered recently that a totally sedentary lifestyle is as much of a risk factor for chronic disease and death as smoking cigarettes.

4. YOUR EXERCISE PROGRAM SHOULD BE VARIED. It should consist of aerobic exercise, weight training, and stretching. If you don't do all three forms of exercise, you will limit your fitness level, limit the benefits to your brain and nervous system, and create the risk of injury.

Aerobic exercise should be an important part of your program, because it directly benefits the brain and nervous system. However, virtually all aerobic exercise should be preceded by stretching. Stretching is critically important for avoiding injuries. It's also the best possible preventive measure for back pain, which is the most common avoidable type of chronic pain.

Weight work can be used to add to muscle mass or to tone muscles. The importance of improving muscle function is obvious, since *all* exercise requires muscle. Mild weight work is also extremely helpful in treating arthritis, which strikes virtually all people in their later years.

Two patients of mine typify the wide variations possible in successful exercise programs. One patient was Darren, a massive, six-foot-three professional athlete who badly injured his back in an exhibition game. The other was Tiffany.

Tiffany's exercise program was relatively mild, consisting mostly of gentle exercises in a warm therapy pool, along with stretching and yogic mind/body exercises.

Even mild exercise was enough to evoke the training effect in Tiffany. Her severely injured body had lost much of its muscle tone, and mild exercise was taxing for her.

Every time her face flushed with improving circulation, though, she felt better. The exercise was good for her mood chemistry, and gave her a neurochemical "shield" against pain that lasted for hours. In addition, exercise made her begin to feel whole and strong again.

Darren, who was twenty-seven, at first refused to exercise, because he was in terrible pain. When I first met him, he was marbled with fat from stress-eating, and his big, blocky face often had that chalky, bloodless color that people get when they are in constant pain. He told me that almost every time he moved, it felt like someone was whipping his back with a lash.

Darren was willing to go on a very aggressive program, because his life had become utter misery. Before he'd begun his program, he'd lived from one injection of pain medication to the next, and had been reduced to a humiliating dependence upon others. He'd given up doing all the things that gave him pleasure—fishing, hiking, bowling, and even sex. He couldn't even sit in a theater long enough to watch a movie.

He responded remarkably well to acupuncture, though, and that gave him enough hope to endure the difficulty of a strict weight-loss diet.

By the time he dropped sixty pounds, he was a different man. The worst of his pain was gone, and he'd regained enough mobility to exercise vigorously. I couldn't ascertain whether his weight loss had helped his pain go away, or whether the loss of his pain had helped his weight go away—and, frankly, I didn't care. All that mattered was that Darren had changed a downward spiral into an upward one.

By the end of his first year on my pain program, Darren was doing a strenuous weightlifting routine that would have killed a lesser man. Every so often, though, while he was lifting, his eyes would freeze, and his face would go white with pain. But then he would breathe through the pain, his color would come back— and he'd laugh and grab another weight.

You do not have to be like Darren, though, to benefit from weight training. Even a very casual program can help—regardless of your current level of strength. This was proven in a recent study done at Tufts University. In that study, fifty frail men and women in their eighties and nineties doubled their strength after ten weeks of weight work. They also developed significantly more mineral density in their bones. Mineral density in bones is extremely important, because it is impossible to remain pain-free without a healthy musculoskeletal system. Unfortunately, though, many people forget that their bones are living, changing structures, and they therefore neglect the health of their bones. When bones are not strengthened with exercise, they deteriorate rapidly. Just two weeks of bed rest causes a 7 percent decrease in the density of vertebrae.

One unfortunate result of lax strength-training habits among older people is that one-fourth of all people over sixty suffer from a crushed vertebra. Also, one-third of all people who live to be ninety break a hip.

To get started on your own weight program, don't buy a fancy machine. Just buy a couple of barbells at a discount store.

Don't worry about doing a complex series of weightlifting exercises. Just do the few simple exercises I describe in Appendix II, "Strength Training."

When you do begin to exercise regularly, it's possible that you'll do a little too much, and feel sore. Don't passively *accept* that soreness, or any *other* kind of pain. Fight it! Beat it!

One of the best ways to beat it is with massage.

Defeating Pain with Massage

Massage is an excellent therapy for localized muscle pain, but—like most of the important elements of my program—it also has a systemic effect. As you know, I believe the best pain-fighting modalities are those that have far-reaching, multidimensional benefits. To defeat an enemy as vicious as chronic pain, you must mobilize the forces of your entire body, as well as your mind and your spirit. No major war has ever been won on a single battlefield.

The most obvious benefit of massage for pain patients is that it gives the brain a competing source of input. As you probably recall, because pain signals travel more slowly than "touch" signals, it's easy for touch signals to outrun pain, and to create a "traffic jam" at the spinal cord's pain gates.

It's especially easy for touch signals to outrun the signals of chronic pain, because *chronic* pain signals are generally carried by the very slowest type of pain nerve. Chronic, long-standing pain crawls along at about three miles per hour (on C-polymodal nerves), while acute, short-term pain moves much faster. Acute pain travels to the brain at about forty miles per hour (on A-delta nerves).

Because chronic pain travels so slowly, it's often experienced as a dull ache, and can be hard to pinpoint. Acute pain, though, is usually perceived as a sharp, piercing pain, and is much easier to pinpoint.

Touch signals, however, are much faster than even the fastest acute pain signals. They race to the brain at between 180 and 200 miles per hour (on A-beta nerves).

It's a blessing that chronic pain signals are so slow. It makes it easy for you to "beat them to the gate."

There are many ways to take advantage of this phenomenon. You may have noticed that sometimes, before your dentist gives you a shot of novocaine, he pinches your cheek and wiggles it, or presses his finger against your gums. He does this to create touch signals, which keep your nervous system busy. Then, when he gives you the shot, it doesn't hurt as much.

Your family doctor might use a similar technique when he presses on your arm before giving you an injection. When he does this, it decreases your pain by about one-third. Also, the cooling disinfectant he puts on your arms also helps block pain, by crowding your pain gates with signals of coldness.

Farmers often use this phenomenon when they give injections to animals. Just before they give the shot, they slap the animal in the area that's getting the injection. When they do this, the animal usually doesn't notice the shot.

One of the oldest home remedies for migraines also employs this phenomenon. Many people find that if they begin to brush their hair at the first sign of a migraine, their headache will go away.

However, as I said, massage also has systemic effects that extend beyond the reduction of pain in a localized area. Here are the other things massage does:

- It stimulates the release of endorphins.
- It promotes dilation of capillaries, and reduces pain caused by swelling.
- It decreases levels of the stimulating neurohormone cortisol by up to 50 percent. When produced in excess, cortisol can magnify the perception of pain.
- It reduces muscle spasm, stiffness, and tension.
- It temporarily relieves pain, and this relief can help break the cycle of pain.
- It creates a sense of emotional well-being, which dampens the intensity of pain signals.
- It aids the egress of toxins, including tension-created kinins, which inaugurate pain signals.

There are many forms of massage, some of which are rather esoteric. However, some of the simplest types of massage can be the most beneficial.

The most common form is Swedish massage, which involves light stroking and kneading, with extra pressure on tight muscles. In Swedish massage, muscles are often gently pulled away from bones, then squeezed or tapped.

Almost any family member or friend should be able to perform Swedish massage, and it is also done by professionals.

Other, more complex types of massage and physical therapy are done almost exclusively by professionals. Many of them can be extraordinarily effective against chronic pain. What follows are descriptions of three of the most popular techniques. To find practitioners, see Appendix III.

MYOTHERAPY

This form of massage was developed by prominent physical therapist Bonnie Prudden. It is sometimes called "trigger point" therapy, because it involves pressing on small, constricted, sore points that trigger pain in areas away from the points. For example, a tense, painful knot of muscles in the neck might cause pain in the head.

The existence of trigger points is widely accepted.

Prudden believes trigger points are created by injuries, muscle strain, and emotional stress, and that they can remain for years. Sometimes, she says, the trigger points lie dormant, and don't cause problems until they are activated by additional physical or emotional stress. When activated, they cause the muscle in which they're located to spasm. This spasm then creates a cycle of pain, which often is not localized in the specific area of the trigger point.

To end the pain, Prudden and other myotherapists press against trigger points for about seven seconds with their elbows, then slowly release the pressure. They press with about fifteen to twenty pounds of pressure; you can ascertain approximately how much pressure this is by pressing on your bathroom scale. Trigger points in the hips may require up to forty pounds of pressure, while trigger points in the face may only require about six pounds.

Trigger points can be located only by feeling for them. They will be in different places on different people. In theory, pressure on the trigger point causes it to relax by depriving it of oxygen. When the trigger points are eliminated, stretching exercises can keep them from returning.

Myotherapy, as you probably noticed, is somewhat similar to acupressure. However, it is based upon the manipulation of muscles rather than nerves or energy meridians.

Prudden has documented many dramatic successes with this therapy.

Many doctors also achieve success by injecting trigger points with a local anesthetic called lidocaine, which is similar to novocaine. I'll tell you about that procedure in chapter 4.

ROLFING

This therapy, also referred to as Structural Integration, is a form of deep muscle massage that once had a fearsome reputation as being quite painful. In recent years, though, many professional "rolfers" have modified the therapy, and made it far more comfortable. The therapy was developed in the 1970s by a biochemist, Ida Rolf.

Like myotherapists, rolfers believe that localized muscle tension can last in the body for many years. In fact, rolfers believe that tense muscles can literally become "cemented"—with connective tissue—to tendons, ligaments, and other muscles. When this happens, the body becomes permanently misaligned, stress is "locked in," and correct posture is destroyed. This disruption can create chronic musculoskeletal pain.

Rolfers forcefully pull "cemented" muscles back into their proper positions, and break the adhesions that have kept these muscles out of place.

In general, about ten sessions are required, which will cost about $1,000 total. Some health insurance policies may cover the cost.

I have seen some dramatic improvements caused by rolfing. It can help people progress from constant stiffness and awkwardness to fluidity and grace.

THE TRAGER APPROACH

This method retrains the brain and body to move in ways that relieve stress and pain.

Trager therapists methodically move patients' bodies in specific patterns, to teach their brains and muscles new ways of moving. This therapy is rather more neurological than physical.

As the therapy restructures bodily movements, it encourages patients to find healthier ways to deal with stress. It can be very helpful for people with chronic back pain.

My own clinical experience with this approach is very limited. However, anecdotal evidence appears to support its effectiveness. Scott was one patient of mine who enjoyed its benefits.

Obviously, the physical therapies listed above are most appropriate in the treatment of chronic musculoskeletal pains, including back pain, osteoarthritis, tension-related headaches, fibromyalgia, TMJ pain, and carpal tunnel pain.

However, achieving optimal function of the musculoskeletal system can be of great benefit to a patient with *any* type of pain. Why? Because the musculoskeletal system is an important part of the entire physical system, profoundly affecting the rest of the body. The body, in turn, affects the mind and spirit. Remember, you are a whole being—not just a collection of unrelated parts. To think that structural therapy helps only the musculoskeletal system is as foolish as thinking that nutritional therapy helps only the digestive system.

If you are trying to recover from chronic pain, you should follow the same basic advice I gave Tiffany: To heal your pain, heal your whole life.

Now let's take a moment to consider one of the most popular forms of physical therapy: manipulation therapy.

The Best Structural Therapy

Manipulation therapy, consisting of osteopathic and chiropractic manipulation, is one of the most popular forms of physical therapy for the simple reason that it often has immediate, profound effects.

Chiropractic manipulation and osteopathic manipulation are rather similar. Both forms help restore the balance, efficiency, and function of the body's skeletal structure. Osteopaths, however, generally have a broader education than chiropractors. Osteopaths receive the same medical training as M.D.s, in addition to their osteopathic training. Nonetheless, most chiropractors are adept at structural manipulation.

For many years, chiropractic physicians, and sometimes osteopaths, endured skepticism and scorn from medical doctors, but that attitude has largely changed. Now most medical doctors recognize that manipulation therapy generally offers the best possible treatment for back pain, one of the most common forms of chronic pain.

Virtually all patients with chronic pain can benefit from manipulation therapy, because it improves overall structural health. Also, many experts on holistic health believe that chiropractors and osteopaths generally offer the most progressive health care available, because their treatments often include a variety of adjunctive modalities, such as nutritional therapy, exercise therapy, massage, and homeopathy.

In 1992 the Rand Corporation "think tank" issued a major report indicating that for treatment of certain types of back pain, manipulation therapy was generally superior to drugs or surgery. More recently, a study by the U.S. Department of Health and Human Services concluded that for patients with back pain, manipulation therapy should be pursued *before* surgery is considered.

The study outlined in the graph below, conducted by the California Workmen's Compensation Agency, indicates that manipulation therapy generally speeds recovery from a certain back injury faster than treatment by a medical doctor.

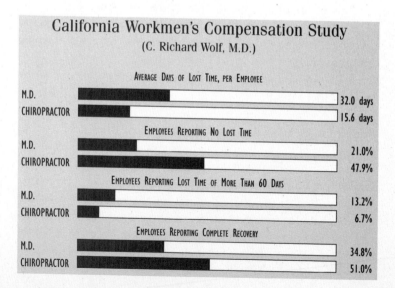

California Workmen's Compensation Study
(C. Richard Wolf, M.D.)

AVERAGE DAYS OF LOST TIME, PER EMPLOYEE

M.D.	32.0 days
CHIROPRACTOR	15.6 days

EMPLOYEES REPORTING NO LOST TIME

M.D.	21.0%
CHIROPRACTOR	47.9%

EMPLOYEES REPORTING LOST TIME OF MORE THAN 60 DAYS

M.D.	13.2%
CHIROPRACTOR	6.7%

EMPLOYEES REPORTING COMPLETE RECOVERY

M.D.	34.8%
CHIROPRACTOR	51.0%

Chiropractic is the most common form of manipulation therapy. Currently, chiropractic physicians perform 94 percent of all spinal manipulation procedures; 4 percent are performed by osteopaths, and 2 percent are done by medical doctors.

Back-pain patients, for the most part, prefer manipulation therapy to treatment by a medical doctor. In a recent study, 66 percent of back-pain patients said they were "very satisfied" with their treatment by chiropractors, compared with just 22 percent who said they were "very satisfied" with the treatment of their back pain by medical doctors. In this same study, patients treated by chiropractors missed an average of just 10.8 days of work, while patients treated by medical doctors missed an average of 39.7 days of work.

The fundamental goal of most manipulation therapy is to correct the position of spinal vertebrae that have been pulled out of place. When this displacement occurs, most often as a result of physical trauma, the area around the vertebrae becomes inflamed, nerves are impinged upon, and muscles go into spasm.

Manipulation therapists correct this vertebral misalignment by carefully stretching the tissue surrounding the vertebrae beyond its normal range of motion. When this is done, the vertebrae often "pop" back into place. Generally, this makes a "clicking" sound, which is apparently caused by gases escaping from the joints.

Many manipulation therapists believe that misaligned vertebrae do more than just cause back pain. They maintain that because the spinal column is the site of the body's primary nerve bundle, anything that harms the function of the spinal column will also harm the body's overall nerve transmission; for example, if there's a misalignment in the area that services the kidneys, kidney function may be impaired.

According to this theory, spinal misalignments are a significant contributor to a wide variety of physical problems. This theory has not been proven, and is disputed by many medical doctors. I believe, though, that there is a powerful element of common sense to it. Whether or not this theory is correct, it is still wise to protect and nurture the spine. The spine is a strong and yet delicate structure, beautifully constructed, pulsing with energy, and has been revered by every healing tradition throughout history. For many people, the best way to take care of your spinal column is with the regular care of a manipulation therapist.

Two more physical interventions against pain work on the same theory as massage: One of the best ways to defeat pain is to beat it in the race to the brain.

Heat and Cold Therapy

When Napoleon's doctors had to perform surgery during the winter campaign against Russia, they laid the injured soldiers in the snow and waited for their bodies to grow numb, which greatly reduced the soldiers' pain. This was hardly the first time cold was used to fight pain: Ancient Egyptian physicians performed their surgery in "cold rooms," dug hundreds of feet into the earth. Even before that, Chinese healers used cold to soothe inflammation. Like touch signals, cold signals travel faster than pain, and can help "crowd out" pain signals. Sufficient cold can cause nerves to go numb.

Cold also fights pain in the following ways:

- Cold stimulates endorphin release.
- Cold constricts blood flow to distressed areas, thereby relieving inflammation, and reducing the influx of pain-causing chemicals (such as kinins and lactic acid).
- Cold relieves muscle spasms.

Cold is generally applied topically, in the form of ice bags or cold packs. It's commonly used for arthritic pain, bursitis, dental pain, and muscle pain, and also for migraines. In one study, cold-pack therapy reduced migraine pain in 80 percent of patients.

Application of heat is also a time-tested remedy for many types of pain. It is particularly effective at promoting relaxation of muscles, and is commonly used for arthritis, back pain, and fibromyalgia. Like cold signals, heat signals travel faster than pain, and they also stimulate release of endorphins.

Heat is usually applied with hot packs, heating pads, and hot baths. Recently, pain therapists discovered that when heat and cold are *alternated* during the same session, it's more effective than either one used alone.

Another recent innovation, which is somewhat similar to application of heat and cold, is the use of a device that produces mild electrical stimulation. The painless electrical current that comes from this device "outruns" pain signals, and jams pain gates. It also causes release of endorphins.

This device, called TENS—for "transcutaneous electrical nerve stimulation"—is quickly being accepted by mainstream pain specialists. Patients using a TENS unit place small electrodes on the area where their pain is, and control the power of the unit themselves. Often the electrodes are placed on acupuncture points adjacent to the painful area.

These units are inexpensive, safe, and effective. For more information about them, consult your physician.

Magnetherapy for Pain

Another technological innovation that is quickly gaining adherents is the use of special magnets for pain control. My patients who have tried this fascinating therapy have responded quite well, and some consider it to be an extremely important part of their pain program.

When I first heard about using magnets to control pain, I thought it sounded futuristic and farfetched. However, as I investigated this approach, I found that the research done on it indicates that it is something that should be taken seriously.

Although there are several sensible theories about how a magnetic force can stop pain, no one is really certain how this therapy works. The most plausible theories are that (1) magnets increase blood flow to the treated areas of the body, possibly by attracting the iron molecules in blood; (2) they influence the bioelectric charge that is present in all living cells; and (3) they stimulate nerve endings and enhance the release of painkilling enkephalins, which are similar to endorphins.

To me, the theory of increased circulation seems quite plausible. Increased circulation helps remove pain-causing lactic acid from muscle tissues, inhibits swelling caused by inflammation, and helps stop calcium ions from migrating to arthritic joints.

The theory of increased circulation is bolstered by the fact that magnets not only appear to reduce pain, but also seem to speed healing. At the University of Miami Medical School, one of a number of research facilities studying magnetherapy, doctors noted that one patient, who suffered from a severe gunshot injury to a bone, fully recovered in five weeks instead of the two to three months that is the norm for recovery from that type of injury. Another patient using magnetherapy fully recovered from bonegraft surgery in five and a half weeks instead of the expected three months.

One very dramatic research photo depicts the abdominal area of a patient who used this therapy to help recover from liposuction surgery. Doctors from Mount Sinai Medical Center in New York placed a large pad containing magnets over this patient's abdomen, following the surgery. In the photo, the area that had been covered by the pad is relatively free from bruising, discoloration, and swelling, while the area outside the pad is a mess of discolored blotches.

This photo was taken during a study of the use of magnetherapy for postsurgical healing. Researchers found that in 75 percent of twenty-one patients, use of magnetherapy greatly reduced pain, discoloration, and swelling.

Another recent study, conducted at Baylor University, indicated that magnetherapy was quite effective for controlling pain in patients with post-polio syndrome. In this controlled study, 76 percent of the patients experienced a significant decrease in pain, compared with 19 percent of a control group treated with sham magnetherapy. The magnetherapy took only forty-five minutes to provide significant relief.

Among the most ardent supporters of magnetherapy are professional golfers on the PGA Senior Tour. Golf can be very damaging to the back, because of the twisting movement of the golf swing. The popularity of magnetherapy among senior golfers began when the therapy was tried by golfer Jim Colbert, who had been forced to retire from the tour because of a degenerative condition in his lower back. Colbert responded quickly and dramatically to magnetherapy, and became the Senior Tour's leading money winner in 1995. Shortly after that, Colbert noted that "half of the men on the Senior Tour are now using magnets." Among those who began using magnetherapy was another Senior Tour top money winner, Bob Murphy, who had previously been forced to retire because of crippling arthritis. Other well-known golfers who have used them include Arnold Palmer and Raymond Floyd.

Not all pro golfers using magnetherapy are seniors, however. Donna Andrews, a star of the Ladies' Professional Golf Association Tour, who is in her mid-thirties, began using them after suffering a severe back injury. Andrews, who regained her success after using magnetherapy, had previously failed to recover from her injury, even though she had participated in a relatively comprehensive pain program that included exercise, nutritional therapy, chiropractic, and pharmacology.

For the most part, the uniquely designed magnetic devices that are used in magnetherapy are worn directly over the part of the body that is experiencing pain. They can also be worn in shoe insoles, wrist splints, or compression sleeves. Sometimes they are placed in mattress pads, in car seat covers, or in chair pads.

The magnets that are used are different from ordinary magnets, which have not been proven to be therapeutically effective.

Like most new technologies, magnetherapy is now being exploited by a few unethical companies that are making cheap, ineffective products. Therefore I urge you to consult Appendix III, which has information about the companies producing the magnets that are now being tested at medical centers.

Even high-quality magnetherapy products are relatively inexpensive. These magnets produce no known side effects.

Magnetherapy is most commonly used for musculoskeletal pain, including such conditions as arthritis and carpal tunnel syndrome. However, it appears to provide pain relief for a wide variety of conditions.

Now let's look at another important new physical therapy that has been widely used for only about fifteen years.

Light Therapy for Building the Pain Threshold

As I've mentioned repeatedly, one of the most important things you can do to cure chronic pain is to increase and stabilize your levels of the neurotransmitter serotonin. If you have low or unstable levels of serotonin, you will be vastly more vulnerable to chronic pain, in the event that you develop a degenerative condition, or suffer an injury. In addition, low serotonin levels appear to directly influence the onset of migraines, clinical depression, PMS symptoms, and fibromyalgia, and may also cause irritable bowel syndrome in some people.

One of the best ways to ensure having an abundant, stable supply of serotonin is with light therapy.

It has been very well documented that low levels of light—most often caused by short winter daylight hours—contribute significantly to low levels of serotonin. The depressive disorder known as seasonal affective disorder, or SAD, has been directly linked to inadequate levels of light.

Light is needed in order for the body to effectively switch from melatonin production at night to serotonin production during the day. Melatonin is important for initiating and perpetuating sleep, but if melatonin production continues throughout the day—because of a lack of light—it decreases the amount of serotonin that can be produced. This often causes many of the classic symptoms of a serotonin deficit, including depression, lethargy, impaired cognitive function, a craving for sweets, and a reduced libido.

In addition, a serotonin deficit lowers the pain threshold, and magnifies the presence of all existing pain.

This problem is very common, especially in the regions of the world where daylight hours are very short in winter. For example, in Washington State, an estimated 10 percent of all people are severely affected by a lack of light, and another 20 percent are moderately affected. In contrast, in sunny Southern California, only about 3 percent are severely affected, and 10 percent are moderately affected. Even in sunny climates, people who are almost always indoors can be affected.

Women are especially vulnerable to this problem during certain times in their menstrual cycles, when their serotonin levels may already be low. Serotonin levels generally drop near the middle of the menstrual cycle, to allow ovulation to occur, and then remain low for about two weeks. Then, just before menstruation, levels drop even further. During these times a lack of light can significantly exacerbate the difficult symptoms of premenstrual syndrome, which include increased perception of pain. In fact, SAD and PMS share many symptoms.

One reason this problem is so common is that there are such wide differences between the amount of sunlight on a bright, sunny day, and the amount that is commonly found indoors. Note in the following chart how dim a "normally lit room" is.

For full-spectrum light to trigger the release of serotonin, it must be at least 2,500 lux. To achieve serotonin release with artificial light that is not full-spectrum, the light intensity must be at least 10,000 lux.

As you probably know, most indoor lights are not full-spectrum lights, which carry all of the sun's various wavelengths. The only full-spectrum lights that are in common use are the "grow lights" that many indoor gardeners use to stimulate growth of plants and flowers.

Most researchers believe that light therapy is best achieved with full-spectrum lights. Full-spectrum lights have many advan-

Variations in Light Intensity

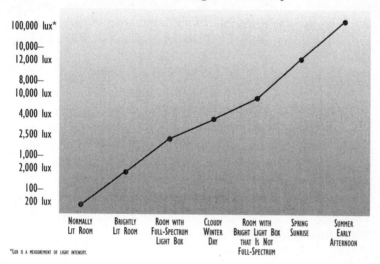

NORMALLY LIT ROOM	BRIGHTLY LIT ROOM	ROOM WITH FULL-SPECTRUM LIGHT BOX	CLOUDY WINTER DAY	ROOM WITH BRIGHT LIGHT BOX THAT IS NOT FULL-SPECTRUM	SPRING SUNRISE	SUMMER EARLY AFTERNOON

100,000 lux*
10,000–12,000 lux
8,000–10,000 lux
4,000 lux
2,500 lux
1,000–2,000 lux
100–200 lux

*LUX IS A MEASUREMENT OF LIGHT INTENSITY.

tages over standard lights. They do not have to be unusually bright, which can strain the eyes. Furthermore, various wavelengths found in full-spectrum lights trigger beneficial biochemical actions. For example, as you may know, ultraviolet light rays activate the synthesis of vitamin D. These rays also appear to decrease serum cholesterol, stimulate the thyroid gland, and increase the levels of estrogen. In fact, every vitamin, mineral, and enzyme in your body uses at least one specific wavelength of light.

The health benefits of full-spectrum light appear to stimulate increased longevity. In one animal experiment, animals exposed to only standard fluorescent lights lived 8.2 months, while those exposed only to full-spectrum artificial lights lived 15.6 months. Animals exposed only to natural sunlight lived 16.1 months. This indicates not only that full-spectrum light is beneficial, but also that artificial full-spectrum light is almost as beneficial as natural sunlight.

Researchers are currently uncertain about exactly how light does trigger certain biochemical reactions, including the release of serotonin. For most of the past fifteen years, it was widely accepted that light changed brain chemistry by entering the eye. Recently, though, researchers found that brain chemistry could be altered by light that was directed only at the skin. The only certain thing is that these alterations in brain chemistry do occur.

You can begin light therapy by purchasing full-spectrum lights at a hardware store. Higher-quality lights, designed specifically for light therapy, are available from a company listed in Appendix III. These lights have a number of advantages, and are more likely to improve your serotonin levels than standard, hardware-store lights.

If you use full-spectrum lights, you should have at least four forty-eight-inch lights, and should sit near them for at least an hour, when you wake up in the morning.

Aromatherapy

Until recently, I'd had no clinical experience with aromatherapy. When I first heard about it, I thought it seemed unscientific and unusual. However, anecdotal evidence indicates that this therapy may be of value for some patients.

Aromatherapy consists of simply inhaling the scents of various herbs and plants. These fragrances appear to trigger specific moods.

It has long been accepted that the sense of smell plays a powerful role in evoking memories. The sense of smell is unique in one very interesting way: All of the other senses must go through a filtering process in the brain that is governed by an area called the thalamus. This filtering process helps screen out sensory input that is nonsensical or extraneous. However, the sense of smell bypasses the thalamus and goes straight to the brain's limbic system, which controls memory and emotion. Therefore, smell has a peculiarly strong ability to evoke memories and emotions.

According to practitioners of aromatherapy, particular smells not only evoke particular moods, but also cause secretion of the brain chemicals that are associated with those moods. Following are fragrances that are often used in aromatherapy, along with the moods and neurochemicals these fragrances trigger. These fragrances are the ones that are most likely to be of value to pain patients.

These fragrances, which may be purchased as oils from most health-food stores, can be used several ways. They may be added to boiling water, to produce an aromatic steam, or to bathwater; they may be heated in a type of lamp called an aroma diffuser; or worn on the skin.

The use of aromatherapy has helped a number of my patients to relax and feel more comfortable.

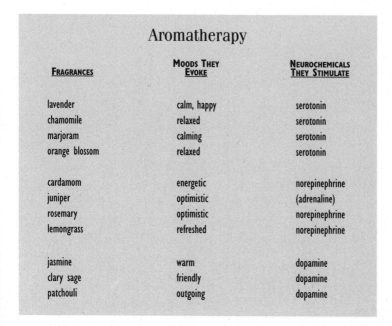

Aromatherapy

FRAGRANCES	MOODS THEY EVOKE	NEUROCHEMICALS THEY STIMULATE
lavender	calm, happy	serotonin
chamomile	relaxed	serotonin
marjoram	calming	serotonin
orange blossom	relaxed	serotonin
cardamom	energetic	norepinephrine
juniper	optimistic	(adrenaline)
rosemary	optimistic	norepinephrine
lemongrass	refreshed	norepinephrine
jasmine	warm	dopamine
clary sage	friendly	dopamine
patchouli	outgoing	dopamine

Don't Be Overwhelmed!

Before we move on to one final form of physical therapy—one that I consider to be the most effective of all, I want to offer you a word of encouragement. By now you may be thinking, "Gee, I'm only about halfway through this pain program, and already this doctor has told me to try about *292 different things.* I'm overwhelmed!"

Don't be. Just do the things that you have the time and energy to do, and don't even *try* to be a "perfect patient." If you get obsessed with perfection, it will just make your pain worse.

The fact is, there *are* a lot of things for you to try, and you won't know which of them will help you most until you *do* try them. We're all quite different, and different things work for different people.

So you'll just have to be patient, and persevere.

Soon, though, you'll find several modalities that *really work* for you, and when you do, you can focus on them. They'll quickly become a natural part of your daily routine.

When you reach that stage—and you will reach it—my program will feel very simple and uncomplicated.

That's what happened to Tiffany when I introduced her to the therapy I'm going to tell you about next. At first this form of therapy seemed difficult and strange to her, because she'd never tried anything quite like it before. Soon, though, it was a normal part of her everyday life.

It was, in fact, the element of my program that turned her life around.

Mind/Body Exercises: Tapping the Power of the Brain

Several thousand years ago—long before anatomists charted the structure of the nervous system—Asian healers discovered that they could influence their patients' health by helping them channel their internal energies. The healers taught patients techniques that enabled them to channel energy from one part of the body to another, and from the body to the brain. We now call these techniques "mind/body exercises." They are a combination of yogic movements, postures, and meditations.

The people who performed these exercises thousands of years ago apparently experienced dramatic increases in mental energy and physical well-being. Since then, countless millions of people have used them.

A form of kundalini yoga, these exercises were widely introduced in the United States in 1969, by Yogi Bhajan, the leader of the Sikh religion in America. Sikhism is an uncomplicated religion that believes there is one Creator, and that people can attune themselves to this Creator by striving to be kind, decent, happy, and healthy. Kundalini mind/body exercise, combined with meditation, is a tool used to achieve health, happiness, and spirituality. When I became a Sikh, about twenty years ago, I experienced profound benefit from these exercises, which I still practice virtually every day.

The current Western interpretation of the mind/body exercises is that they facilitate the transport of nerve energy from outlying peripheral nerves, to the spinal cord, to the brain.

The ancient interpretation of the mind/body exercises was that they facilitated the transport of life-energy, or kundalini, from the body's lower energy centers, or chakras, to the higher energy centers in the brain. When this occurs, healing and regeneration are promoted on all levels: physical, mental, and spiritual.

Having studied the subject for the last twenty years, I have come to believe that there is truth in both these interpretations. Neither one alone, I believe, represents the full truth.

Mind/body exercises are still widely practiced in Asia, and are practiced by hundreds of thousands of people in the West. The popularity of these exercises endures simply because they work. If they didn't, people would have abandoned them centuries ago.

Each of the mind/body exercises has a specific effect: some promote increased cognitive energy; some create increased physical energy; others cause profound relaxation; and some help block pain.

I taught several of the pain-blocking exercises to Tiffany. I also taught her exercises designed to stimulate mental energy. Both helped her body to launch its counterattack against pain.

The most important mind/body exercises for raising the pain threshold are described in Appendix I. In addition, that section includes mind/body exercises that are particularly appropriate for arthritis, back pain, headaches, and fibromyalgia. You will find these exercises relatively easy to perform; they're certainly no more difficult than aerobic exercise or weight training. They are very self-motivating, because the payoff from them is often immediate. For example, my polymyositis patient, Scott, needed no encouragement at all to do the exercises, because he felt that doing them was similar to, as he put it, "getting a shot of the best possible pain medication—without the side effects."

I strongly believe that mind/body exercises exert the greatest power when they are done in the morning, as part of a regular health-building routine. I call this routine "Wake Up to Wellness." When performed properly, it activates endocrine secretions that energize the mind and body, and help protect it against stress for the entire day. The routine varies from one patient to another, but always includes meditation, mind/body exercises, good nutrition, and cleansing.

I begin my own routine by stretching in bed, and taking at least twenty-six long, deep breaths. Before I even get out of bed, I can feel blood pulsing throughout my body, recharging every cell with oxygen and energy.

I take a pleasant shower, and then cool the water temperature at the end. The bracing stream of cool water is invigorating.

I usually drink at least one glass of water with lemon juice.

As I prepare to do my mind/body exercises, I pray to the God within me and the God that is outside of me. I ask for the blessings of mental, physical, emotional, and spiritual health, and for happiness, prosperity, grace, and joy. I ask for the blessings of my family, my children, and my patients. I ask for the loving, healing energy of God to flow as freely through me as my breath flows through my body.

Then I do my mind/body exercises, meditate, and eat a power-packed breakfast. By that time I feel prepared for any possible challenge.

When Tiffany began doing the mind/body exercises, she had a startling reaction to them. She began to experience enhanced nerve transmission to her lower body. In fact, so much of her feeling returned that she became uncomfortably aware of the rods that had been inserted along her spine.

As her healing progressed, the sensation of the rods became so bothersome that she underwent surgery to have them removed. Her doctors noted that Tiffany healed from this surgery much faster than most patients do, and that she was able to control her nervous system's reaction to painful procedures almost at will. They were amazed at this ability, which Tiffany credited mostly to her mind/body exercises and meditation.

After the rods were removed, she began to feel even better. She had greater flexibility, and her muscle tone became firmer. Her pain continued to decline in intensity, duration, and frequency.

The better she felt, the more involved she became with all areas of her life. She deepened a relationship with a very nice young man, and started to focus on the future instead of the past.

Then, one day, she came to her appointment wearing leg braces.

With difficulty, she stood and took several tentative steps toward me.

I was not surprised by this achievement, because she had been working toward it steadily.

But when she took those steps, her eyes held the light of the sun in them, and I was very moved.

I saw Tiffany again recently, just before Cameron Stauth and I finished writing this book, and I was amazed at how radiant and filled with life she was. She told me she is still in her wheelchair most of the time. But it no longer seems to devastate her, as it once did, because she looks at her life so differently now. Now she seems to regard her wheelchair not as something that imprisons her, but as something that empowers her.

Her physical therapy and her pain program are both going extremely well, and she hopes to be able to someday walk without any physical aids.

She told me that she is getting married soon, at a lovely resort in West Palm Beach, Florida, and that she plans to take her vows in a beautiful pool, where she'll be able to walk to the altar easily and unaided.

I was overjoyed to hear about her plans, and was touched when she asked me to present a blessing at the wedding.

The healing of Tiffany's legs still continues.

The healing of her life is complete.

4

Level Three: Medication

Although the world is full of suffering,
it is full also of the overcoming of it.
—HELEN KELLER

Martha's niece, who was also her caregiver, lifted her aunt out of a handicap-equipped van, and helped her shuffle into my office. Leaning on a walker, Martha slowly made her way to a chair, with her back and neck bent forward.

She collapsed into the chair, and fought to catch her breath. As she gulped air, she shifted fitfully, as if looking for a comfortable position she knew she'd never find.

Even in the chair, Martha's neck was still hunched downward. She had to lift her eyes to see me.

Martha's niece bent over her. "What can I get you?"

"Aspirin."

Martha looked up at me with pain-shadowed eyes. "Thank God for aspirin," she murmured.

"Do you take a lot of it?" I asked.

"I *live* on it."

"Any stomach problems?"

"Not yet, knock on wood," she said. "But my arthritis specialist told me it's just a matter of time; he says aspirin gives you ulcers."

Martha, seventy-five, had severe arthritis. She also had a joint disease called ankylosing spondylitis, which had caused the tendons in her neck and spine to freeze into rigidity.

"If you're taking a *lot* of aspirin," I said, "it may be doing more than just causing ulcers. It's probably making your arthritis worse."

"Worse?" Martha's jaw dropped. "Aspirin is the only thing that stops the pain."

"I can give you other things for pain," I said. "But aspirin can damage cartilage."

I picked up a model of a spinal column and pointed at the small pads of cartilage between the vertebrae. "Your cartilage," I told Martha, "is like a sponge that keeps your bones from touching. But, to do that, it has to absorb water. Aspirin slows down this absorption, and makes your joints hurt even worse."

"That's a new one on me," Martha said glumly.

"It's a new one on everybody. Doctors didn't know about this until just a few years ago. Some still don't seem to know about it."

Martha looked defeated. Her tormented eyes went glassy with tears. "Then what can I *do?*" She almost started to cry, but then stopped. Martha was tough. If she hadn't been tough, she'd have been in a nursing home by this time, bedridden, and on narcotics.

"There are *dozens* of things you can do for your pain," I said. "Some involve medication, and some don't."

"Don't worry, we'll handle it," her niece said softly, as she patted her aunt's hand.

Family members who serve as caregivers are extraordinary people. They give their hearts *and* their help, and those are the two most precious things a person can give.

As I looked at these two brave women, joined together in love and suffering, I promised myself I'd find a way to help them.

I began to tell them about my own approach to medication, in which I use three basic types:

1. PAIN MEDICATION. Some of the pain medications I use are available only by prescription, and some can be purchased over the counter. Unlike many pain specialists, however, I recommend not only such common over-the-counter medications as acetaminophen and ibuprofen, but also powerful herbal and homeopathic medications.

2. COGNITIVE-ENHANCEMENT MEDICATION. Because pain is in the brain, the better the brain works, the more effectively it will control pain. To build the power of the brain, I advise my pain patients to use some of the same cognitive-enhancement medicines that I prescribe to my brain longevity patients. Medications such as deprenyl boost the ability of the brain to launch a strong counterattack against pain.

3. CONDITION-SPECIFIC MEDICATION. These are medications that treat the *root causes* of specific conditions, such as arthritis or migraine. As I've mentioned, integrative medicine is often more effective than conventional medicine at reversing long-standing degenerative conditions, such as arthritis. When those conditions cause chronic pain, any improvement in the condition can significantly reduce that pain. Therefore, some of the medications I prescribe to pain patients are not intended to directly relieve their pain, but to improve the underlying conditions *causing* their pain.

After my initial meeting with Martha, I consulted regularly with her for the next few months. She participated in a full-spectrum pain program, and responded remarkably well.

At the outset of Martha's program, I helped relieve her pain with acupuncture, anti-inflammatory nutrients, herbal medications, homeopathic remedies, and various forms of bodywork.

Some of these modalities were new to her, and some were similar to things she'd already tried. Previously she had been treated by a doctor who had employed herbology, acupuncture, and a form of yoga. These therapies had been somewhat effective, but had not cured Martha's pain. It appeared to me that they had failed because they had not been integrated into a comprehensive, coordinated program, in which every level of the program synergistically supports every other level. To be effective, a program must be more than merely a smorgasbord of natural therapies.

As Martha responded to her pain management program, I was able to reduce drastically her use of aspirin.

One level of her program, of course, was medication. The medications that had the most profound effect upon her were condition-specific medications: hormonal replacement agents that opposed the root cause of her arthritis.

I prescribed two hormones to Martha—pregnenolone and human growth hormone. Although these two hormones are not widely used for arthritis, I have found them to be extremely helpful for some patients.

Pregnenolone is a hormone that the body converts into steroidal hormones, such as estrogen and testosterone. Steroidal hormones help arthritis by reducing inflammation, and by supporting the health of cartilage. Though many doctors give arthritis patients *synthetic* steroidal hormones, such as cortisone or prednisone, these have a host of negative side effects. Pregnenolone is much safer, and has fewer potential side effects.

The other hormone I gave her, human growth hormone, is not yet widely used by most doctors, but its popularity is beginning to increase. It has the general effect of stimulating biochemical youthfulness, through a cascade of chemical mechanisms. Because of its "re-youthing" effect, I find human growth hormone helpful for a variety of age-related conditions, including arthritis.

Martha also responded very favorably to nutritional therapy. She took abundant amounts of two nutrients that help cartilage absorb water: chondroitin and glucosamine. As these nutrients helped thicken her cartilage, her pain subsided.

In less than six months, Martha overcame the worst symptoms of her arthritis and her ankylosing spondylitis. Her mobility and flexibility increased dramatically, and her pain became very manageable. The ligaments in her spine and neck normalized, greatly increasing her ability to stand straight and walk normally. She no longer required any assistance with her daily tasks. This was a blessing not only for Martha, but also for her niece.

In fact, Martha became an avid swimmer.

These days I enjoy stopping by Martha's southwestern home, which has a lovely swimming pool, and watching her swim laps. It reminds me of how far she has progressed from the day when her niece helped her hobble into my office.

Currently, when Martha has a flare-up of joint pain, I advise her to take a helpful, almost "magical" medication: *aspirin.*

I'll tell you why.

Aspirin and Similar Medications

When used properly, aspirin is a superb drug: fast, safe, and effective. It's no wonder that it is by far the most popular pain drug in the world. Unfortunately, though, aspirin is improperly used in a staggering number of cases. For the most part, the misuse consists of taking *too much* aspirin, which can cause internal bleeding, particularly in the stomach. It's estimated by the U.S. Food and Drug Administration that each year excessive use of aspirin and drugs like it (such as ibuprofen) causes approximately 200,000 cases of gastrointestinal bleeding, and several thousand deaths.

Because aspirin is so widely used—and abused—it's the first medication I want to tell you about. After we discuss aspirin and ibuprofen, we'll look at the two other major types of over-the-counter anti-pain medications that I use: homeopathic remedies and herbal medications.

Then we'll examine prescription painkillers, and cognitive enhancement medications.

The only medicines we won't discuss much in this chapter are the condition-specific medications. We'll look at those in the chapters on specific conditions.

Please note that *any* of the medicines I mention in this chapter might help you—regardless of the source of your pain—because all of them are part of my *general program* for pain. Their actions are universal, and will help you fight many kinds of chronic pain that have become "embedded" in your nervous system.

The active ingredient in aspirin, salicylic acid, has been used for thousands of years. Early Chinese healers gave their patients salicylic acid in the form of willow bark, which is the richest natural source of the substance. They even used it as part of a powerful anesthetic potion that kept patients unconscious during major surgeries. In the West, though, the medicinal use of willow bark wasn't discovered until 1758, when a doctor named Edward Stone found that it reduced pain and fever in his patients.

One reason aspirin is so popular is that it has three major actions: it relieves pain, reduces fever, and decreases inflammation.

Because aspirin reduces inflammation, it is part of a class of substances known as nonsteroidal anti-inflammatory drugs. As the name indicates, these drugs fight inflammation, as steroids do, but don't have any of the other properties of steroids. The acronym for this class of drugs is NSAID, which is pronounced "in-sed."

There are more than twenty different NSAIDs. Some are over-the-counter drugs, and some are only available by prescription. Here are some of the most widely used NSAIDs (their generic names are given first, with the most common brand names in parentheses):

- aspirin
  (e.g., Bayer, Anacin, etc.)
- ibuprofen
  (e.g., Advil, Motrin)
- naproxen
  (e.g., Anaprox, Aleve)
- indomethacin
  (e.g., Indocin)
- tolmetin
  (e.g., Tolectin)
- phenylbutazone
  (e.g., Butazolidin)
- diclofenac
  (e.g., Voltaren)
- diflusinal
  (e.g., Dolobid)
- piroxicam
  (e.g., Feldene)
- oxyphenbutazone
  (e.g., Oxalid)
- sulindac
  (e.g., Clinoril)
- fenoprofen
  (e.g., Nalfon)

NSAIDs reduce inflammation by blocking two important inflammatory chemicals—prostaglandins and arachidonic acid. As you probably remember, I mentioned them in the chapter on nutrition, because you can also block them with nutritional therapy.

Other than NSAIDs, there is only one other common anti-pain, or analgesic, drug that's sold without a prescription. This drug, however, does *not* relieve inflammation. It is acetaminophen; the most popular brand is Tylenol. Acetaminophen, like NSAIDs, relieves pain and reduces fevers, but has no effect on the chemicals that cause inflammation. Therefore, it's not as effective as aspirin or other NSAIDs for inflammatory conditions.

It may surprise you to know that we doctors aren't entirely sure why aspirin and other NSAIDs stop pain. Of course, relieving inflammation helps stop pain, but these drugs also stop pain when no inflammation is present.

One current theory is that aspirin and other NSAIDs amplify the brain's counterattack on pain by improving the function of the "descending pathways" that go from the brain to the site of pain. This theory is probably accurate, but no one is certain.

Although it may seem odd to you that doctors aren't sure how aspirin works, this really isn't very unusual; dozens of drugs work in ways that doctors don't fully understand. By the same token, many of the modalities of Eastern medicine, such as acupuncture, are also rather mysterious.

It may also surprise you to learn that many doctors prescribe NSAIDs for pain, but do not prescribe them for inflammation. This is a mistake. Inflammation should be treated, with NSAIDs, even when it's not causing significant pain. When inflammation is *not* treated, it can grow worse and become embedded in the nervous system as chronic pain. By the time that happens, it may be too late to cure inflammation with a simple therapy like use of NSAIDs.

Therefore, if you sprain your ankle—or incur inflammation for any other reason—use NSAIDs as soon as possible, even if you don't feel much pain. Remember, though, that acetaminophen doesn't stop inflammation, so don't rely on it to treat your sprained ankle.

For a similar reason, acetaminophen is also a less effective medication for menstrual cramps. Menstrual cramps are caused, in part, by excessive production of prostaglandins in the uterus. Because NSAIDs block prostaglandin production, NSAIDs are the appropriate medication for menstrual cramps. Of the various NSAIDs you could use for cramps, studies indicate that ibuprofen is generally the most effective. Therefore, for menstrual cramps, I recommend ibuprofen.

A reasonable dosage of ibuprofen for menstrual cramps, as well as for inflammation, is 400 mg every four hours. When you first suffer an inflammatory response, though, you can take up to 800 mg; this should help prevent the onset of severe inflammation. Your *daily* intake of ibuprofen should not exceed 2,000 mg. If you use ibuprofen or any other NSAID every day, you should take even less than 2,000 mg. All the NSAIDs may have negative side effects when used in high dosages on a long-term, daily basis.

Here are the worst problems associated with improper use of NSAIDs:

GASTROINTESTINAL BLEEDING

When NSAIDs block prostaglandins, they can cause stomach problems, because one of the functions of prostaglandins is to manufacture the mucus that coats the stomach lining. Even a few weeks of regular NSAID use can cause ulcers and gastrointestinal bleeding, particularly in people older than sixty.

This problem often goes undetected, though, because NSAIDs block most of the pain from it. About 4 percent of all patients who regularly take high dosages of NSAIDs develop ulcers, but more than half of them don't know it until they experience a potentially life-threatening event, such as a perforated ulcer, or massive internal bleeding.

If you're routinely taking NSAIDs to control chronic pain, you are 650 percent more likely than the average person to be hospitalized for gastrointestinal distress. If you do experience NSAID-related gastrointestinal distress, don't try to treat it with antacids, because that won't work. Your problem is not simple hyperacidity. If you develop an ulcer from taking NSAIDs, you can heal it with an ulcer medication such as Tagament, but this medication will *not* prevent future ulcers.

To help prevent gastrointestinal distress caused by NSAIDs, ask your doctor about a relatively new drug called misoprostol, or Cytotec. It will help protect your stomach lining and stop problems before they start.

LIVER AND KIDNEY DAMAGE

Kidney damage is the second-most-common problem caused by NSAIDs. The kidneys are vulnerable because they filter NSAIDs out of the blood. Some studies indicate that 7 to 10 percent of all terminal kidney diseases may be related to excessive use of NSAIDs. If you already have kidney damage—or if you have congestive heart failure, or high blood pressure—significant use of NSAIDs can be very dangerous. In some cases it can cause total kidney failure in less than a week. People taking diuretics are also at increased risk.

Another group of people who are especially vulnerable to the side effects of NSAIDs are people with autoimmune disorders. People with rheumatoid arthritis, lupus, and other autoimmune diseases should be particularly cautious about controlling their symptoms with NSAIDs.

Until recently, it was believed that the NSAID known as sulindac caused the least damage to kidneys, but now it appears as if excessive use of sulindac contributes to kidney stones.

The liver also removes NSAIDs from the bloodstream, and can therefore be damaged by them. If you regularly take large amounts of NSAIDs, you should periodically have your liver function monitored by blood tests. Alcoholics, whose livers are already under stress, are particularly vulnerable to liver damage from NSAIDs.

NERVOUS SYSTEM DAMAGE

NSAIDs, which appear to act on the central nervous system, can interfere with normal nervous system function. The greatest risk to the brain and nerves occurs when you take high dosages for extended periods. This can cause confusion, agitation, ringing in the ears, memory loss, insomnia, depression, and even hallucinations and seizures. Sometimes, when older people taking high dosages of NSAIDs have mental problems, their families and even their doctors wrongly assume that they are suffering from early symptoms of Alzheimer's.

Another nervous system problem that NSAIDs can cause is, ironically, a lowering of the pain threshold. When high dosages are taken for a long time, the nervous system loses some of its ability to fight pain on its own. The brain, in effect, becomes dependent upon NSAIDs to help launch the counterattack against pain.

This problem is *magnified* when NSAIDs start to lose their "punch" because of overuse. When this happens, you *really* need your own natural pain-fighting ability. But if it's been weakened by NSAIDs, you'll be caught in a bind. You'll be tempted to take higher and higher dosages of NSAIDs, but when they wear off, you'll be in more pain than ever. The pain that results from overuse of NSAIDs is sometimes called "rebound pain."

Another side effect of NSAIDs, which is partly related to nervous system disruption, is skin rash. Approximately 3 percent of all people who take NSAIDs develop a rash, or report itching. The NSAIDs that generally cause the worst skin reactions are phenylbutazone, sulindac, and piroxicam.

AGGRAVATION OF ARTHRITIS

Although doctors have long encouraged arthritis patients to use NSAIDs, it now appears that excessive use of NSAIDs can actually exacerbate arthritis.

Most arthritis is caused by damage to cartilage—the spongy padding between joints—and NSAIDs can contribute to this damage. To work well, cartilage must absorb water, but NSAIDs slow down production of the molecule that holds water in cartilage. When cartilage gets too dry, it doesn't protect joints, and symptoms of arthritis appear. Even if you don't have arthritis now, you should be aware that high regular dosages of NSAIDs might contribute to its later development. I'll tell you more about this problem in chapter 6.

I hope I haven't gotten you so apprehensive about NSAIDs that you'll never again take an aspirin. Aspirin and other NSAIDs are *terrific* drugs, when used properly. In fact, there's considerable evidence that taking about 80 mg of aspirin each day can help protect you against cardiovascular disease, because of its anti-clotting effects. Aspirin is especially valuable for people who have already had one heart attack and are trying to prevent another.

Wise use of NSAIDs can also help *prevent* chronic pain, by stopping it before it has the chance to create a recurring cycle. For example, one forty-eight-year-old patient of mine experienced severe back pain every time he played his favorite sport, racquetball. The more he played, the worse his pain became. He was gradually developing chronic back pain. His orthopedist told him that continuing to play would be crazy. But I recommended that before every game he should warm his back muscles with hot water, do stretching exercises, and take 400 mg of ibuprofen and 500 mg of aspirin. I also advised him to take pregnenolone, which synergistically improves joint function when taken with NSAIDs. This regimen totally eliminated his pain.

Obviously, for inflammation, NSAIDs can be a godsend. When you use them regularly as analgesics, though, they can be hazardous if you're not prudent.

Now that you know how NSAIDs can be dangerous, you'll probably have a better appreciation for the other two widely used types of nonprescription analgesics—homeopathic remedies and herbal preparations. They are *much* less likely to cause negative side effects, and they often work extremely well. Frequently they are far more powerful than NSAIDs.

The Power of Homeopathics

It astonishes me that so many American M.D.'s know so little about homeopathic medicine. There's really no excuse for it.

This healing tradition has been widely used for almost two hundred years. Earlier in this century, there were almost as many homeopathic colleges in America as there were medical schools. Hundreds of fine homeopathic products are available in this country, and dozens of well-documented articles about homeopathy have appeared in the medical literature. Nonetheless, most American M.D.'s don't know very much about homeopathy, and don't appear to be interested in it.

I can certainly understand why a medical doctor would not want to abandon his or her own current approach and embrace only homeopathy. But I cannot understand why a doctor wouldn't want to investigate this approach thoroughly.

The primary goal of all physicians should be to *relieve the suffering of patients,* and physicians have an obligation to investigate anything that's been convincingly shown to relieve suffering. Homeopathy, without a doubt, has been shown to relieve suffering. It merits more attention from the orthodox American medical community than it has thus far been granted.

Homeopathy is particularly effective at helping to stop pain. As you may know, homeopathy works on a principle somewhat similar to that of immunization. In homeopathy, patients take extremely small dosages of substances that stimulate the healing responses of their own bodies.

Two basic strategies are used. One is to give the patient small dosages of substances that evoke the symptoms the patient is trying to cure. For example, to cure an allergy to wheat gluten, patients might be given a pill containing a tiny amount of gluten.

The other basic homeopathic strategy is to give patients tiny dosages of substances that *oppose* symptoms. For example, to cure insomnia, a patient might be given a pill containing a tiny amount of a sedative herb.

Thus, the theory behind homeopathy is that extremely small amounts of substances are even better than large amounts for stimulating the body's *own* healing responses.

Homeopathy was created in Europe, and is still employed more widely there than in America. For example, in England, an estimated 42 percent of all medical doctors refer patients to homeopathic physicians. As you may have heard, England's royal family has for many years been routinely treated by a homeopathic physician. It's also interesting to note that the leading remedy for influenza in France is a brand-name homeopathic medication called Oscillococcinum, and it is rapidly becoming popular in America. I use Oscillococcinum myself at the first sign of a cold, and find that it often stops the cold immediately.

Recently, the prestigious *British Medical Journal* published a major review of studies done on homeopathy. Of the 107 clinical trials that were reviewed, 81 showed positive results achieved by homeopathy.

As part of this review, twenty studies of pain and physical trauma were examined. Of those, eighteen showed positive results.

Here are some examples:

• In a study of fibromyalgia, twice as many patients improved on a homeopathic medicine as on a placebo.

• In a study of migraines, patients on homeopathic medications reduced their number of headaches per month from an average of 10 to an average of 1.8. These patients also experienced a considerable reduction in the *intensity* of pain. A control group of patients on a placebo showed negligible improvement.

• In a study of sprained ankles, more than two-thirds of patients using the homeopathic formulation Traumeel were pain-free within ten days, compared with one-third of patients on a placebo.

I have often prescribed Traumeel in my own practice, and have found it to be generally quite effective. For example, when one of my patients pulled a major tendon in his leg, I prescribed Traumeel, along with a topical herbal analgesic called Narayan oil. The patient, an avid tennis player, had previously pulled the same tendon—the plantaris—which runs down the back of the leg from the knee to the ankle. The second injury was more severe than the first. When the first injury had occurred, the patient had received only orthodox medical care, and had been incapacitated for six weeks. However, with the homeopathic remedy and the topical herbal treatment, the patient was playing tennis again within seven days.

It's quite possible that this patient prevented lifelong chronic pain by aggressively treating his second injury. Often an acute injury like this develops into chronic pain, especially if the injury recurs. *Approximately 20 percent of all serious injuries result in chronic pain.*

One extremely interesting study, though, showed that only about one-fifteenth of all seriously injured patients who are financially well off develop chronic pain, compared with *one-half* of all injured patients who are poor. What I infer from this study is that most well-off people have the money and the time to properly *treat* their injuries, while most poor people must simply *endure* them. The lesson from this is clear: If you suffer a serious, painful injury, *don't* ignore it—*treat* it.

If you want to find a homeopathic remedy that will help control your chronic pain, the best approach would be for you to consult a doctor trained in homeopathy. Physicians who practice *only* homeopathy are relatively rare in America, but many naturopaths and chiropractors are trained in homeopathy, and so are some M.D.'s. The help of a trained professional can be important, because these people will know about various substances that can interfere with homeopathic remedies. For example, camphor can interfere with arnica.

One way to find a doctor trained in homeopathy is to get a referral from the National Center for Homeopathy (see Appendix III).

You can also find homeopathic medicines by simply visiting a health-food store. There you will see individual homeopathic remedies, as well as formulations of combined remedies. The package of every *individual* homeopathic remedy will clearly state the condition the remedy treats. It will also recommend the proper dosage.

Formulations of combined remedies are also clearly labeled, carrying such designations as "Arthritis Formulation" or "Stress Formulation," among many others.

Here are some of the most popular individual homeopathic remedies for pain and a brief description of some of their benefits. Of course, you should become familiar with their contraindications and possible side effects. As with any medication, it is also important to consult your doctor before taking multiple remedies in order to understand how they interact with one another.

- *Arnica* 6x. One of the most widely known homeopathic pain remedies, Arnica is effective for acute pain, and helps prevent acute pain from becoming chronic pain. The formulation Traumeel contains this remedy.

- *Aconitum* 12x. This can help reduce severe pain, such as postsurgical pain or burn pain. Most effective when used immediately after an injury, it is also helpful for arthritis.

- *Chamomilla* 3x. Derived from the calming herb chamomile, this remedy helps with low-level chronic pain, and has a mild sedating effect.

- *Apis* 12x. Helpful as an anti-inflammatory agent, this is often used to treat insect bites and beestings.

- *Arnica* 3x. This will help reduce the swelling, discoloration, and stiffness that results from a bruise, particularly if taken shortly after the injury occurs.

- *Hypericum* 6x. This is often prescribed for cuts and abrasions.

- *Rhus tox* 6x. Many fibromyalgia patients, as well as other people with muscle pain, gain relief with this remedy. It can also help with any form of pain that responds well to heat.

• *Pulsatilla* 6x. Most often used to treat pain caused by premenstrual syndrome, this remedy is also effective for pain in the lower back. It is sometimes effective for arthritis pain.

It's possible that you may benefit more from a formulation than from an individual remedy, because the formulations contain a variety of synergistic and complementary ingredients. For example, a popular product called "Injury and Backache," distributed by Nature's Way, contains Arnica 6x, Hypericum 6x, Rhus tox 6x, Bellis perennis 3x, Ruta grav 3x, and Phosphorus 12x. Another popular homeopathic formulation, the insomnia product Calms Forté, also contains a wide variety of various homeopathic medications.

To find high-quality formulations, visit your local health-food store, or consult with a doctor trained in homeopathy.

If you have children, you may find that homeopathic remedies may be the safest medication currently available. The pills are easy to take because they're quite small—about one-third the size of a pencil eraser. They have a pleasant, sweet taste. In addition, they're ingested by dissolving them under the tongue, so they quickly melt in the mouth, and can't cause choking.

Two of the most popular homeopathic pain medications were designed specifically for children. Made by the Hyland company, they are used to treat infant colic and teething. Parents who have used both of these medications have told me that they are extraordinarily effective, and are easy to give to children, and even infants.

Most medical consumers use homeopathic medications without seeking a doctor's advice. However, for best results, and to promote safety, you should consult with a health professional about this form of medication, as well as all other medications.

Some physicians who use homeopathy believe that it is counterproductive to simultaneously use both homeopathic remedies and standard, symptom-suppression medicines. The standard medicines, they believe, will negate the effects of homeopathy. Other doctors, however, combine the two approaches, as I do myself.

Herbal Medications for Pain

Herbs are the single most common source of modern medication. One-third of all prescription medicines are derived from plants. Herbs also constitute the largest category of natural medication. In Traditional Chinese Medicine, the pharmacopeia is mostly herbal.

My pain patients have responded wonderfully to herbs. For example, a seventy-year-old patient of mine named Rebecca gained great relief from severe arthritis in her knee by taking two Chinese herbal formulas—"Meridian Circulation" and "Dynamic Warrior"—made by the K'hn Herbal Company. Prior to using this herbal formulation, Rebecca had lost so much of the function of her knee that her physician had recommended knee replacement surgery.

However, Rebecca responded positively to a combination of herbal therapy and electroacupuncture. She soon no longer needed the surgery, and for the past four years her knee has functioned normally.

Herbs are generally milder in action, and therefore safer, than most pharmaceutical drugs. Their effects are often more subtle, with far fewer side effects. Like most medicines, though, herbs can sometimes be harmful, if taken in excess. I recommend you use herbal medicines only under the care of a health professional trained in herbology.

Following are some of the herbs that are most commonly used for pain. All of them are probably available at your local health-food store. As a rule, they are ingested as hot tea, or may be taken in capsule form. The package containing the herb will give you directions for use, and dosages.

ARNICA. As you'll recall, minute dosages of this herb are used as a homeopathic preparation, but arnica can also be helpful in large dosages. It helps alleviate most types of pain, by soothing the nervous system. It can be ingested as a tea, taken in capsule form, or used topically in a cold, damp compress. It is available as a salve or ointment.

CHAMOMILE. This pleasant-tasting herb is an effective anti-inflammatory agent, and a mild sedative. It also helps relieve muscle spasm. It can be taken orally, or used topically in a compress. A chamomile compress is soothing for the facial nerve pain known as trigeminal neuralgia. To make a chamomile compress, boil chamomile in water, allow it to cool, pour it into a cloth, and apply the cloth directly to the painful area.

WINTERGREEN. This herb, like willow bark, contains salicylates, the active ingredient in aspirin. Therefore it can be helpful as both an anti-inflammatory agent and as an analgesic. It is used topically, not orally.

GINGER. This herb, which I mentioned in the chapter on nutritional therapy, is a powerful anti-inflammatory agent. It works best when it is dried and taken in capsule form; fresh ginger is not as strong.

CAYENNE PEPPER. For centuries, people have relieved pain by rubbing distressed areas with either cayenne pepper (also called capsicum) or red chili peppers. When these substances are applied topically, the warmth to the skin that they provide gives the brain a competing source of neurological input. As you may remember, heat signals "outrun" pain signals in the race to the spinal cord's pain gates, and thereby block pain. Cayenne pepper, used externally, helps prevent the production of the pain-carrying chemical called substance P. It is particularly effective for stopping the nerve pain that results from herpes zoster, or shingles.

CALENDULA. This herb is used topically for skin pain, including the pain of sunburn. Many commercial sunburn products contain calendula.

ALOE VERA. This herb has mild analgesic qualities, and can be soothing for an open wound, for skin irritation, or for lesions in the digestive tract. It's commonly applied topically to sunburn, cuts and abrasions, herpes lesions, and ulcerated sores. It is also taken orally to help speed the healing of stomach ulcers, an irritated stomach lining, or inflammatory intestinal disorders such as colitis and diverticulitis. Aloe vera penetrates tissues extremely well, and is therefore often combined with other anti-pain substances, in order to help transport them to distressed subdermal tissues.

PASSIFLORA. This mildly sedating herb combats some of the characteristics of chronic pain syndrome, such as insomnia, anxiety, and agitation. In so doing, it indirectly helps relieve pain. It is also useful for reducing muscle spasm. A teaspoon of liquid extract of passiflora can help pain patients fall asleep, even when they're distracted by pain.

Like homeopathic medicines, herbal medications are sold not only as individual herbs, but also as formulations that contain several herbs. At your health-food store you will find a number of different herbal formulations that are intended for various conditions. Often these formulations are more effective than individual herbs.

There is a tremendous range of time-tested formulations of Chinese analgesic herbs. To find them, you will probably have to go to a specialty herb store instead of a health-food store. Licensed acupuncturists also often sell them.

A few examples of such formulations are Corydalis Yan Hu Suo, which is used for pain in internal organs; Yunnan Paiyao, which is used for inflammatory pain; Qi Ye Lien, which is used for muscle and joint pain; and Xiao Yao Wan, which is used for muscle pain and spasm.

Chinese herbs generally have a mild, subtle effect, and usually cause few significant side effects. However, you should use them under the care of a health professional. As a rule, acupuncturists know more about these herbs than any other type of health-care professional, with the exception of physicians trained in Traditional Chinese Medicine.

As you can see, there are dozens of excellent pain medicines that you can purchase yourself, without a doctor's prescription. In fact, these herbal, homeopathic, and over-the-counter analgesic medications are usually the first line of defense against pain; as such, they are used by pain patients far more often than prescription pain drugs. When used intelligently and in proper combinations, such nonprescription medications are extremely powerful. Frequently a synergistic combination of nonprescription medications can be even more powerful than a prescription medication.

Of great importance, these nonprescription medications are also generally safer than prescription medications, so they can often be used over a longer period.

Prescription medications, though, can also be of tremendous benefit when used properly, so let's now take a look at some of them. First we'll examine some prescription analgesics. Then I'll tell you about prescription drugs that enhance brain power. It's possible that either of these two classes of medication—or *both*—will soon help you conquer your pain.

Prescription Medications that Stop Pain

Prescription drugs are the "big guns" in most pain-management programs. They can be incredibly powerful, and sometimes have almost instantaneous effects. Many pain doctors rely more on prescription drugs than any other modality, because the effects of these drugs are so profound and so predictable.

I rely on them less than do most pain doctors, because I have strong concerns about their side effects. I believe it makes more sense to use combinations of safer therapies than to rely primarily on just one prescription "magic bullet."

Even so, I have prescribed prescription drugs to thousands of patients, generally with very positive results. If used cautiously, prescription drugs can be a valuable modality in a comprehensive pain-management program.

Following are the major categories of the prescription drugs that are commonly used to fight pain. If it sounds as if one of them might be appropriate for you, consult a physician. As a rule, a doctor who specializes in pain will know more about these drugs than a doctor who is not a pain specialist.

OPIOIDS

These drugs, also called narcotics, are usually derived from the opium poppy plant. Opium has been used as a painkiller since at least 1500 B.C. It was commonly used as an analgesic by ancient Egyptian, Chinese, and Mesopotamian healers.

Usually, because of fear of addiction, opiates are given only for short-term, acute pain (such as postoperative pain) and for pain caused by late-stage terminal illnesses. However, the most recent research indicates that the fear of addiction may be exaggerated. In fact, most people with serious chronic pain do *not* become addicted to opioid drugs, because these drugs have a different effect on pain patients than on healthy people. Pain patients usually do not feel euphoria when they take opiates, presumably because the drugs get "used up" fighting the patient's pain.

Another reason why doctors often avoid long-term administration of opiates is that patients tend to build up tolerance to them, needing higher and higher dosages to kill pain. In my practice, though, I've gotten good results with very careful administration of certain opiates. For example, I successfully prescribed opiates to a patient of mine who had a form of central pain called reflex sympathetic dystrophy, which he developed after dropping a heavy rock on his foot. Even after the injury healed completely, this patient—a logger named Chuck—still had excruciating pain in his foot. The stimulating sympathetic branch of his nervous system was grossly overactive, due to the presence of a deeply embedded cycle of pain in his brain and nerves.

I tried acupuncture on Chuck, but it only worked temporarily. Then I gave him a series of local injections, called nerve blocks, but they also failed to stop the pain permanently. A surgeon then operated on Chuck, cutting the pain nerves that were overactive. But the nerves soon grew back. At that point, Chuck's doctor wanted to amputate part of his foot.

I feared, however, that amputation would not work, because so much of Chuck's pain was already embedded in his nervous system, and I suspected that even if part of his foot were to be amputated, he would still experience "phantom pain" that would feel as if it were coming from his foot.

Despite my misgivings, Chuck's surgeon went ahead and amputated part of Chuck's foot. Unfortunately, my fears were well founded; the operation did not stop the pain. Chuck's suffering continued.

Throughout this process, Chuck was courageous, but he was beginning to develop several of the characteristics of chronic pain syndrome. The quality of his life was quickly being destroyed.

Finally I treated Chuck with a form of opioid therapy called a Fentanyl patch. Worn on the skin, a Fentanyl patch delivers the opiate Fentanyl, which is ten times more powerful than morphine. The patch almost immediately took away Chuck's pain, and kept it away. Chuck again became happy, productive, and active. He never experienced euphoria or any of the other characteristics of opioid intoxication, such as lethargy or confusion. The patch didn't even make him feel sedated. It just made him feel *normal.* This non-euphoric reaction to opiates is common among people with severe pain. It has been several years since Chuck began using the Fentanyl patch, and he is still doing extremely well.

Opioid use, as mentioned above, is especially helpful for anyone with a late-stage terminal illness, because drug dependence is usually not a major concern of people who are dying. However, even many terminal patients still resist becoming dependent upon opiates, because of the stigma our society places on drug dependence. This attitude causes millions of terminally ill people to suffer unnecessarily.

For over a hundred years, this distaste for drug dependence has interfered with the proper use of opiates. In fact, the drugs chloroform, nitrous oxide, and ether were shunned by the medical community for many years, even after doctors knew that they were effective analgesics. During this time, in the mid-1800s, these three drugs were relegated to "back alley" use, and were commonly taken as intoxicants by the general public. In England, a group of physicians urged that chloroform be used to alleviate pain during childbirth, but they were opposed by the Anglican church, which espoused the biblical injunction that women should "bring forth children in sorrow." This unenlightened philosophy reigned until Queen Victoria requested chloroform during the birth of her child. After that, the practice became common, and analgesics became far more widely accepted by doctors.

Even if you have severe chronic pain, your doctor may not prescribe one of the strong opiates—such as morphine, Dilaudid, or Demerol—for the reasons just mentioned. It's possible, though, that from time to time your doctor may prescribe one of the milder opiates, such as codeine. This may be appropriate for occasional, intense flare-ups of your pain.

If your doctor does prescribe codeine, you should know that it generally works best when it is combined with a nonprescription analgesic such as acetaminophen. An example of this type of combined medication is "Tylenol with codeine."

ANTIDEPRESSANTS

I once had a fibromyalgia patient who flatly refused to take antidepressants, because she thought I was implying that her pain was "all in her mind." For years, she told me, her husband, who was a psychotherapist, had tried to convince her that her pain was, as he put it, a "neurotic manifestation of unresolved conflict." Obviously this guy knew how to spout psychological jargon, but he didn't know much about the origin of pain. In fact, pain that is totally created by the mind, which is called *psychogenic* pain, is exceedingly rare. It accounts for fewer than one out of every thousand cases of chronic pain, and is most often associated with conditions of frank mental illness, such as schizophrenia.

Psychosomatic pain—pain that is partly influenced by the mind—is vastly more common. In fact, virtually all chronic pain is at least partly psychosomatic, because negative thoughts always make pain worse, and it's impossible to have chronic pain without occasionally having negative thoughts. In fact, it's impossible to be *alive* without occasionally having negative thoughts.

My fibromyalgia patient with the aversion to antidepressants undoubtedly did have some psychosomatic pain, but the origin of her pain was physical, not mental. Why then, she asked me, did I want her to take antidepressants?

I wanted her to take antidepressants because they often have a strong effect on the physical transmission of pain, first by slowing the release of pain chemicals in nerves, and, second, by helping to stop pain from reaching the brain. Thousands of pain patients who were not depressed have benefited from antidepressants.

There are two primary types of antidepressants: tricyclic antidepressants (including Elavil, Desyrel, and Pamelor), and selective serotonin reuptake inhibitors (including Prozac, Paxil, and Zoloft). The tricyclics usually work better for pain than the Prozac-type drugs. As a rule, pain patients require lower dosages of antidepressants than patients with depression.

As I've mentioned, though, many pain patients do suffer from depression, and they, too, can benefit from antidepressants. In one study, 66 percent of pain patients were found to be suffering from depression. In this study, researchers found that the patients with depression were more sensitive to pain, more irritable, and more pessimistic about treatment than nondepressed pain patients.

Tricyclic antidepressants are also widely used to prevent insomnia, which can significantly exacerbate chronic pain. In general, though, I prefer to treat insomnia with the sleep-inducing hormone melatonin, which is popular among many pain patients.

If you are suffering from clinical depression, you might benefit tremendously from antidepressants. Curing your depression might be pivotal in taking control of your pain.

ANTICONVULSANTS

Anticonvulsants are typically used by epileptics to prevent seizures, in which nerve and brain cells fire spontaneously, triggering uncontrollable responses. As you know, some kinds of chronic pain are also a result of spontaneous firing of nerve cells. Pain nerves can "get in the habit" of firing, as a result of an injury or illness. In effect, they get stuck in the "on" position. Anticonvulsant drugs stop not only the spontaneous firing that causes seizures, but also the spontaneous firing that causes some forms of chronic pain. They do this mostly by improving the "insulation" of nerves. Poor insulation of nerves is often the primary cause of spontaneous firing.

Because anticonvulsants act directly on nerve cells, they are most effective for nerve pain, or neuralgia. Nerve pain is often experienced as a sharp, stabbing pain. It feels sharper than other types of chronic pain simply because it originates in the nerve, and therefore has a "straight shot" to the spinal cord and brain.

Two of the most common nerve pains are trigeminal neuralgia, a shooting pain in the face, and postherpetic neuralgia, a piercing pain originating from nerves that have been infected with the herpes virus. Both of these conditions are sometimes improved with administration of anticonvulsants.

Anticonvulsive drugs are powerful and can have debilitating side effects, including sedation, confusion, and loss of balance. Therefore, if your doctor prescribes them, he or she will start with a very low dosage, and slowly increase it until it achieves the desired effect. If you take anticonvulsants, you will probably experience their side effects before you experience pain relief, so try to be patient.

Cancer patients are sometimes given anticonvulsants when tumors invade nerves. In such situations, opioids are often administered simultaneously.

The three most commonly used anticonvulsants are valproic acid, carbamazepine, and phenytoin.

Steroids

Steroids are wonderfully effective at reducing inflammation, and are extremely valuable in a medical crisis, but they can have terrible side effects during long-term use, and are therefore generally inappropriate for ongoing chronic pain.

Pain patients who use steroids for extended periods frequently suffer from skin reactions, organ breakdown, psychological and cognitive disorders, bloating, and bone loss.

As you'll recall, my polymyositis patient, Scott, was taking steroids when I first met him, and he hated their side effects even more than he hated his pain.

Because of the side effects, most doctors refuse to prescribe steroids for long-term pain control. However, the majority of doctors do approve of occasionally injecting steroids into an area near the spinal cord, when that area becomes inflamed. Inflammation of this area, called the epidural space, can cause great pain.

Epidural injections are generally safe and effective. Because epidural injections deliver the medication directly to the distressed site, injected dosages are far lower than oral dosages, and this helps prevent side effects.

Nerve Block Injections

If you've ever gotten a novocaine shot from your dentist, you've experienced a nerve block. This procedure—done by injecting a local anesthetic into a nerve—is often perfect for acute, short-term pain, and can sometimes help chronic pain.

Nerve blocks can help stop chronic pain by breaking the cycle of pain long enough for the nervous system to normalize. I've noticed that for some patients, the temporary relief from nerve blocks gets longer and longer each time the blocks are administered. Each successive shot helps destroy the nervous system's ingrained "memory" of the pain.

Sometimes, when pain is severe and intractable, doctors attempt to block signals permanently from the overactive pain nerve by cutting it, freezing it, or destroying it with chemicals. However, in most cases, the nerve grows back, and the pain returns. If the regrowth of the nerve is imperfect, it causes a new type of pain, usually a tingling, burning sensation, similar to the feeling you get when your foot falls asleep.

Even when the procedure is successful, the results usually don't last long. As a rule, doctors only expect a so-called permanent nerve block to last for about six months. Permanent blocks rarely last longer than two years.

Even if nerves do not regrow, the pain from a distressed area often shifts to another nerve. For terminal patients, though, permanent nerve blocks can provide great relief.

A procedure that is in some ways similar to a permanent nerve block is the implanting of an electrode that blocks pain. Like a permanent nerve block, this procedure requires surgery. The electrode, implanted in the patient's brain or spinal cord, sends out a small current of electricity when activated, usually by the patient. This electricity blocks pain signals, and also stimulates endorphin production.

Often this procedure is initially effective, but fails to provide long-term relief.

MUSCLE RELAXANTS

Ironically, these medications don't directly affect muscles. Instead, they appear to act on the central nervous system, causing general relaxation. This general relaxation allows tight muscles to loosen, and reduces spasm in muscles.

Muscle-relaxing medications—which include cyclobenzaprine, carisoprodol, and methocarbamol—can be helpful for people with fibromyalgia, back pain, and other disorders that create muscle pain.

Muscle relaxants are generally effective only when used occasionally, and are not considered appropriate for long-term use. In my experience, they have been overused by physicians who are unfamiliar with non-drug pain treatments.

MINOR TRANQUILIZERS

These medications have no direct analgesic effect. However, they can reduce some of the characteristics of chronic pain syndrome—such as depression, anxiety, and insomnia—and *indirectly* relieve pain.

Minor tranquilizers include popular drugs such as Valium and Xanax. Their side effects can include lethargy, dizziness, constipation, and nausea. In some people, minor tranquilizers do not improve depression, but make it worse. Furthermore, these drugs can be very addictive.

Despite their obvious hazards, though, these medications can be valuable. They often give patients temporary relief from some of the most debilitating mental aspects of chronic pain syndrome. Sometimes this encourages patients to participate more actively in their pain programs.

Cognitive-Enhancement Medications

Now let's look at one final class of medication that can help you defeat pain: prescription drugs that *improve brain function.*

If you have read *Brain Longevity,* you know that I have a high regard for several cognitive-enhancement medications. In my clinical practice, I have used these drugs to help patients fight terrible brain disorders, including Alzheimer's disease. The results were often remarkable. In many cases, patients achieved things that were thought to be impossible.

Cognitive-enhancement medications have also helped patients

with *mild* cognitive impairment. These patients have not only overcome their difficulties, but have also reached new, previously untapped levels of brain power. They've shown remarkable increases in memory, concentration, learning ability, and mental energy.

The same medications often help pain patients. Because pain is in the brain, any medicine that improves cerebral function will boost the ability of the brain to defeat pain.

I recently treated a fibromyalgia patient whose muscle pain was so severe that she was almost an invalid. Virtually every time she moved, it aggravated her pain. Because of this incessant irritation, her face was a constantly shifting mask of suffering. Her expression repeatedly metamorphosed from a grimace to a wince, to a scowl, and then back to a grimace again. She rarely smiled. She was very depressed, and told me her mind felt "foggy."

She began a full-scale, four-level pain cure program, and seemed to benefit from many of the modalities. However, one modality appeared to have the most immediate positive effect: administration of the cognitive-enhancement drug piracetam. When she started taking piracetam, her depression lifted, her mental clarity returned, and she experienced considerable relief from pain.

Piracetam increases the energy level in the brain, and optimizes general cerebral function. For this patient, that was vitally important because it helped her brain to launch a stronger biological counterattack against her pain.

As you know, you can also increase brain power with other modalities such as nutritional therapy and exercise therapy, but for dramatic, immediate results, it's hard to beat the effects of prescription brain-enhancement medications.

Here are the best ones:

PIRACETAM

This remarkable medication, developed in Europe, has been shown in controlled clinical trials to help improve the mental abilities of Alzheimer's patients, as well as the mental abilities of people with only very mild cognitive impairment. Piracetam increases levels of the primary chemical carrier of thoughts and memories. This chemical is a neurotransmitter called acetylcholine.

When people don't have enough acetylcholine, it's harder for them to create new memories, and to concentrate; their cognitive ability is significantly diminished. Piracetam rebuilds acetylcholine levels, and helps restore cognitive strength. When acetylcholine levels are restored, patients generally enjoy a resurgence of energy. Although piracetam is not a stimulant, it definitely increases mental energy, and this in turn usually sparks a feeling of physical energy. Some patients taking piracetam have told me that they no longer need minor stimulants, such as caffeine.

Piracetam can even help the two hemispheres of the brain to work together more efficiently. It does this by improving the function of the band of nerves that connects the two hemispheres, the corpus callosum. Because piracetam improves hemispheric coordination, it has a reputation for increasing creativity. In Europe, piracetam is widely used by writers and artists.

Piracetam has been prescribed by doctors in Europe for a number of years, but has not yet gone through the lengthy approval process of the U.S. Food and Drug Administration. However, it can still be legally obtained by U.S. citizens, from a European "buyers' club" such as those listed in Appendix III.

If you wish to import medications that have not been approved by the FDA, you must meet the following criteria: You must comply with all applicable state and local laws, and must import only an amount appropriate for personal use. Also, you must import only medications that do not pose significant safety risks, and that are intended for a serious medical condition. If you do choose to import any medications, I strongly urge you to do so only with the advice and supervision of a physician.

Many studies have been done on piracetam, and it has thus far shown no significant side effects. An appropriate dosage for a person in good health is 600 mg daily. People with age-related cognitive decline generally require a higher dosage, in the range of 1,800–2,400 mg daily. Pain patients often require a larger dosage than healthy people do. Occasionally, some of my patients take up to 3,200 mg daily, and report no significant side effects.

DEPRENYL

This drug has been widely used for many years in America and elsewhere as a treatment for Parkinson's disease, the nervous system disorder that causes loss of muscular control.

Parkinson's disease is primarily caused by depletion of the neurotransmitter dopamine, which controls physical movement. Dopamine levels decline in all people as we age. The decline starts at about age forty-five, and continues at a rate of about 13 percent per decade. Therefore, by age eighty, most people have only about half as much dopamine as they did when they were younger.

Although dopamine is mostly used for muscular coordination, it has other important functions. It is the most important neurotransmitter in sexual function, and it also affects cognitive ability, and immunity to disease.

Deprenyl restores dopamine levels, and improves coordination, concentration, memory, mood, and sex drive. It has an especially positive effect on depression. In one study, 60 percent of patients with clinical depression—all of whom had failed to improve while taking other drugs—responded positively to deprenyl. In my practice, I've noted that patients who did *not* have depression responded to deprenyl with increased mental energy and physical vitality.

Deprenyl can help pain patients by increasing mental energy, and by decreasing depression. Recently it was tested in a landmark study on Alzheimer's, in which researchers found that the progress of the disease could be slowed significantly with deprenyl and vitamin E.

Deprenyl can be purchased through an overseas buyers' club, or it can be obtained with a prescription from a doctor. If you do purchase it from a buyers' club, I strongly recommend you consult with a doctor about it.

When I prescribe deprenyl, I almost always start my patients on very low dosages—about 4 mg three times weekly. If this does not appear to be effective, I increase the dosage gradually. In patients with moderate cognitive decline, I prescribe up to 5–6 mg daily. Patients with severe cognitive decline receive 7–10 mg daily. The dosage range for pain patients generally ranges from 3 to 8 mg daily.

Deprenyl has been shown to be a safe, well-tolerated drug. Deprenyl is contraindicated when patients are taking antidepressant medications, however. Because deprenyl tends to increase energy, most patients prefer to take it in the morning. Taking it at night sometimes causes insomnia.

Hormonal Replacement Medications

As we age, the levels of our hormones begin to decrease. This contributes to cognitive decline, lower energy levels, decreased immunity, mood disorders, cardiovascular diseases, and various ill effects of aging, such as joint deterioration and loss of muscle mass. *All* of these conditions can radically increase vulnerability to pain.

In recent years the medical community has taken enormous strides in recognizing the value of hormonal replacement therapy. When hormones are replaced to normal levels, patients often experience a "re-youthing."

Many of my pain patients have responded exceedingly well to hormonal replacement therapy. I've already mentioned one patient whose arthritis improved immeasurably after she began hormonal replacement therapy. Other patients, with a variety of pain problems, have responded equally as well.

For example, I administered hormonal replacement therapy to one middle-aged male patient with back pain, and he soon noticed a sharp improvement in his condition. The hormonal replacement therapy increased his cognitive function, improved the function of his joints, and elevated his mood. Each of those factors played a role in his ability to conquer his pain.

Two hormones that I administer frequently are DHEA and pregnenolone, both of which are converted by the body into steroidal sex hormones, such as estrogen and testosterone; for this reason they are known as "precursor hormones." The beauty of these two hormones is that they are used by the body according to its own needs. Thus, these precursor hormones take advantage of the "wisdom of the body."

DHEA has recently been touted by the media as a new "wonder drug," and it deserves the attention it has received. It has astonishing properties. It appears to slow the biological symptoms of aging and to help prevent arthritis, cancer, osteoporosis, viral and bacterial infection, obesity, and high blood pressure. It boosts cognitive ability and can help relieve depression.

To determine an appropriate dosage, I test existing levels of DHEA. This can be done by any medical laboratory, with a simple blood test. Then I prescribe a dosage that will restore the DHEA level to the level it would have been during the patient's late twenties, when DHEA levels peak.

Some doctors restore the DHEA level only to the average level of the patient's current age group. I think that's insufficient. Patients do best when doctors restore DHEA to *youthful* levels.

The dosage can range from 10 mg to 200 mg daily. The 200-mg dosage would be for an older person with an extremely low DHEA level. I often start patients on 10 mg daily, and increase the dosage gradually if necessary.

Although long-term studies have not been done, DHEA currently appears to have no significant side effects when used properly. It should not be used by men who have prostate cancer, because it can elevate sex hormones that may exacerbate the cancer. Also, it should not be used by people in their twenties, because their levels are already high. Young bodybuilders, who already have high DHEA levels, sometimes take extra DHEA to increase muscle mass. This is a serious mistake. It's similar to taking steroids.

When I prescribe DHEA to men, I always order a PSA test, to screen for prostate abnormalities, and I ask their family doctor or a urologist to perform a prostate examination. I also recommend that all men who take DHEA use saw palmetto, an herb that is very effective at supporting prostate health.

Pregnenolone, the other hormone I routinely recommend, is similar to DHEA. DHEA is made from pregnenolone, as are all other steroidal hormones. Thus, pregnenolone sits at the top of the sex-hormone "pyramid." Because pregnenolone is used to make many other hormones, it helps the body and brain adapt to their changing hormonal needs.

Pregnenolone, like DHEA, has a wide range of positive effects. It improves cognitive function, relieves depression, and has a general "re-youthing" effect. These qualities make it valuable to pain patients.

Pregnenolone also helps prevent the progression of arthritis. In fact, the hormone was commercially developed as an arthritis treatment in the 1930s, but its popularity declined when synthetic hormones were invented.

Dosage varies from patient to patient. I often start pain patients at 50 mg daily, and increase the dosage gradually if necessary. The highest dosage level that I recommend is 100 mg daily.

Pregnenolone is generally free of side effects, although occasionally it may make a patient feel edgy. Like all medications, it should be used cautiously, under the direction of a physician.

Another hormone I commonly recommend is melatonin. Melatonin is the hormone, produced by the pineal gland, that helps control the body's sleeping and waking cycles. The body's level of melatonin generally increases in the evening, and helps induce sleep. Sleep, of course, is very important for pain patients, because lack of adequate sleep drastically lowers the pain threshold. Unfortunately, as we age, the pineal gland tends to atrophy and produce less melatonin. This often accounts for the tendency of older people to sleep less than younger people.

A reasonable daily dosage of melatonin, taken in the evening, is .5–3 mg.

In addition to these hormones, I also prescribe testosterone to some patients. As you may know, testosterone is the sex hormone that is most abundant in males, but it is also present in females. When testosterone levels decline during the aging process, both men and women are affected physically and emotionally. Low levels of testosterone, in both males and females, are relatively common among people fifty years of age or older, and can cause depression, weight gain, loss of muscle and bone mass, decreased oxygenation of cells, and reduced libido. Several of these characteristics can contribute to increased chronic pain. To determine your current level of testosterone, your doctor may order a standard hormone blood assay test.

Dosages of testosterone vary considerably. The hormone may be taken orally, by injection, with a patch, or in a cream. There is some evidence, though, that oral testosterone causes liver damage in some patients. To determine your proper dosage and the appropriate method of application, consult your physician.

A final hormone that is helpful for many patients is human growth hormone, or HGH. Unfortunately, though, HGH is quite expensive, costing as much as $12,000 per year.

HGH is the hormone that triggered your growth when you were a child, and it is still responsible for inaugurating a significant degree of healing and regeneration within your body. HGH helps your body to repair muscles and other tissues, and promotes the proper function of the kidneys, the heart, and the immune system. It seems to have a powerful "re-youthing" effect upon many people, and has notably improved mood and cognitive function in a number of my patients.

If you have fibromyalgia, you may have a deficit of HGH; for more information on this, please read chapter 9.

To determine whether you are a candidate for HGH replacement therapy, consult your physician.

Those are the medications that can help you overcome your pain.

Once again, you may feel overwhelmed by your number of options. But don't be disheartened. It's *great* that there are so many things that might help you. If you try several of these medications, you will probably discover that one or more of them will help you.

In all likelihood, you will soon be using at least one medication from each of the major categories: synthetic over-the-counter medicines, herbal preparations, homeopathic remedies, prescription analgesics, hormonal replacement agents, and cognitive-enhancement medicines. Taken properly, each of these will synergistically increase the power of the other medications.

Furthermore, your menu of medications will work synergistically with the other three levels of your pain program.

Even though we have discussed only three of the four levels of your program, you already have a vast and powerful arsenal of anti-pain modalities at your disposal.

Now it's time to enlist the power of your two greatest assets: your *mind* and your *spirit.*

Onward—and upward!

5

Level Four: Mental and Spiritual Pain Control

If suffering alone taught, all the world would be wise.
To suffering must be added love.

—ANNE MORROW LINDBERGH

I'm going to tell you something that you may not want to hear:
Your personality is probably causing a lot of your pain.

If you have chronic pain, you probably have a "pain personality," characterized by anxiety, depression, anger, and rigidity. These traits intensify and perpetuate pain.

This probably sounds like an accusation, but it's not. It's a statement of clinical fact.

During my many years of clinical work with pain patients, I have found that most of them have a pain personality to some degree. It is extremely common.

Pain patients, however, generally *hate* to be told that their personality is part of their problem. Why? Because too many of their friends and family members—and even their doctors—have told them that their pain is "all in their mind." Pain patients can't stand to hear this, because it's condescending, unsympathetic, and almost always untrue.

Pain virtually never exists *solely* in the mind. That type of pain, called "psychogenic pain," generally occurs only among highly delusional psychotics. It's extremely unlikely that your pain is "all in your mind."

However, a person's mental outlook can partly contribute to the onset of chronic pain. Many pain patients have a pain personality *before* their pain starts, and this personality makes them more vulnerable to the onset of chronic pain.

Also, a person's *reaction* to chronic pain can create a pain personality. Most pain patients develop pain personalities as a *result* of their pain. This change in their personalities greatly magnifies their existing pain. This phenomenon is so common that it is often considered normal.

Because your mind does play an important role in your pain, it's vitally important that you address the mental aspects of your pain. If you ignore the role that your mind plays in your pain, you might be in pain for the rest of your life.

In this chapter I'm going to tell you how you can move beyond your pain personality. You will learn how to respond to pain in a way that is far healthier than the "normal" response.

Even if you don't have a pain personality, this chapter will still be of great value. You will learn how to kill pain just by focusing the forces of your mind and spirit. If you work hard, you'll soon have stunning mental control over your pain. It may even be equal to the mental control of yogic masters.

In many ways, this is the most difficult level of my pain program. When you're working on this level, you can't just take a nutrient or do an exercise, and then go about your business. Instead, every day you must dig deep within your psyche and your soul, and grapple with the demons your pain has spawned. This will be a monumental fight. But that's the beauty of it! This battle will offer you the rare opportunity to discover *exactly who you are,* and what you have inside.

That knowledge will do even more than just help stop your suffering. It will bring you closer than you've ever before been to your true self. You will grow wiser. Your spirit will blossom.

You will become the person you've always hoped you could be.

That's the challenge of this final level—and that's the reward.

* * *

Thus far, in our discussions of the brain, we've focused mostly on the brain's automatic, involuntary functions, viewing it as the body's "master housekeeper." Now it's time to look at your brain as the site of your mind and your spirit.

I guarantee you that you will need *both* your mind and your spirit to cure your pain. It's difficult to cure most chronic health problems when you ignore the mind and spirit, as orthodox, mechanistic doctors often do, and it's virtually impossible to cure chronic pain if you ignore the mind and spirit.

Pain is one of the most intense of all human experiences, and therefore *demands* meaning, which only the mind and spirit can provide. If you fail to find a positive meaning for your pain, your interpretation of your pain will almost certainly be negative. Unfortunately, this negative interpretation will greatly increase your suffering.

If you've ever felt pain for more than just a few days, I'm sure you've asked yourself, "What's going *on*? What does this *mean*?" If you failed to come up with a good, positive answer, you probably felt scared, angry, and anxious. You probably began to develop some of the negative emotional characteristics of a pain personality.

Every time you experienced these negative emotions, they touched off a biological assault on your nervous system. They created the biological "stress response." Your heart beat faster, you secreted stress hormones, your brain pumped out excitatory neurotransmitters, your muscles tensed, your blood vessels constricted, and your brain was deprived of its glucose "fuel." *All* of these biological reactions heightened your pain, lowered your pain threshold, and decreased your brain's ability to launch a counterattack against your pain.

In addition, these negative emotions probably caused you to adopt some of the lifestyle traits of chronic pain syndrome. Your anger, depression, and anxiety probably made you want to withdraw from life. You may have backed away from your work and hobbies, or limited your contact with other people. Your eating and sleeping patterns probably changed, and you may have begun to depend on painkilling drugs.

Chronic pain syndrome, combined with a pain personality, is usually present—to some degree—in most pain patients. Both of these phenomena reinforce each other, and perpetuate each other.

Unfortunately, they both make pain far worse. They are the "dynamic duo" of suffering.

When I treat patients who clearly have a pain personality, it's usually hard for me to tell whether their personality caused their pain, or whether their pain caused their personality.

In many patients, *both* of these things happen. For example, in migraine patients, excessive anxiety generally exists *before* patients begin to suffer from migraines, and excessive depression usually starts *afterwards*.

I don't really worry about which came first, though, because it has little bearing on my treatment. The same basic mental techniques work in both situations.

My primary concern is simply helping patients to realize that there *is* such a thing as a pain personality. To do that, I sometimes present them with the following statistics, which were gleaned from major studies:

* Fifty-eight percent of all migraine patients suffer from high levels of anxiety; this includes 59 percent of all females with migraines, and 55 percent of all males.

* Nineteen percent of migraine patients suffer from clinical depression.

* Nineteen percent of osteoarthritis patients have symptoms of clinical depression.

* After psychological counseling, pain patients reduce their number of annual doctor visits by an average of 38 percent.

* Twenty-five percent of fibromyalgia patients suffer from at least one other stress-related condition, including irritable bowel syndrome, chronic headaches, or dysmenorrhea (painful menstruation).

• Thirty-three percent of all chronic pain patients have a serious psychiatric disorder.

Another way in which I sometimes help patients to understand that their mind and spirit affect their pain is to describe how people from different cultures react to pain. Theoretically, since the human nervous system is virtually identical among all people, people around the world should respond to pain similarly, but they don't.

For example, people from Nepal appear to have the world's highest pain threshold, probably because of their country's harsh living conditions, and because of their culture's emphasis on spirituality.

Similarly, in other Asian cultures, where pain is often embraced as a path to spirituality, people tolerate it much more readily than do most people in Western cultures. Hindus, for example, perceive pain as just a transitory condition that will pass during the soul's immortal journey. To defeat pain, Hindus focus on their spirit, which they believe is invulnerable to pain. In fact, Hindus are so adept at dispelling pain with mental and spiritual pain-control techniques that they resist taking any analgesic medicines that might dull their cognitive powers. For them, painkillers often *increase* their perception of pain.

Two other cultures with elevated resistance to pain are Native Americans, and Mediterranean people of Jewish origin. Both of these cultures stress finding *meaning* in pain, rather than trying to end it as quickly as possible. Also, there appears to be an element of sheer toughness or survivalism in these cultures. In one interesting experiment, a group of Christian Protestants and a group of Jewish people were tested for their tolerance to pain. After the test, both groups were told that the other group had shown a higher tolerance. They were then tested again. In the second test, the Protestant group produced the same results as in the first test. But the Jewish group showed a far higher tolerance for pain. Their social conditioning had apparently motivated them to "dig deeper" for resistance to pain.

In European cultures, Irish males tend to react to pain by withdrawing, while Italian people generally seek comfort from friends and family.

Christians often tend to see pain as punishment from God, and this negative outlook frequently increases their perception of pain. In fact, the English word *pain* is derived from the Greek *poine,* which means "punishment."

I do not believe that any of these psychological and spiritual reactions to pain are more morally correct than the others. However, some are more *therapeutically valuable.* In general, reactions that involve acceptance of pain, and the search for meaning, help people to recover from pain more quickly and more completely.

You certainly don't need to accept the beliefs of another culture, though, to gain relief from pain. All of the best mental and spiritual control techniques for pain now exist in the context of our own Western culture. These techniques are (1) a form of goal-setting called "psychic clustering"; (2) a form of psychotherapy called "cognitive therapy"; (3) visualization; (4) a type of psychotherapy known as "behavioral therapy"; (5) stress reduction; (6) meditation; and (7) spiritual searching.

Those are the techniques I most often use in the mental-control level of my pain program. They are extremely effective, and when they are applied in conjunction with the other levels of my pain cure program, they bring pain relief to the vast majority of patients.

Let's now begin one of the most important journeys of your life: a journey into your own mind and spirit.

Psychic Clustering

Before you begin this journey into your mind and spirit, you should decide what you want your destination to be. This destination will be the ultimate goal of all your pain-control work.

When I first ask patients what their ultimate goal is, most of them answer, "To be free of pain." After we do a goal-setting exercise that I call "psychic clustering," though, they generally realize that being free of pain is not their ultimate goal.

What almost all of them really want, more than anything else in the world, is to have a happy life. This is quite understandable, of course, because that's what almost all of us truly yearn for. Having a happy life is a simple, common goal, but an extraordinarily ambitious one—a goal that's far easier to desire than to achieve. However, when we're temporarily in the midst of a great challenge—such as overcoming pain, or striving for success—we often become fixated on this immediate, lesser goal. But this lesser goal is usually just a means to an end. What most of us really crave, above all, is a happy life.

Some patients are flabbergasted when they realize that they want their life to be happy even more than they want it to be free of pain. Having been focused so long and hard on fighting pain, they have forgotten that simply being happy is almost always the most important thing of all.

Many of my patients don't realize that their ultimate goal is happiness until they perform the exercise of psychic clustering. It's a wonderfully effective exercise because it's highly personal, and very simple. Here's how to do it.

Take a blank sheet of paper, and begin to jot down all of the things that you deeply desire. Place these desires, or goals, in general clusters of related categories. For example, make one cluster of *work-related* goals, such as to get a promotion, to make more money, or to work fewer hours. Try to link these goals loosely in a logical sequence; for example, link together getting a promotion with making more money.

Then make a cluster of *family-related* goals, such as to spend more time with the kids, to be a better spouse, or to go on a family vacation.

Then make a cluster of health goals, spiritual goals, social goals, or any others that are important to you.

Jot down anything that comes to mind. Don't write down what you think you *should* want; write down what you really *do* want. There are no right or wrong answers. The primary purpose of the exercise is simply to give you greater clarity about your true goals in life. The secondary purpose is to remind you that there is much more to your life than just overcoming your pain.

You'll probably find that some of your clusters and goals are interlinked. For example, the work-related goal of working fewer hours might link up to the family-related goal of spending more time with your kids.

The following page shows an example of a typical patient's psychic clustering chart. As you can see, this patient—after doing a couple of preliminary charts—eventually placed happiness at the center of his chart. Most patients do, after giving it some thought.

When pain patients compile this simple psychic clustering chart, and become explicitly aware of their deepest desires, it often has a profound effect upon them. It gives them a feeling of mental and emotional clarity, and heightens their state of consciousness. It helps them to realize that there is so much more to their existence than just fighting pain. They often realize that there is an eternal—or divine—aspect of their being which is impervious to their pain. They often realize that their pain is just ephemeral and sometimes even, to some extent, illusory.

When they begin to reach these realizations, it endows them with a special dignity—one that is sometimes not present in people who do not suffer. They walk tall. They act with purpose. They become better prepared to do the hard mental and spiritual work that is necessary to conquer pain.

Most of all, they move closer to becoming their true selves—and casting off their pain personalities.

When this point of clarity arrives, it's time for them to begin using various mental and spiritual techniques that stop pain.

Let's take a look at those techniques.

First we'll examine the mental and psychological programs that help control pain. Then we'll go even deeper, and look at the most potent pain-fighting force in the universe: the realm of the spirit.

This will be an exciting journey. Let's get started!

Psychic Clustering Chart

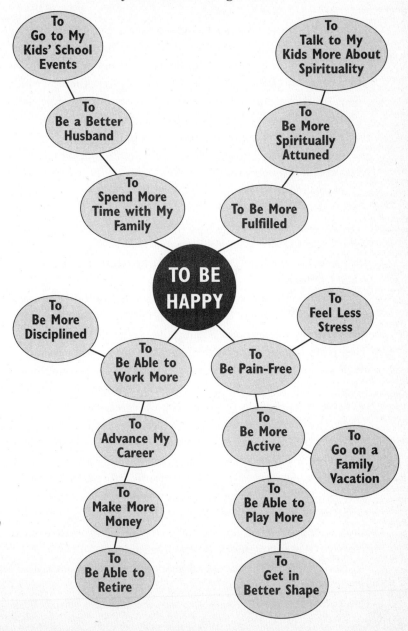

Controlling Pain with Cognitive Therapy

Cognitive therapy is a superb psychological technique for fighting chronic pain. It's a relatively new form of psychotherapy that consists of confronting negative thoughts cognitively, or rationally, instead of emotionally. Unlike older forms of psychotherapy, which focus on processing painful memories, cognitive therapy deals mostly in the here and now. The goal of cognitive therapists is to improve a person's current mood and behavior *by changing faulty thinking*. Cognitive therapy helps people see the world more realistically and less pessimistically.

According to cognitive therapists, many people perceive the world as far more difficult and negative than it really is. One major reason for this negative outlook is that people get in the habit of seeing things in absolute, black-and-white terms. Often they become rigid perfectionists, and generate a great deal of stress for themselves.

In addition to causing stress, this absolutist attitude leads people to adopt a variety of faulty styles of thinking. Often they overgeneralize, and believe that *one* negative event reflects *all* of reality. They jump to conclusions, thinking things are far worse than they really are. In addition, they overpersonalize events, blaming themselves every time something goes wrong. Cognitive therapists call all these forms of faulty thinking "cognitive distortions."

People who have many cognitive distortions often develop the characteristics associated with a pain personality, even before they begin to suffer from chronic pain. Their absolutism leads to rigid, compulsive behavior, and makes them suffer from anxiety and depression. When this happens, they are relatively more vulnerable to the onset of chronic pain. If they suffer a serious injury or develop a degenerative disease, they are more prone than most people to develop pain that lingers indefinitely.

Also, many pain patients adopt negative, rigid personalities *after* they have begun to suffer from chronic pain. Their pain is so traumatizing that it changes the way they see the world. They begin to believe ideas that seem reasonable at the time, but are really illogical and self-destructive.

Many of these illogical and self-destructive ideas contribute to chronic pain syndrome. For example, many pain patients begin to think that if they can't do their work as well as they once did, they'd rather not do it at all. Others think that they'll feel better emotionally if they pull away from other people, when what they *really* need is love and help.

Even if these patients don't develop full-blown chronic pain syndrome, they still often develop many of the characteristics of a pain personality.

Often, when pain patients begin to have a pain personality, they gradually go onto "automatic pilot," and stop engaging in the ongoing examination of life that enables people to sort out the good from the bad, and to find meaning in daily living. Instead, these people become fixated on their pain, and turn their lives into a one-note symphony of suffering. Ultimately, this makes their pain almost unbearable, because of the biological consequences of depression and anxiety. This outlook on life is extremely alienating, and often forces away friends and family.

To find out if a pain patient might benefit from cognitive therapy, I often ask him or her these ten simple questions:

1. Do you think about daily activities mostly in terms of how much pain they cause?

2. Do you often think there's nothing worse than chronic pain?

3. Did a number of your friends begin to avoid you after your pain started?

4. Do you frequently let people do things for you that you could do for yourself?

5. Do you look forward to taking analgesic medications?

6. Do you get angry with yourself because pain has limited your abilities?

7. Do you ever think that dying will actually be a relief?

8. Is it hard for you to go a day or two without mentioning your pain?

9. Is it important to you to have the very best doctor in your area?

10. Do you often think about how much you could achieve if you weren't in pain?

A "yes" response to any of these questions is an indication that your belief system is, to at least some extent, rigid, self-destructive, irrational, or absolutist.

If you answered yes to only one or two questions, you have a basically healthy, realistic, flexible outlook, and may not benefit very much from cognitive therapy.

If you answered yes to four or five questions, your belief system is probably contributing significantly to your pain, and you should strongly consider cognitive therapy.

If you answered yes to between six and ten questions, you have an essentially unhealthy outlook, which is almost certainly intensifying and perpetuating your pain. In all probability, you could benefit greatly from cognitive therapy.

Don't feel bad if you got a high score. The majority of my patients do, when they first begin their programs.

If you do need to do some work on your personality, embrace this as an *opportunity for healing*. Be *glad* that there's something you can do to feel better. After all, there's nothing worse than hearing a doctor say, "I'm sorry, there's *nothing* I can do for you."

If you do begin cognitive therapy, you'll probably make quick progress, because most patients do. As a rule, most patients see a therapist for less than three months.

To find a psychologist who practices cognitive therapy, consult your telephone book's Yellow Pages, or ask your family doctor for a referral. Some psychologists specialize in this type of therapy, but a doctor can employ cognitive therapy without specializing in it. In fact, I use this therapy myself with some of my patients.

One of my patients who benefited greatly from therapy was a forty-two-year-old screenwriter named Dale, whose life was being ruined by migraines. When Dale first bustled into my office, he seemed preoccupied and in a hurry, even though he was early for his appointment. He fidgeted in his chair and sipped coffee from a Styrofoam cup. "Hope you don't mind the coffee," he blurted in a staccato rush of words, "but days like this, when I don't have to work, are the only times I can get away with drinking it. If I drink it while I'm working—boom!" He pantomimed hitting his head with a hammer.

Immediately I suspected that stress played a primary role in Dale's debilitating migraines. If a nutritional trigger of migraines is active only at certain stress-related times, such as during work, it indicates that stress is a major factor in the problem.

Dale was scared. He was on the verge of losing a job worth $250,000 for a script rewrite because of his headaches. He'd missed several deadlines because of disabling headaches, and the movie's producer had told him that if his undependability continued, he would cancel his contract and get someone else to do the job.

Dale's migraines had transformed about ten of his days each month into sheer hell. When he should have been working, he found himself vomiting brown bile into a toilet and trying to escape from all noise, which was impossible in his Santa Monica apartment. Dale, who had a vivid imagination, told me that his headaches were like "having a pincher-bug inside my ear, eating its way toward my brain."

Dale had many of the characteristics of a pain personality, and had moderate chronic pain syndrome. He was a total perfectionist. He told me that he drove himself crazy with perfectionism, but even so, he thought this trait was the source of his success. The more I talked with him, though, the more I became convinced that his *creativity* was the main source of his success, and that his perfectionism actually worked against him, by stifling his creative instincts. When I mentioned this to him, he said I might be right, but that he didn't know how to change.

I put Dale on a full-spectrum program, and it was difficult for him. Before his program had begun, he'd indulged in a careless diet, had smoked cigarettes, and had been sedentary, all of which had contributed to his migraines. The cigarettes were particularly harmful, because smoking disrupts brain biochemistry and markedly impairs circulation, thus lowering the pain threshold. But it was hard for him to give up these things, because they helped relieve his stress. Dale considered life inherently difficult, and embraced any indulgence that gave him temporary refuge.

Even though Dale's program included a good diet, herbal therapy, yoga, meditation, mind/body exercises, and acupuncture, he was not making much progress. He still had a very high stress level, but was reluctant to abandon his rigidity and negativity.

One day, however, while I was giving him an acupuncture treatment, he told me that he thought his perfectionism stemmed from a traumatic experience in his childhood. When he was seven, his three-year-old brother choked to death while he was playing with him. Since then, he had felt guilty about not saving him. After that incident, he said, he'd always been hard on himself, to make up for his failure.

He'd had psychological counseling, so he knew it was foolish for him to blame himself for his brother's death, and to try to be perfect to make up for it. But just *knowing* this hadn't really helped. The insight hadn't "sunk in" enough to change his outlook or behavior.

I decided to try cognitive therapy with him.

I asked him to begin a new habit: to tell himself, every single day, several times a day, that he had *not* been responsible for his brother's death, and that trying to be perfect was *not* the proper response to this tragedy. I also urged him to tell himself, several times a day, that his perfectionism was not the source of his success, and that he'd be even more successful if he'd just loosen up and let go.

I hoped that this daily self-talk, as cognitive therapists call it, would change Dale's outlook. It would not give him more insight into himself than he already had, but it would *drive home* his existing insights.

It worked! In a matter of weeks, Dale's stress subsided dra-

Ten Cognitive Distortions

(adapted from the work of cognitive therapist Dr. David D. Burns)

1. *All-or-nothing thinking.* This type of faulty thinking consists of viewing the world in absolutist, black-and-white terms. Perfectionists often think this way.
2. *Overgeneralization.* This happens when you think one event represents all of reality.
3. *Mental filter.* This means focusing on just one negative aspect of a larger situation. For example, if you win the lottery, all you do is worry about the taxes.
4. *Disqualifying the positive.* This happens when you fail to see most of the good things around you. If there's one cloud in the sky, you call it a cloudy day.
5. *Jumping to conclusions.* Before all the facts are in, you assume the worst. Often this becomes a self-fulfilling prophecy.
6. *Magnification and minification.* This happens when you exaggerate bad things and downplay good ones. If you're the type of person who can never accept a compliment, it may be because you downplay your good qualities and magnify your bad ones.
7. *Emotional reasoning.* This faulty thought style consists of mistaking your emotional reaction for objective reality. For example, if someone hurts your feelings, you take that as proof that they are cruel. You allow your emotions to determine reality, instead of your rational thought processes.
8. *Labeling.* This happens when you decide someone or something has a particular quality, and then you refuse to budge from your opinion. You fail to realize that people and things often change.
9. *Personalization.* This occurs when you think that everything happens because of something you did.
10. *Obligatory thinking.* This occurs when you become fixated on what you *should* do, instead of what you would really like to do. It makes you feel pressured and resentful.

matically. His demeanor became much more placid, and he seemed to feel more secure. His headaches soon diminished in intensity, frequency, and duration. In less than two months they were no longer a major factor in his life.

Dale finished the script rewrite and was assigned another job, for even more money. He lost about thirty pounds, stopped smoking, and became more physically active. For the first time in his adult life, he felt great.

The last time I saw Dale, which was the day he received another script rewrite contract, he bounced into my office with such zest that I told him he looked as if he felt like a kid again.

"I feel *better* than that," he said with a grin. "I feel like a *rich* kid!"

Cognitive therapy can be a powerful tool for reducing stress, and for diminishing the damage that's done by a pain personality, and by chronic pain syndrome.

But cognitive therapy can do far more than even that. Applied properly, it can help produce thoughts that *directly kill pain*.

With proper training, you can learn to generate thoughts that will have the same painkilling power as the most effective analgesic drugs.

These thoughts relieve pain by unleashing the force of one of your most powerful allies in your war against pain: the mind-power effect.

> **"It doesn't hurt when you're winning."**
>
> —Baseball player Pete Rose, commenting on his broken toe

Mind Over Matter: Harnessing the Mind-Power Effect

Once, an elderly arthritis patient of mine began to cry when she started telling me about her last visit to her family doctor. Her eyes—which had that hard, wide look that people get when they're in severe pain—were dry one minute, and floating in tears the next.

"I told my doctor I was taking *these*," she said, pulling a small vial of a homeopathic remedy from her purse. "And he said, 'You're wasting your money! These are just placebo pills. They won't help!'

"But they *do* help," she said to me, "and I told him so. But he wouldn't listen, even after I got upset. He told me that if I wanted to take quack medicine, I should find another doctor."

"Where did you get these?" I asked. To me, it looked as if they were the wrong medication for her problem. I agreed with her doctor's opinion of the medication, but I totally disagreed with his psychological approach.

"My daughter gave them to me," she said.

"You'd be crazy not to take these," I told her. "I think I can find you some even better medications, but if these help, they help. And *you* know if they're helping a lot better than your doctor does."

"Oh, thank you," she said. She was so grateful that she stood up and gave me a hug. She was sweet. But it made me sad. How could her doctor have been so cold? And how could he, after four years of medical school, have been so ignorant about the value of a positive belief system in the treatment of chronic pain?

Obviously this woman believed these pills were helping her—possibly because she associated them with the love and concern of her daughter. Her doctor had blundered in not clinically *employing* the power of her belief. Because homeopathic remedies are harmless and inexpensive, her doctor easily could have prescribed *other* therapies to be used *with* this particular homeopathic remedy. Instead, he subverted her positive belief system, and sent her away in pain.

Unfortunately, her doctor's approach is very common. Many medical doctors are uninterested in the role that the mind plays in disease and discomfort. Because this role is often mysterious, many doctors consider it to be unscientific, and therefore of little significance.

Because we doctors are scientists, we love it when we can reduce medical problems to clear, biochemical, one-on-one, cause-and-effect relationships. This reductionist approach is the foundation of the scientific method. However, as you know, it is my firm belief that almost all chronic, degenerative conditions have multiple causes, and require multiple therapies. One of the most important therapies is *psychological* therapy. In the treatment of chronic pain, when the patient's psychological outlook is ignored, the treatment often fails. The mind, as I've shown, can intensify and perpetuate pain. And the mind can take pain away. The *primary* way that the mind can take pain away is by activating the force that I call the "mind-power effect." In fact, the mind-power effect is simply another phrase for the "placebo effect." I often avoid the word *placebo,* though, because it has a negative connotation among most patients, and most doctors. As a rule, doctors and patients don't even know what this word means.

Most people think that *placebo* means "fake." It does not. *Placebo* is a Latin word that means "I will please." Thus, placebo refers to the pleasing, positive psychological effect that is caused by *any* therapy. Even therapies that are biologically *effective* usually have a placebo effect, and so do therapies that are biologically *ineffective.*

The placebo effect, or mind-power effect, is strongest in patients who are most responsive to the power of suggestion. It is also much stronger among patients with overall positive belief systems, since these patients are more likely to tell themselves that a therapy is helping.

As a rule, patients who respond well to biologically effective drugs also respond well to biologically *ineffective* drugs. For example, one study showed that morphine was approximately 95 percent effective for relieving pain among patients who had previously responded positively to biologically ineffective drugs. But morphine was only about *50 percent effective* among patients who had *not* responded positively to biologically ineffective drugs.

This is a powerful reminder that no matter how biologically effective any pain therapy is, patients still need to *believe* in it to obtain the highest level of healing.

Another interesting study that shows the importance of the mind-power effect was one that examined the effectiveness of various surgeries. Researchers found that in the early years of *ineffec-*

tive surgeries, which were later discredited, patients enjoyed a 70 percent *success* rate. However, as doctors and patients began to lose faith in these surgeries, the positive response rates began to plummet.

In most ways, the effects of the inactive placebo drugs mimic the effects of biologically active drugs. Like active drugs, inactive, placebo drugs have time-effect curves, as well as peak, cumulative, and carryover effects.

In clinical trials of most new drugs, biologically inactive drugs usually elicit a positive response rate of about 33 percent. This is impressive; it's a rate equal to that of some very effective medications. However, in the treatment of chronic pain—which has a *major* mental component—biologically inactive drugs are even *more* effective. In studies of the mind-power effect in pain treatment, the positive response rate to inactive drugs was found to be as high as 60 percent.

Furthermore, researchers found that the power of inactive drugs could be increased dramatically with proper presentation. Inactive drugs were far more likely to be effective if the doctor was attentive and concerned, if the setting was comfortable, and if the patient had the expectation of recovery.

One reason the mind-power effect is so powerful against chronic pain is that the nervous system's transmission of pain is so inefficient. Chronic pain travels *slowly*. Carried by thinly insulated nerves, chronic pain crawls along at only three miles per hour, while other nerve signals, such as touch signals, travel at about 200 miles per hour. Because of this relative lack of speed, the signals of chronic pain can be thwarted by "crowding" the brain with competing sources of input—including positive *thoughts.*

Besides providing a competing source of neurological input, positive thoughts also kill pain by altering the body's biochemistry. As you know, stressful, agitated thoughts create the biological stress response, which heightens pain. However, calm, soothing thoughts—including those created by inactive drugs—have the opposite effect. They cause the body to secrete chemicals that block pain.

The most important painkilling chemicals released by the placebo response, or the mind-power response, are endorphins. Researchers recently proved that placebos stimulate endorphin release. They proved this in a study of people who'd had their wisdom teeth extracted. After the extraction, some of the patients were given morphine, and some were given inactive placebos. As expected, about one-third of the group who'd been given placebos felt no pain. Then, however, the patients on placebos were surreptitiously given a drug that blocks the release of endorphins. When they took this drug, 100 percent of them began to feel pain.

The other chemicals that are secreted in response to the soothing mind-power effect are the calming neurotransmitters serotonin and GABA. Serotonin, as I've mentioned, is probably your body's most powerful painkiller. GABA also soothes nerves. Furthermore, when GABA and serotonin are *both* simultaneously present in abundant quantities, they stimulate the release of endorphins.

Obviously the mind can create positive physical changes in response to any treatment. However, if the patient believes the treatment is *harmful*, this response can be negative. This negative response—the opposite of the placebo effect—is called the "nocebo" effect. *Nocebo* is a Latin word that means "I will cause pain."

The nocebo effect not only makes existing pain worse, but can create new pain.

In a survey of pain treatment studies reported in the *Journal of the American Medical Association*, an average of 19 percent of all chronic pain patients suffered pain due to the nocebo effect. Most of those patients were ones who'd been given a harmless, inactive drug. They had been told that the drug would probably help them. Sadly, though, they refused to accept this positive reassurance. After they took the drug, they became convinced that it had caused them to feel more pain. In some cases the patients claimed their pain had been made *permanently* worse, even after they'd been told that they had been given only a harmless, inactive substance.

Healthy people can also suffer from the nocebo effect. In one study, 70 percent of a group of healthy students suffered headaches after a fake, nonexistent electric current was applied to their heads.

One of the most powerful creators of the nocebo effect is a negative experience with a doctor. In one study, a doctor noted the clinical responses of two groups of patients who all had similar mild ailments that he thought would normally go away in about one or two weeks. The doctor told one group that he knew what they had, and that they would soon be better. He told the other group that he couldn't diagnose their problem, and couldn't help them. Two weeks later, 64 percent of those he'd "diagnosed" were better. But only 39 percent of the patients he'd said he *couldn't* help got better. He attributed their poor recovery rate to their negative encounter with him, and the negative expectations it caused.

As you can see, the mind-power effect can be a powerful weapon in your battle against pain. So let's look at how you can *activate* it.

One of the best ways is with cognitive therapy. You must tell yourself, at least several times every day, that you believe in the effectiveness of your pain program. Tell yourself that it has helped hundreds of people who had pain that was similar to yours, and that it will help you, too.

To strengthen your belief in your program, it may help if you skim through this book repeatedly, on a regular basis. Look at all of the studies that I present, and reread some of the case histories. This will help you to build a rational basis of belief in your program.

Similarly, you should research chronic pain in other sources. Check Appendix III for good books on the subject. The more information you have about chronic pain, the less likely you will be to engage in faulty thinking about it. You'll break free of the cognitive distortions that make your pain worse.

It's also important that you dispel any cynicism you may have about the mind-power effect. Don't think of it as a means of "fooling yourself," but as a force that literally puts mind over matter. The mind-power effect is very real, and when it helps kill your pain, your relief will be real, too.

When you do this self-talk, be honest with yourself. Don't tell yourself something you don't really believe. It won't work, because you're too smart to believe your own lies. Lying to yourself will just undermine your faith in what you really do believe.

You may also want to consult a cognitive therapist, and have him or her help you create several "self-talk" phrases that will activate the mind-power effect. In addition to using the techniques of cognitive therapy to elicit the mind-power effect, there is another very effective technique for achieving a positive mind-power response.

That technique is visualization.

PLACEBO FACTS

- Large capsules are better placebos than small capsules.
- Yellow placebos are most effective as stimulants, and white placebos are most effective as painkillers. Green placebos are best for anxiety.
- Injections are better placebos than pills.
- Placebos achieve their most pronounced effect among people who have severe anxiety about their conditions.
- Taking two placebo pills works better than taking one.

PLACEBO FICTION

- Taking a placebo is the same as doing nothing.
- Placebo effects are usually short-lived.
- People who respond to placebos didn't have anything wrong with them to begin with.

Visualizing Pain Relief

Thus far, the mental control techniques I've described consist of presenting your mind with *ideas*. In visualization—in which you close your eyes and "picture" pain relief—you not only present your mind with ideas, but also with *images*. These images have a neurological impact that's different from the impact of ideas.

Verbally based *ideas* are processed primarily in the left hemisphere of your brain, while visual *images* are processed primarily in the right hemisphere. As you probably know, your left hemisphere is somewhat more involved with logic, reasoning, and detailed thinking than your right hemisphere, which is rather more involved with intuition, emotion, and "big picture" thinking. Therefore, when you engage in visualization—and focus on both images *and* ideas—you involve both hemispheres more completely in the fight against pain, and get a "double dose" of cognitive control.

Because of this unique neurological effect, visualization is particularly powerful in altering perception. It literally "reprograms" the brain's cortex.

In addition, visualization usually has a powerful temporary sedating effect, and therefore creates biochemical changes in the body. It stimulates the production of endorphins and calming neurotransmitters, including serotonin. Thus it helps break the cycle of pain, and can have effects that last long after the session of visualization ends.

I've noticed that my patients often respond to visualization with dramatic improvements, and studies done at major pain clinics confirm its effectiveness. At the UCLA Medical School, where I learned medical acupuncture, a study showed that 60 percent of patients with chronic headaches learned to relieve their pain with just one training session on visualization. At another major pain clinic, 20 percent of patients with severe chronic pain achieved total relief after just four weeks of visualization.

Because visualization is so effective for "programming" the brain, many athletes use it. Jack Nicklaus visualizes every one of his golf shots before he swings. Arnold Schwarzenegger visualizes lifting a weight before he actually lifts it.

Artists and inventors also use it. Nikola Tesla, the electrical engineer who designed over seven hundred inventions, was trained in imagery, and visualized all of his inventions in detail before he built them. Author Thomas Wolfe visualized scenes before he wrote them; he said he could visualize a scene so vividly that he could "see it just the way it was."

Visualization is very easy, and requires little training. As patients do it repeatedly, it becomes even more powerful.

A session of visualization usually lasts ten to twenty minutes. To do it, lie down in a comfortable, quiet place, free of distractions. Close your eyes, breathe deeply, and relax as much as possible. Then begin focusing on an image of pain relief. As you picture this image, tell yourself what the image means to you; try to use a simple, repetitive phrase, such as "My pain is shrinking."

It usually works best to visualize symbolic images rather than literal ones. For example, instead of visualizing that the swelling in your arthritic hand is going down, create a *symbol* for your swollen hand—such as a balloon—and imagine that the air is slowly leaking out of it. Symbolic images will more effectively hold the attention of your mind, because they are usually more vivid than literal images. Also, literal images of painful conditions often evoke stress.

Several categories of images that seem to be the most helpful:

IMAGES OF POWER. Many people imagine that they are a powerful figure, such as a warrior, and that they are easily overpowering their pain, which is symbolized by a weak figure, such as a young boy or girl.

IMAGES OF PLEASURE. Some people like to visualize a beautiful place, or situation, which their pain cannot enter.

IMAGES OF RECOVERY. Patients often see themselves getting stronger and healthier. They tell themselves, "I'm feeling better every day."

IMAGES OF THE PAST. Most pain patients are comforted by specific images of happy events that occurred before their pain began. Many of these images come from memories of childhood.

IMAGES OF THE FUTURE. Patients often enjoy visualizing how good they will feel in the future, after they have cured their pain. Sometimes, patients like to visualize specific upcoming events, such as a vacation.

It's important, though, that you create your *own* special images. Only you truly know what you need. If you focus hard enough on your image, you'll be surprised at how real it will feel.

Sometimes, pain patients benefit from just *stating* how they want to feel. These statements are called "affirmations." In effect, an affirmation is a "verbal visualization." Affirmations can be combined with visualization, or used by themselves. The great thing about affirmations is that you can do them anytime, anyplace.

Here are some of the affirmations that my patients have used:

- "I'm not *afraid* anymore. Now I *understand* my pain."
- "*I'm* in power. Not my pain."
- "I love my life, even in pain, and I'm going to *live* it."
- "Pain is a problem, but not a threat. This *isn't* going to kill me."
- "*Everybody* has pain. Not just me."
- "This pain is *not* my fault. It's just bad luck—and luck always changes."
- "My healing's already begun."

Cognitive therapy, visualization, and affirmations can change the way you think. However, to gain full control over pain, you need to change more than just how you think. You also need to change how you *act*.

To do this, you may need to engage in behavioral therapy.

Behavioral Therapy for Pain Patients

Most pain patients need to make changes in the way they live. The majority of pain patients regularly indulge in self-destructive behaviors that make their pain worse. Cognitive therapy helps patients recognize their unhealthy behaviors, but cognitive therapy alone won't automatically *change* all of them. Often these behaviors need to be *directly confronted*. The type of psychotherapy that directly confronts negative behavior is known as "behavioral therapy."

Behavioral therapy consists of trying to stop a self-destructive behavior without delving into the deep-seated cause of that behavior. Behavioral therapy is particularly appropriate for pain patients, because many don't have any deep neurotic cause behind their negative behavior. Frequently they begin to engage in self-destructive behavior simply because their pain causes them to develop some bad habits. Patients often develop these habits thinking that the habits will be helpful, not harmful.

Sometimes, patients don't even realize the habits are harmful until a pain specialist tells them.

As you know, I don't believe in using single, isolated therapies, so I generally recommend behavioral therapy as just one aspect of a multifaceted program. It's usually most effective when it is combined with cognitive therapy and other forms of mental control. In one study, 65 percent of patients using a *combination* of cognitive therapy and behavioral therapy experienced a marked reduction in their perceptions of pain.

Behavioral therapy is extremely beneficial for patients who have severe chronic pain syndrome. As you probably remember, chronic pain syndrome is a set of behaviors that includes being sedentary; limiting work and hobbies; withdrawing from friends and family; relying too much on medication; and eating a poor diet.

Each of these behaviors can be seductive, but each significantly *increases* the perception of pain. Behavioral therapy helps patients refrain from these behaviors, and thereby decreases their pain. If you are having a hard time getting over any negative, pain-causing behaviors, you would probably benefit from consulting a behavioral therapist.

Even without a behavioral therapist, though, you can still employ many of the basic techniques of behavioral therapy. These techniques are simple to understand. The hard part is *doing* them.

For the most part, the techniques consist of learning coping skills that stop negative behavior.

Here are some of the most commonly recommended coping skills:

DISTRACTION. When you're tempted to indulge in a pleasant, harmful behavior, treat yourself to a pleasant, *healthy* behavior. This could include eating something good, going to a movie, taking a hot bath, or doing anything else that helps you forget your temptations.

ELIMINATING TRIGGERS OF NEGATIVE BEHAVIOR. Many harmful behaviors are triggered by external stimuli. You need to avoid the things that trigger your negative behaviors. For example, if you're dieting, you shouldn't keep fattening desserts in your refrigerator.

ASKING FOR HELP. An astonishing number of people suffer in silence when they're trying to control an urge to indulge. Speak up! Tell people the behavior you're trying to avoid, and most people will be extremely helpful. Almost everyone likes to help people who are trying to help themselves.

DETACHMENT. When you get an urge to indulge in a negative behavior, don't assume that the urge represents the "real you." The urge is just an impulse, and it will pass, as all impulses do. Learn to observe your urges with a detached frame of mind. If you do, your urges will lose power, and you will gain power.

ACHIEVING BALANCE. It's extremely hard to eliminate self-destructive behaviors if your overall life is out of balance. Learn to balance all of the negative elements in your life—stress, sacrifice, drudgery, and so on—with positive elements. Learn to balance work with play, and tension with relaxation. If you don't, you'll always be looking for avenues of escape, and many of those avenues will be harmful.

These coping skills are the foundation of behavioral therapy. I know you have the power to learn them. *Use this power.* When you do, your power over your pain will grow even stronger.

Now let's move on to one of the most *pleasant* aspects of mental control: stress reduction. Stress-busting techniques are vitally important—and extremely effective—in overcoming pain.

Stress Reduction = Pain Reduction

For most pain patients, chronic pain *is* chronic stress.

Before my patients begin their programs, almost all of them find it impossible to experience pain without feeling stressed by it. Every pain sensation they feel triggers the stress response.

Unfortunately, when they experience the stress response, it makes their existing pain even worse, and creates new pain.

Stress keeps a pain patient's cycle of pain circulating in an endless downward spiral of stress hormones, excitatory neurotransmitters, impaired circulation, tense muscles, constricted breathing, and decreased cognitive power.

But this downward spiral can be stopped. Stress can be *arrested* and, with effort, this downward spiral can actually be *reversed* and transformed into a positive upward spiral. This occurs when the stress response is replaced with deep relaxation.

Deep relaxation is not the same as simple relaxation. Deep relaxation can be achieved only through a simple technique called "voluntary relaxation," in which patients actively strive to create physical conditions in their bodies that are the exact opposite of the conditions created by the stress response. Because these physical conditions are the exact opposite of those of the stress response, they have a profound biological impact—one that is much more far-reaching than the physical impact of simple relaxation.

When deep relaxation is achieved, the following changes take place: the production of stress hormones decreases; calming neurotransmitters are released; cognitive power is elevated; muscles relax; circulation is improved; heart rate slows; breathing becomes slower and deeper; immunity is enhanced; the nervous system is no longer dominated by the excitatory sympathetic branch; blood pressure drops; and the mind stops racing with thoughts.

Every one of these actions decreases pain, for reasons I've already described.

Here's *how* to achieve deep relaxation:

1. Find a quiet place where you'll be undisturbed.
2. Close your eyes and focus on relaxing your whole body, one area at a time.
3. Breathe deeply and adopt a calm, passive attitude.
4. In your mind, say a simple, comforting word or phrase to yourself, over and over.
5. When thoughts intrude, let go of them and return to your phrase.
6. After ten to twenty minutes, open your eyes, and sit quietly for a few more minutes.

Voluntary relaxation is a valuable technique, but there is another method of using the mind to control pain that is even more valuable: meditation. I believe this is one of the most important things you can do to overcome your pain.

The Language of Healing Is Silence

Many times, I have seen patients who were in great pain become tranquil, strong, and happy when they meditated. Often, when patients with severe pain made the effort to meditate virtually every day, they developed the ability to completely rise above their pain, and soon considered themselves cured of chronic pain, even when some of their physical discomfort remained.

Meditation is a wondrously powerful medical modality. In a Harvard University study, over 60 percent of pain patients who had not been helped by the best drug and physical therapies improved significantly after learning to meditate. In another study, 72 percent of pain patients reported a dramatic decrease in pain after learning how to meditate.

But meditation is even more than a potent medical modality; it is also a means of reaching within yourself, and finding the "real you" that has been twisted and distorted by pain. Furthermore, many people—including myself—believe that meditation is also a means of reaching the divine spirit, which, I believe, lives in all of us.

As you know, I think that one of the best ways to rise above pain is to increase your mental energy. When you do this, your brain can launch an effective counterattack against pain. Furthermore, when you build your mental energy, you can become so focused and "mentally tough" that your remaining pain feels like nothing more than a minor distraction. Meditation is a superb way to increase this mental energy, because it directly confronts the mind's tendency to drift and disperse its energy. It is a practical, viable method of tapping into the mysterious, cosmic ch'i or kundalini energy that constantly flows around us and through us. When you do tap into this cosmic energy, you'll *know* it; it will be like the feeling you get when you unfurl the sail on a skiff, and catch the wind.

Part of the power of the type of meditation that I teach my pain patients stems from the fact that this style of meditation is not solely a *mental* activity, but a mental *and* physical one—a mind/body activity—because it enlists the natural energy of the body in the meditative process.

When meditation is done properly, it brings patients to an extraordinary mental, physical, and spiritual condition that I call the "sacred space," a state of pure awareness and absolute calm, devoid of thoughts and words. Sometimes it is referred to as the "space between thoughts." In the sacred space, the body has amazing powers of healing and regeneration. Western doctors who have observed accelerated healing in patients who reach this state ascribe its healing power to a shift in the function of the endocrine system. Eastern healers attribute it to the improved circulation of ch'i, or kundalini, within the patient.

As a doctor of integrative medicine, I believe that both of these perspectives are valid.

Now I will tell you exactly how I teach my pain patients to meditate. As you'll note, the meditation that I teach employs not just patients' mental energies, but also their physical energies. This meditation was adapted from the ancient healing science of Sat Nam Rasayan, as taught by Guru Dev Singh Khalsa.

Often, patients combine this form of meditation with specific mind/body exercises. When these two healing forces are combined, they can be incredibly powerful, and can literally work miracles. I have seen this happen many times.

How to Meditate

To begin, find a quiet, comfortable place where you will not be interrupted. You may sit on the floor or in a chair, but try to sit up straight.

Close your eyes and drift into a meditative state, devoid of thoughts and words. When thoughts intrude, let go of them, and return to your meditative state. Breathe deeply.

To help focus the physical energy of your brain, place the thumb of your left hand on your forehead, between your eyebrows. This is near the area of your brain called the prefrontal cortex, where your highest thought processes occur; the Eastern healers have long referred to this area as "the third eye." Then, with your thumb still touching your forehead, make a fist, but leave your little finger extended. Grasp your extended little finger with the palm of your right hand, and extend the little finger of your right hand.

Holding that position, breathe deeply for three minutes.

Then inhale deeply, and put your hands down. You should already feel somewhat more centered, focused, and aware.

Begin to repeat a simple, spiritual phrase, or *mantra,* to yourself, such as, "I am truth." Your mantra will help keep thoughts away, and will remind you that we live in a sacred, mysterious universe.

Breathe deeply and slowly, and begin to focus on your immediate environment. Listen to everything around you, as you pay attention to the sounds entering each ear. Become aware of everything: the feelings of touch and warmth on your skin, the sensations of sun or wind, the taste in your mouth, the smells that enter your nose.

Do not place more attention on one sensation than another. All are equally important, and equally unimportant. Do not reject any of them as negative. Do not embrace any of them as positive. Assume a neutral state of mind. Detach yourself from all judgment.

If you have pain, begin to focus on it intently. Note how it sometimes shifts from place to place, and waxes and wanes. If your pain is too disturbing, soothe it with slight movement, and try to "breathe through" the pain.

Become aware of the part of your mind that registers pain and is hurting. Focus on it. Realize that your pain is not just in your body, and not just in your mind. Your pain is a mind/body phenomenon. It's also in your spirit. Focus on the part of your spirit that is in pain. Realize how intimately your mind and body and spirit are connected.

Find the areas of your mind, body, and spirit that are not in pain. Focus on the comfort in them, and the health. Recognize this comfort as a real sensation, as real as your pain.

As you explore your body, mind, and spirit—without words and without thoughts, deeply relaxed and fully aware—you may begin to drift into the sacred space where your healing will take place. Don't strive for the space, or even try to occupy it. Let it occupy you.

As you begin to feel increasingly strong and centered, inhale deeply. Stretch your arms out straight in front and stretch your thumbs out. Your middle finger and ring finger are then separated. Open your eyes and focus on the tip of your nose. Breathe deeply through your nose and follow your breath for about ten more minutes. Focus your attention on the sacredness of your life, and of all life. Become aware of your ability to make sacrifices, for yourself and for others.

Then begin to scan your body. Find any tightness or tension that still remains. Let the peace of your mind and spirit wash away this tension.

After about ten more minutes, inhale deeply, put down your hands, and close your eyes.

Allow yourself to exist in a state that is pure awareness—not negative, not positive, just pure awareness. With your neutral state of mind, be aware of how you feel, but don't be judgmental about it. Don't become attached to comfort, or repulsed by pain. Just accept yourself, exactly as you are.

Begin to emerge gradually from your reverie. Open your eyes, see the beauty of the world around you.

You will feel wonderfully relaxed. You will also feel a new power over your mind, your body, and your spirit. You will realize more fully that healing your chronic pain depends largely upon where you place your awareness.

As my teacher, Yogi Bhajan, once said, "Now is the time you must face yourself, to heal yourself by finding the God within."

If you can do that, you will have a way to heal your pain.

You will hear the healing message that is meant only for you.

You will hear it in a new language—the language of healing.

The language of healing is silence.

Breathing Away Pain

During the course of a busy day, when you don't have the opportunity for either meditation or the relaxation response, you can still help achieve cognitive control over pain just by breathing deeply.

Deep breathing is most effective when it's combined with meditation or voluntary relaxation, but it can be of considerable value by itself.

Many chronic pain patients gradually develop the bad habit of taking about twenty short, shallow breaths per minute. They do this in response to the stress caused by chronic pain. Shallow breathing is a classic response to stress.

Unfortunately, this type of breathing tends to reinforce stress and to heighten anxiety, and it generally increases sensitivity to pain.

I advise all my pain patients to do a deep-breathing exercise several times each day. This very simple exercise intervenes in their ongoing cycles of stress and pain.

I also advise patients to breathe deeply any time their pain begins to "spike."

Deep breathing consists of taking only *five to ten* breaths per minute.

When patients consciously slow their rate of respiration, it invariably eases their pain. It also gives them a greater sense of control over their pain.

One reason why deep breathing alone reduces pain is that it helps shift brain waves away from the excitatory beta brain-wave frequency to the calming alpha frequency. Interestingly, virtually all intense pain is experienced when our brains are operating in the beta-wave frequency. A shift to the alpha-wave frequency—which also occurs during meditation and the relaxation response—significantly reduces the brain's perception of pain.

A session of deep breathing can be of great value, even if it lasts only one minute. Its calming effects may linger for hours.

Breathing also causes other biochemical changes in the body. Besides supplying oxygen and removing carbon dioxide from our cells, the respiratory system helps regulate our body's acidity and alkalinity, and helps eliminate water, hydrogen, and small amounts of methane. If you do not expand your lungs to their full capacity, the small air sacs in the lungs (the alveoli) cannot clean their mucus lining properly, and toxic irritants will build up in the body. This can lead to an increase in the inflammation process, and can sensitize nerves.

To take a full yogic breath, start by relaxing your abdominal muscles, and then fill your abdomen with air. After your abdomen is full, fill your chest. As you exhale, let the chest deflate first, then pull in your abdomen as far as possible.

By taking deep, yogic breaths, you can expand the air sacs in your lungs by up to eight times their usual size.

If you establish a habit of breathing slowly and deeply, you will greatly enhance your nervous system's ability to fight pain.

We are very near the end of my basic program for chronic pain. By the end of this chapter, I will have presented the entire program. The remaining chapters will cover special techniques for particular conditions, including migraine, arthritis, back pain, and fibromyalgia.

Thus far, you have learned to marshal the power of your body and mind to defeat pain, but you have one more powerful resource that we have not yet fully discussed. That resource is your own spirit.

When your body, your mind, and your spirit are all working together—focused on the same foe, united in the same fight—your strength will be incredible.

You *will* be able to rise above your pain.

You will, in fact, be able to live a life so rich in power and meaning that someday—when you are once again at peace—you will be *grateful* for the foe that forced you to unite your being.

To achieve this, though, you must fully use the most powerful force you have: your own inner spirit.

Rising Above Pain with Spirituality

"I'm a *scientist*," snapped Constantina, a forty-eight-year-old biologist with crippling fibromyalgia. "I don't *believe* in faith healing." I had just told Constantina that she needed to address the spiritual aspects of her pain. But when I said that, she became angry. She thought spiritual healing was quackery.

I decided to appeal to her logic. "Science and spirituality *do* have *one* important thing in common," I said. "They're both trying to find an answer to the same question: *Why?* Scientists like you try to understand why things happen in a physical sense. Spiritualists also try to understand why things happen, but in a larger sense."

"What if there *is* no larger sense? What if things . . . just happen?" she said, as she shifted painfully in her chair. "That's how *I* think the world works."

"Maybe things *do* just happen. But I'll bet you're not sure about that. As a scientist, you know there's no definitive answer. In fact, you've probably searched for the larger meaning of your pain a lot of times. I'll bet I even know what you asked yourself."

"What?"

" 'Why me?' "

She smiled tightly. "Well, of course I asked myself that," she said. "But I didn't come up with some pat religious answer."

"I've always thought that spirituality is more about questions than answers," I said. "My only spiritual advice to you is this: Just keep asking yourself 'Why me?' "

"That's all?"

"That's a *lot.*"

She looked relieved. Maybe she'd thought I was going to ask her to wear a turban, or go on a pilgrimage.

It seemed to me, though, that the most practical way to reach Constantina's inner spirit was to ask her to do some self-examination. She was *very* self-absorbed, and I hoped she would welcome the chance to focus even more on herself.

I thought that if she did find herself, she would also find her own sense of spirituality.

This search, though, would not be easy. Constantina had a classic pain personality. She was terribly frightened by the intensity of her pain; her jaw was habitually locked tight with tension. However, she had been too pessimistic to try to overcome her pain. She'd read in a medical journal that the muscle pain of fibromyalgia is essentially incurable, so she'd allowed this scientific "fact" to feed her negativity. Even when promising experimental approaches to fibromyalgia had been developed, she'd still clung to her hopelessness.

It seemed to me that her reluctance to try to heal herself stemmed from her low self-esteem. Even as a child, she told me, she had felt like "a loser," even though she'd been very bright. During my initial four-hour consultation with her, I learned that neither of her parents had given her the unconditional, uncritical love that creates self-esteem, confidence, and optimism. She told me that her parents hadn't wanted her to think she was a "privileged character."

As an adult, she had become an intellectual perfectionist. But there was something cold in her. I first noticed it when I happened to mention that I'd been forced to skip lunch, and was hungry. She looked at me with genuine puzzlement, as if to ask, "So? How does that affect *me*?"

Still, she was married to a warm, supportive man—a fellow doctor, who had referred her to me—and I believed that, with his help, she could overcome her suffering, if she could just find a way to focus the full power of her being on recovery.

The *full* power of her being, though, meant more than just the energy of her mind and body. It also included her spirit. If she couldn't get in touch with her spirit, I did not think she would be able to recover.

In fact, I don't think *any* pain patient ever fully recovers from chronic pain until he or she addresses the spiritual elements of pain.

When I tell this to patients, some of them become confused. Some tell me that they are not even sure what spirituality is. They think it must be some kind of church thing, or New Age thing. But I don't think that's true.

To me, spirituality is simply *the search for meaning*.

I think that is the most encompassing concept of spirituality, and also the most accurate.

If, indeed, spirituality is the search for meaning, then all pain patients *must* address their pain on the spiritual level, because pain *demands* meaning.

Pain demands meaning for one essential reason: pain is one of the most intense of all human experiences.

All humans have an innate, immutable need to understand the meaning of life's most intense experiences. This need is so strong, and so relentless, that sometimes it feels like a curse. But this strong need for understanding is the most profound blessing of the human condition; it is the force that compels us to seek knowledge of ourselves—and of the infinite.

It is the force that links the soul and the mind.

It is also, in my opinion, the force that occasionally allows us to glimpse the nature of God.

The human need for understanding is also the force that allows us to finally *rise above our pain*. With our bodies and minds, we can usually overcome most of the pain that haunts us. But we can almost never overcome *all* of it. Most chronic conditions simply don't work that way.

However, when we *understand* our pain—when we can find a *meaning* in it—we can transform this remaining pain in our lives into an entity that is *not* painful. This new entity—which once was pain—might be merely a physical sensation. It might be a moderately uncomfortable feeling that's mostly a reminder of how bad things *used* to be. Or it might be a "good" hurt, like the fatigue and sore muscles you get after a day of play.

The search for the meaning of pain will bring relief, though, only when you find a *positive* meaning for pain. An interpretation of pain that is negative will only heighten your stress response, and decrease your cognitive control over pain.

I'm not saying, though, that you will be able to find a meaning for your pain that is *completely* positive. I just don't think that's realistic.

However, just as pain is never all *good*, it's also never all *bad*. You *can* find good things in your pain, if you look hard enough.

When you do find those good things, you've got to *focus* on them. You've got to *embrace* them. They are your allies. They are the component of your pain that will help end your suffering.

When you focus on the positive elements of your pain, and distance yourself from the negative elements, you will nurture your body's nervous system by decreasing your stress response. You will also invigorate your mind, because your mind won't be preoccupied with thoughts of danger, punishment, mortality, regret, and fear.

You will also energize and empower your spirit, as you become ever more adept at perceiving the tremendous force that lies within you. Whether this force is the divine spirit or the human spirit, it is the force that sometimes enables you to "do the impossible." The more you *use* this force, the stronger it will become.

In my own practice, the pain patients who did address the spiritual aspects of their pain definitely seemed to fare better than those who didn't. This phenomenon is common, not only in pain treatment, but also in the treatment of a wide variety of other conditions. In fact, researchers have compiled more than 250 separate medical studies indicating that spirituality is a positive factor in recovery from disease.

There is debate, of course, over whether this enhanced recovery rate stems from psychological or theological factors, but there is general agreement that the enhanced recovery rate is genuine.

One medical condition that appears to be particularly responsive to spirituality is heart disease, probably because the mind plays a major role in its development. More than fifty-five studies of heart attacks, angina, and other serious heart ailments indicate that people who have strong, positive spiritual beliefs suffer markedly less heart disease than nonspiritual people. This holds true regardless of age, sex, or religious affiliation. In fact, Dean Ornish, M.D., the creator of the world's most popular program for heart disease, includes, as an integral part of his program, "opening your heart to a higher power," and "opening your heart to others."

One of the most therapeutically valuable practices of spiritual people is prayer. More than 150 medical studies indicate that prayer, which is a form of meditation, promotes health. All of those studies were randomized, controlled, prospective, and double-blind.

In most of those studies, prayer was proven to be beneficial when the patient prayed for himself or herself. Interestingly, though, in a number of studies, prayer appeared to help patients even when the patients were not aware that someone else was praying for them. For example, in one study of eighteen children with leukemia—in which neither the patients, the parents, nor the physicians knew that prayer was the subject of the study—prayer appeared to confer therapeutic benefits. After fifteen months of prayer, seven of the ten children who had been prayed for still survived, compared with just two of the eight children who had not been prayed for. Similar results have occurred in other studies of patients who did not know they were being prayed for.

In an incident in my own practice, I had a patient named Richard who employed prayer to achieve an "impossible" recovery. When Richard checked into the hospital where I was working, he was suffering from horrible abdominal pain caused by a swollen spleen. The medical diagnosis was idiopathic thrombocytopenic purpura, a potentially fatal condition in which the spleen destroys the blood's ability to clot.

His surgeon wanted to have Richard's spleen removed immediately, because the surgeon thought there was no reasonable possibility that the organ would normalize. But Richard resisted his doctor's strong warnings. He postponed the operation while he remained at the hospital, under observation.

Every day, Richard's friends came to his room and prayed fervently for his relief from pain, and for his recovery. Each of these intense sessions had an almost electrifying effect upon him. I saw Richard every day at the end of the prayer sessions, and his eyes were wide with excitement and hope. Sometimes he would be so infused with positive energy that it almost seemed as if his hair were standing on end. At these times, pain was the *last* thing on his mind. I was able to drastically reduce his analgesic medication for hours after the prayers ended.

Within a week, blood tests indicated that Richard's spleen had begun to heal. Soon he was completely well.

I met with him again, after he'd been discharged, and he told me that the experience had made him feel "reborn." Several times he referred to his luck, once calling himself "the luckiest guy in the world."

He didn't mean that he was lucky to recover. He meant he was lucky to have been sick.

Here is a prayer that was taught to me by Yogi Bhajan. It is a prayer for relief from suffering. As you can see, embodied in the prayer are directions for breathing. Thus, the prayer is one that involves the body, the mind, and the spirit.

Inhale and hold your breath, for the peace of the world,
for the health of all,
to make everybody happy,
so those who are lonely may have their partner
and God may find mercy on everybody,
on each individual.
Say this prayer on this breath and please exhale. This is the
    charity of the breath.
Inhale again.
Pray for all the dear ones, related ones, known and unknown,
on the whole planet—for those who are sick, those who are
    unhappy, unhealthy, or need spirit.
Send this thought, by doing a prayer on this breath.
Let the breath go.
Inhale deeply again to end all causes and effects, which affect
    all men and make them unhappy or in pain.
For anything that brings war and destruction.
For anything that brings hatred and jealousy.
Say a prayer on this breath, and let it go.

Constantina's Story

I'll always remember the last time I saw Constantina. She was so different from the person who'd first walked into my office.

Her program had been brutally difficult for her. When she'd begun, she had suffered from unpredictable, excruciating jolts of pain that had shot through her shoulders, arms, abdomen, and back. She had been in the throes of major depression, and had considered suicide.

I had treated her aggressively with antidepressants, nutritional therapy, specific medicinal nutrients, acupuncture, Chinese medicinal herbs, and massage therapy. In addition, she had consulted a psychologist who had helped her confront her low self-esteem. She had also learned to meditate, and she had regularly performed mind/body exercises.

Each element of her program had potentiated and reinforced every other element, and gradually her pains had begun to subside in frequency and intensity. Each improvement, in turn, facilitated other improvements, as her cycle of pain slowly began to fracture, and finally dissolve.

Many times, before her recovery had begun to gain momentum, she had despaired. But each time she'd pulled through, and had emerged stronger than ever. Her husband, my physician friend, had been instrumental in helping her endure. He had been warm and loving, and had countered her despair with optimism and her rigidity with good humor.

As we sat talking for the last time, I mentioned the role her husband had played.

Just the mention of his name made her face go soft and bright. "He was the *key*," she said. "I really feel like his love was what healed me. I know that's not scientific," she said quickly, "but . . ." She just shrugged, and let it go.

"You know," she said, "early on, you told me I should figure out 'why me?' Well, I think I did.

"You told me I should come up with a positive meaning for my pain. At first, I thought, what on earth is *positive* about feeling like your muscles are on fire? It just seemed stupid. No offense. But then I got to thinking about my husband—about how he was so good to me for so long, and how that had changed me.

"And here's what I figured out.

"If you suffer, but don't get any love, it just makes you bitter.

"If you never suffer, though, I think it makes you shallow.

"But if you suffer—and get love while you're suffering—you learn compassion. You learn to love—even in pain—and that's the most beautiful love of all.

"I *needed* to learn compassion. And, in my pain, I finally did.

"That's 'Why me?' "

Constantina smiled, and it lit up the room, and it lit up my heart.

PART THREE

Curing the
Pain of Specific
Conditions

6

Curing
Arthritis Pain

In our sleep, pain, which cannot forget, falls drop by drop
upon the heart, until, in our own despair, against our will,
comes wisdom, through the awful grace of God.

— AESCHYLUS

Please note that although this chapter contains information specifically about arthritis, this material does *not* replace the previous information about my pain program. *All* patients should follow the complete pain program described in chapters 2 through 5. Arthritis patients should *also* follow the advice in this chapter.

Most doctors who practice conventional medicine think arthritis is incurable. *I don't agree.*

I believe arthritis can *often* be cured, particularly in its earlier stages.

However, I believe arthritis can be cured only when it is treated with a comprehensive program of integrative medicine. When doctors use only the conventional symptom-suppression approaches, they invariably fail to cure the disease.

As I stated in chapter 1, one of the best ways to stop pain is to cure the condition causing the pain. Unfortunately, though, conventional medicine is usually not particularly effective at curing chronic, degenerative conditions such as arthritis. However, integrative medicine is frequently *very* effective.

Most degenerative diseases are caused by lifestyle mistakes, such as eating an unhealthy diet, smoking, being sedentary, or experiencing unbalanced, chronic stress. Integrative medicine, which addresses all aspects of lifestyle, *counteracts* the lifestyle mistakes that cause, perpetuate, and aggravate degenerative diseases.

For example, the pain from the most common form of arthritis—which is caused by the deterioration of cartilage—can be temporarily soothed by the most popular conventional therapy: aspirin. However, aspirin *itself* may destroy cartilage. Therefore, many patients get trapped in a cycle of pain/aspirin/pain, and are never cured.

Physicians who treat arthritis with integrative medicine, though, focus on rebuilding cartilage with nutritional therapy, natural medications, and exercise therapy. This, too, stops pain—by reversing the underlying condition. Such an approach can relieve pain *permanently.*

I have treated many arthritis patients who responded wonderfully to integrative medicine. Most of them experienced a significant reduction of symptoms, including pain. Some are still totally free of symptoms, years after their initial treatments.

If you have arthritis, you should carefully follow the advice in this chapter. However, as I mentioned in the opening paragraph, you should use this advice in conjunction with my full, four-level pain cure program. The advice in this chapter complements the complete program.

What Arthritis Is—and Isn't

Arthritis is a group of diseases that cause pain in joints. By far the most common type of arthritis is *osteoarthritis,* which is also called *degenerative arthritis.*

Osteoarthritis is caused by the gradual degeneration of cartilage, which is the "padding" that keeps bones from rubbing together.

The second most common type of arthritis is *rheumatoid arthritis,* which is quite different from osteoarthritis. The only major similarity between the two diseases is that they both afflict the joints. Rheumatoid arthritis appears to be a disorder of the immune system, and is characterized much more by inflammation than osteoarthritis.

The other arthritic conditions are relatively mild, transitory disorders, such as tendonitis and bursitis, or relatively rare disorders, such as lupus and scleroderma.

Osteoarthritis is so common that 80 percent of all people have it by age fifty. Virtually *everyone* has at least minor arthritis by age sixty-five. Worldwide, more than 10 percent of all people now have osteoarthritis. Skeletal remains indicate that even cavemen had it.

Internationally, arthritis treatment generates $50 billion annually, so there is fierce competition among the companies that sell arthritis remedies. This competition sometimes inspires unethical conduct and misinformation; for example, in 1996, the manufacturer of one of the world's most popular nonprescription pain relievers was fined millions of dollars by the U.S. government for providing the public with misleading information about arthritis.

Osteoarthritis almost always occurs in the hands, the spine, or the weight-bearing joints (hips, knees, and feet). Usually the pain is confined to the immediate area, but arthritis can disrupt the body's structural balance and cause pain elsewhere.

Osteoarthritis pain comes mainly from direct contact between bones. Inflammation may also be present. Bones come into direct contact when the cartilage between them deteriorates. Cartilage is a tough, spongy material that is very slick. In fact, it's more than five times as slick as ice. Because it's so slick, bones easily glide across it.

One reason cartilage is so slick is that it is almost 80 percent water. There are only three solid substances in it: (1) collagen, the connective tissue that's found throughout your body; (2) proteoglycans, which are molecules that trap water, and keep cartilage wet and slippery; and (3) cells called "chondrocytes," which manufacture new collagen and proteoglycans.

As we age, our cartilage gradually loses its spongy, slippery strength. It begins to recede and stiffen, and allows the growth of small nubs of bone called "spurs," which often rub against other bones. When this happens, our joints ache, and feel creaky and stiff.

No one is absolutely certain *why* cartilage deteriorates. In all probability it deteriorates for the same basic reason that other parts of our bodies deteriorate—because it doesn't have enough of the proper "building materials" to keep up with the constant rebuilding process. Other factors also appear to interfere with the rebuilding process. These may include poor function of the liver (which helps produce the substances that make up cartilage), poor blood circulation to the joints, and other errors of metabolism, caused by lifestyle mistakes.

Doctors *do* know that arthritis can be triggered by an injury to a joint, or by long-term physical trauma. Athletes often suffer from osteoarthritis. Manual laborers have about 800 percent more arthritis than average. Overweight people are particularly vulnerable to arthritis in their weight-bearing joints.

Conventional wisdom says that osteoarthritis is a "wear and tear" disease. But I don't entirely agree with that. It's clear that arthritis *is* a "tear" disease, because physical trauma and injury obviously contribute to it. But *normal* "wear," in my opinion, probably does *not* significantly contribute to it. In fact, moderate exercise is highly beneficial for joints, and helps *prevent* arthritis.

I believe that metabolic errors, caused by lifestyle mistakes, are the major contributing factor to arthritis. Therefore, I see osteoarthritis as essentially an "error and tear" disease.

Thus, the therapies I recommend are aimed at correcting the errors, and healing the tears.

The modalities I employ most frequently, in combination, are nutritional therapy, mind/body exercise therapy, heat-and-cold therapy, acupressure, homeopathic remedies, herbal preparations, hormonal replacement therapy, cautious use of anti-inflammatory and analgesic medications, and appropriate techniques for the mental and spiritual control of arthritis pain.

For the most part, the modalities I use are similar to those I employ in my standard pain program. However, there are certain specific nutrients, mind/body exercises, medications, and acupuncture points that are especially valuable for arthritis patients, and I'll tell you about them in this chapter and in Appendix I, "Mind/Body Exercise and Meditation."

My pain program, when tailored to meet the specific needs of arthritis patients, has helped many people to conquer their arthritis. In most cases, some degree of mild arthritis has remained, but has not been severe enough to cause significant pain.

Conventional treatment of arthritis is far more narrow, and much less aggressive. The primary therapy is use of nonprescription pain relievers, including aspirin, acetaminophen, and ibuprofen. Conventional treatment also often includes rest, mild exercise, and heat-and-cold therapy.

As you can see, conventional treatment of arthritis is focused mostly on just suppressing pain, instead of reversing the underlying conditions that cause arthritis. However, conventional arthritis treatment falls short even as a *pain control* program. It's very limited, and doesn't fight pain on every level. Therefore it does not cure the pain.

Because conventional arthritis therapy is so limited, most people with arthritis don't get significant help from conventional treatment. Most of them simply suffer in silence, presuming that their situation is inescapable. This suffering is a needless tragedy.

Unfortunately, many doctors believe that because arthritis is so widespread, suffering from it is "normal." I hate that attitude; I don't think there is anything "normal" about suffering. We all deserve to be—and *can* be—healthy and happy, all of our lives, even if our lives contain a limited amount of pain. As I've said many times, life need not be a painful struggle.

The conventional therapy for rheumatoid arthritis is also quite limited, and generally has little therapeutic effect.

As I mentioned, rheumatoid arthritis is an inflammatory disease, apparently caused by a malfunction of the immune system.

When the immune system is functioning properly, it correctly identifies "foreign invaders"—everything from viruses to allergens—and then attacks these invaders. Part of this attack consists of inflammation, which brings extra blood to the distressed area. However, when the immune system *malfunctions*, it identifies *harmless* substances as foreign invaders, and tries to get rid of them with inflammation. This type of malfunction is what appears to cause rheumatoid arthritis.

Some researchers, though, think that the inflammatory response of rheumatoid arthritis is *not* a malfunction of the immune system, but a *proper* response to a real foreign invader, such as a "slow virus."

Regardless of its root cause, rheumatoid arthritis is characterized by an active immune response, which can include fever, fatigue, and emotional malaise.

The inflammation of rheumatoid arthritis strikes joints, settling in the membranes that surround them. Soon it damages cartilage and bone.

Although many people have only very mild rheumatoid arthritis, the disease is frequently horrific. Severe rheumatoid arthritis can turn hands into claws, and can put people into wheelchairs. The pain from it is often torturous.

Rheumatoid arthritis strikes women three times as often as men, and usually begins between the ages of twenty-five and fifty.

The conventional treatment centers on use of anti-inflammatory drugs, including steroids and nonsteroidal anti-inflammatory drugs. This treatment is intended to decrease pain, but not to cure the disorder. No known cure exists.

However, many patients with rheumatoid arthritis have responded dramatically to a program of integrative medicine. This program generally includes most of the same health-building and anti-pain modalities that I use against osteoarthritis. With rheumatoid arthritis, though, special emphasis is placed on improving the function of the immune system, and on "purifying" the body, to rid it of any genuine foreign invaders or any substances that are misidentified as foreign invaders.

Now I'll give you the details on treatment. We'll go through my pain program level by level, and I'll tell you about special modalities that are particularly valuable against arthritis.

Keep in mind, of course, that these special modalities must be used as *part* of my standard pain program. If you apply *only* the modalities I mention in this chapter, you probably won't be able to control your arthritis.

Level One: Nutritional Therapy

Let's start by quickly reviewing the advice I've already given you about nutritional therapy, which comprises the first level of my standard pain program.

In chapter 2, I recommended that you (1) eat nutrients that relieve inflammation; (2) eat nutrients that increase serotonin levels; (3) eat nutrients that boost brain function; and (4) avoid the four classic dietary pain pitfalls: undereating, overeating, eating foods that cause allergies, and eating foods that disrupt hormones.

This is excellent advice for all arthritis patients.

If you have arthritis, though, you should *also* do the following:

USE NUTRIENTS THAT BUILD CARTILAGE. For osteoarthritis, this is the *single most important* element of nutritional therapy.

The four primary nutrients for building cartilage are: glucosamine, chondroitin, SAMe (S-adenosil-methionine), and a recently discovered nutrient, cetyl myristoleate. None of these nutrients is concentrated in any particular food, so they are ingested as supplements.

Glucosamine is the nutrient that's needed to build the water-holding proteoglycan molecules that keep cartilage slippery and strong. If you have arthritis, not having enough glucosamine in your system is the worst mistake you can make. Quite possibly, your deficit of glucosamine is the primary *cause* of your arthritis. Glucosamine, which consists of glucose plus the amino acid glutamine, is a nutritional "wonder drug" for osteoarthritis. Recently, some doctors have begun to refer to powerful nutrients such as glucosamine as "nutraceuticals."

Numerous studies indicate that patients with severe osteoarthritis can often recover completely if they take glucosamine supplements. In one thirty-day study of glucosamine, 73 percent of patients with severe arthritis experienced a good-to-excellent response, and 20 percent became totally free of symptoms.

In a study of the effects of glucosamine on pain, arthritis patients taking glucosamine achieved a significant reduction in pain, after just six weeks of glucosamine use. In this study, glucosamine relieved pain more effectively than ibuprofen.

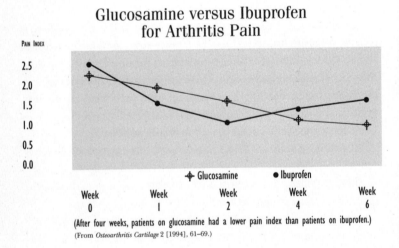

Glucosamine versus Ibuprofen for Arthritis Pain

(After four weeks, patients on glucosamine had a lower pain index than patients on ibuprofen.)
(From *Osteoarthritis Cartilage* 2 [1994], 61–69.)

The typical response to glucosamine is not only speedy, but is long-lasting. Even when glucosamine use is discontinued, positive effects usually linger for six to twelve weeks. When glucosamine use is continued indefinitely, the positive response generally remains.

Chondroitin is a substance that attracts and holds water. Therefore it, like glucosamine, is extremely beneficial to the proteoglycan "water tanks" that keep cartilage strong and supple.

Chondroitin is found in most animal tissues, but is most abundant in cartilage.

Like glucosamine, chondroitin has been thoroughly tested, and has been shown to improve the health of cartilage and to reduce arthritis pain. For example, in one study, thirteen of seventeen patients taking chondroitin supplements experienced a significant reduction in pain.

People with only mild arthritis can also benefit significantly from chondroitin. One very athletic patient of mine, who had developed mild arthritis in his knee, needed only a few weeks of chondroitin therapy to reverse the disorder. During this time he did not even need to alter his exercise program.

Another important anti-arthritis nutrient, SAMe, is a form of an amino acid (methionine) that stimulates production of *both* chondrocytes and proteoglycans. SAMe is very effective for generating new cartilage. It has been extensively tested, and has been found to reduce arthritis pain by building cartilage. In one study of more than 20,000 arthritis patients, approximately 80 percent of those taking SAMe experienced significant reduction of pain, with minimal side effects (primarily mild gastrointestinal upset).

The fourth critically important nutrient, cetyl myristoleate, was only recently discovered, but may prove to be the most helpful of all. Cetyl myristoleate is a form of fatty acid that has extraordinary qualities of lubrication. It enhances the natural lubrication in joints provided by cartilage and synovial fluid. Cetyl myristoleate is present in all joints, but often becomes depleted. Oral ingestion of this nutrient has been shown to compensate for this depletion, however, and improve joint function. In one study of the substance, 63 percent of patients taking cetyl myristoleate alone experienced significant relief from joint pain. It has been found to be even more effective when used with chondroitin, glucosamine, and SAMe. Unlike those substances, however, cetyl myristoleate need not be taken on an essentially constant basis. Its effects tend to endure. Interestingly, cetyl myristoleate has also been shown to reduce the symptoms of rheumatoid arthritis, presumably because it has anti-inflammatory properties.

This new substance is growing in popularity, but can still be relatively difficult to find in the retail marketplace. For access to it, see Appendix III.

At the time of this writing, a new natural nutritional substance for arthritis has just emerged: MSM, or dimethyl sulfone. MSM is a normal metabolite, or by-product, of the nutritional compound DMSO. Several years ago, DMSO gained a great deal of attention as a remarkable natural penetrating agent, which was quite helpful for some people with joint pain. However, DMSO never became widely popular, because it created an objectionable, fishy odor. MSM causes no odor, and appears to have beneficial effects upon arthritis pain and stiffness, with no apparent significant side effects. At a dosage of approximately two grams daily, MSM has been shown in studies to prevent breakdown of cartilage, and reduce joint inflammation. For access to MSM, see Appendix III. The substance can be effective when taken orally, or applied topically. At least one commercially available product contains both cetyl myristoleate and MSM.

A reasonable dosage of glucosamine is 500 mg, three times daily. At this dosage level, there are rarely any side effects, except for occasional mild gastrointestinal upset. As a rule, this quickly passes.

A reasonable dosage of chondroitin can range from 1.5 to 10 grams daily. Side effects are extremely rare, and there is no known toxic level of chondroitin.

A reasonable dosage of SAMe is 600–1,200 mg daily. If gastrointestinal upset occurs, reduce the dosage until the upset no longer occurs.

A reasonable dosage of cetyl myristoleate is 500–1,000 mg daily.

Here are the other important nutritional guidelines for arthritis patients:

USE NUTRIENTS THAT BUILD SYNOVIAL FLUID. Synovial fluid is the liquid that lubricates the membrane that surrounds joints. Called the synovial membrane, this is where rheumatoid arthritis begins its attack on joints. If the membrane does not have sufficient fluid in and around it, it is more vulnerable to the onset of arthritis.

Synovial fluid also seeps in and out of cartilage, and helps lubricate it and nourish it.

The nutrients that are most important in the manufacture of synovial fluid are vitamins A, B complex, C, D, and E, and the minerals calcium, magnesium, and zinc. A deficiency of any of these nutrients can result in a deficiency of synovial fluid. This deficiency can aggravate both osteoarthritis and rheumatoid arthritis.

As I mentioned previously, the emotional stress that is caused by chronic pain can deplete the body's supply of nutrients. Therefore, it would be prudent for arthritis patients to ensure abundant intake of key nutrients by regularly taking vitamin and mineral supplements.

For the proper dosage levels of the most important vitamins and minerals, see chapter 2. The levels recommended in that chapter are appropriate for arthritis patients.

USE NUTRIENTS THAT SUPPORT MUSCLE, BONE, AND CONNECTIVE TISSUE. Cartilage and synovial fluid are not the only parts of an arthritis patient's body that need extra nutritional support. Arthritis starts a chain reaction of structural and biochemical deterioration that soon harms the entire joint, and everything surrounding it, including bones, muscles, tendons, and ligaments.

To repair the damage that's been done by arthritis, and to better resist further damage, you should take vitamins C, A, and E, niacin, pantothenic acid, and the minerals magnesium, calcium, manganese, boron, zinc, and selenium.

Of these nutrients, vitamins C and D appear to be the most important for nourishing bones and connective tissue. The famous Framingham Heart Study showed that people who take higher than average amounts of vitamins C and D are unusually resistant to the progression of arthritis, after it has begun. Researchers believe this is because vitamin D helps bones to repair themselves, and because vitamin C helps regenerate connective tissue.

The antioxidant nutrients—including vitamins C, A, and E and selenium—appear to help stop the breakdown, or oxidation, of synovial fluid. The minerals calcium, manganese, boron, and zinc help build bone strength. When bones begin to "demineralize," they are especially vulnerable to arthritis. Magnesium is vitally important for keeping muscles loose and flexible. This greatly eases the strain on joints.

For protection against arthritis, I strongly urge you to take *all* of these vitamins and minerals. A deficit of any one of them could contribute to arthritis.

AVOID FOODS THAT MAY CAUSE ALLERGIES. This is particularly important for people with rheumatoid arthritis, because that type of arthritis is aggravated by—and apparently caused by—the immune response, which is very similar to the allergic response. Both responses trigger inflammation, as the body tries to rid itself of foreign invaders.

Rheumatoid arthritis patients often feel immeasurably better when they limit their dietary intake to a narrow range of pure, wholesome, whole foods. In fact, some of the most gratifying improvements in patients with rheumatoid arthritis have occurred when patients have gone on juice fasts. This type of internally cleansing fast eliminates virtually all common allergens, such as meat, milk, and wheat.

If you have rheumatoid arthritis, you may well benefit from a five- to seven-day juice fast. During this time you may drink an unlimited amount of fresh or canned pineapple juice, mixed with water and chlorophyll, but should ingest nothing else. This may sound difficult, but many patients really enjoy it. As the fast progresses, the patients usually gain energy, and rarely become hungry or uncomfortable. They also find that the juice drink is truly delicious. At the end of the fast, begin to gradually add foods to your diet, one at a time, and carefully note your response to each food. If you have any allergic symptoms to a food, eliminate it permanently. When you begin adding foods, start with simple, whole foods, such as fresh fruits and vegetables.

As you begin adding foods, you may notice that you have a negative response to the "nightshade" family of vegetables, which includes tomatoes, potatoes, peppers, and eggplants. About 20 percent of all arthritis patients appear to react negatively to these foods, as do many migraine patients. The nightshade vegetables contain a substance called solanine, which can interfere with enzymes in muscles, and can aggravate pain. Also, the nightshade vegetables are highly acidic, and acidic foods often tend to aggravate arthritis.

It's important for rheumatoid arthritis patients to keep their consumption of fats and oils to an absolute minimum. As I stated in chapter 2, most common oils, and all animal fat, heighten inflammation.

One recent study showed how valuable dietary restrictions can be for rheumatoid arthritis patients. In this study, a group of twenty-seven patients with rheumatoid arthritis fasted for one week, and then began eating only fruits and vegetables. After four weeks these patients—compared with a control group of patients on a standard diet—had significantly less pain, more strength, and less swelling in joints.

All rheumatoid arthritis patients should also regularly ingest an abundant supply of the anti-inflammatory nutrients such as turmeric, ginger, boswellin, and EPA. For more information on the anti-inflammatory nutrients, see chapter 2.

Level Two: Physical Therapies

Many of the physical therapies I described in chapter 3 can be immensely beneficial for arthritis patients. All these methods help relieve the pain of arthritis, and some of them can even help cure its underlying causes.

Exercise therapy is probably the most important physical therapy for arthritis patients, because it not only stops pain, but can help reverse arthritis.

Numerous studies have shown that appropriate exercises are directly therapeutic for arthritis. Even when arthritis is severe, exercise can help. For example, in a Harvard study of ninety-year-old patients with advanced arthritis, all of the patients regained a significant degree of mobility after engaging in a weight-training program.

Here's what exercise does for arthritis:

EXERCISE INCREASES THE FLOW OF SYNOVIAL FLUID. Exercise forces synovial fluid to flow in and out of cartilage. The effect of exercise on cartilage is analogous to repeatedly squeezing a sponge in a bucket of water. As I mentioned, synovial fluid nourishes and moistens cartilage, and helps keep it from deteriorating.

EXERCISE STRENGTHENS BONES. Arthritis patients sometimes forget that bones are growing, changing structures that need exercise almost as much as muscles do. Exercise makes bones more dense, and more packed with minerals. This makes them far more resistant to arthritis.

EXERCISE STRENGTHENS MUSCLES, TENDONS, AND LIGAMENTS. This helps hold joints in their proper positions. Having strong, flexible muscles, tendons, and ligaments is especially important in the lower body, where weight-bearing joints are under almost constant physical stress.

EXERCISE HELPS CONTROL WEIGHT. Being overweight is extremely harmful to the weight-bearing joints, and to the spine.

EXERCISE INCREASES CIRCULATION. Good circulation is pivotally important for health in the joints. Blood brings nutrients and oxygen to joints, and carries away toxins and waste.

As you can see, exercise opposes many of the root causes of arthritis. In addition, as I mentioned in chapter 3, exercise relieves pain by increasing the output of three powerful pain-fighting substances: endorphins, serotonin, and norepinephrine.

When these natural pain relievers flood your body and brain, you'll not only feel less pain, but you'll feel more capable of doing the things that you will need to do to overcome arthritis.

I advise my arthritis patients to do any kind of exercise they enjoy, as long as it doesn't strain their joints. If an exercise hurts their joints, I advise them to modify it until the pain goes away.

Some arthritis patients enjoy swimming or water aerobics, because water helps support their weight, and relieves strain on their joints. Many especially like to swim in a warm-water pool, because warm water generally soothes joint pain.

I believe that the best exercises for virtually all pain patients, including all arthritis patients, are the kundalini yoga mind/body exercises. These exercises are especially effective when they are combined with meditation, and performed as part of a daily "Wake Up to Wellness" routine. For mind/body exercises designed specifically for arthritis patients, see Appendix I.

Acupuncture and acupressure are other physical therapies that not only relieve pain, but also help distressed areas regain health. Acupressure may be somewhat less therapeutic than acupuncture, but it is easier to apply.

One advantage of both acupuncture and acupressure is that they can be directed at very specific areas of the body. For example, if you have arthritis in your wrist, there are particular acupuncture points that are directly related to the wrist.

Another advantage of acupuncture and acupressure is that their effects are immediate. Sometimes patients badly need an immediate boost when they are trapped in the negative, downward spiral of chronic pain. This spiral typically includes intense pain, which leads to inactivity, which leads to depression, which leads in turn to even more pain. Acupuncture can intervene in this negative spiral, and give patients an opportunity to create their own *positive*, upward spiral. Acupuncture often immediately improves a patient's attitude, pain behavior, and motivation.

I once had an arthritis patient who was caught in a dangerous downward spiral. Ruth Ann was a sixty-eight-year-old woman with crippling arthritis in her wrists and hands. She'd been in great pain for several years, and it had made her feel despondent, powerless, and pessimistic. When she first began her pain program, she didn't want to change her diet, and hated the idea of exercising. I gave her a series of six acupuncture treatments, which halted much of her pain, and returned some strength to her hands. She became encouraged, and I seized the opportunity to intensify her program. Soon she was taking a large number of supplements, doing mind/body exercises, meditating, and receiving regular treatments of massage therapy.

Her arthritis subsided dramatically, and never returned to its former severe condition. Interestingly, though—even after everything she had done for herself—she still gave credit to acupuncture for, as she put it, "saving my life."

If you have arthritis, I strongly recommend you see a licensed acupuncturist. I personally prefer the style known as medical acupuncture, which is taught at the UCLA School of Medicine, but any of the most common forms—all of which I described in chapter 3—can help.

If you choose to do only acupressure instead of acupuncture, you should still go to a licensed professional, such as a massage or shiatsu therapist. He or she will not only give you a treatment, but will probably also show you the most important acupressure points for your condition, so that you will be able to treat yourself. Following are some of the acupressure points that may help relieve arthritis pain (for information on how to perform acupressure, see chapter 3):

• Point LI-4. Location: at the top of the webbing between the thumb and index finger. For arthritis of the wrist and hands.
• Point LI-5. Location: the inside of the wrist, in the depression between the two largest tendons. For arthritis in the wrist.
• Point ST-35. Location: the depression under the kneecap. For arthritis in the knee.
• Point TH-4. Location: the hollow on the back side of the wrist, behind the index finger. For arthritis of the fingers and wrist.

• Point Li-11. Location: on the inside of the elbow, on the same side as the thumb. For arthritis of the shoulder.

• Point ST-36. Location: in the hollow beneath the kneecap. For arthritis in the knee.

• Point SP-6. Location: four fingers up from the top of the inside of the ankle bone. For insomnia caused by pain.

Another physical therapy that can relieve arthritis pain is heat-and-cold therapy.

Cold therapy, or cryotherapy, is one of the oldest home remedies for arthritis, and is also accepted as a mainstream treatment. Cold decreases inflammation, relieves swelling, and temporarily reduces pain. Patients generally use ice bags, cold packs, or immersion in cold water. The treatment may be continued until the area is moderately numb, but be careful not to induce frostbite with direct application of ice.

A significantly more effective form of cryotherapy is the use of penetrating cooling gels, which I describe in chapter 3. These gels, or liniments, can cause a pleasant feeling of coldness well beneath the skin. They are easier to apply than ice or cold packs, and can be used at virtually any time or place.

Heat therapy is also effective. Like cold signals, heat signals travel faster than pain signals, and can therefore block pain signals from reaching the brain. In addition, heat relaxes muscles, increases blood circulation, and reduces stiffness. I recommend that arthritis patients take frequent hot baths, because moist heat seems to be more effective than dry heat. The effectiveness can often be increased when aromatherapy oils are added to the bath. The aromatherapy tends to increase relaxation and improve mood.

Also, hot tubs and therapy spas can help relieve arthritis pain, and increase mobility.

Recently, when I was a speaker at an international medical conference, I met a health-care practitioner from Europe who had used hydrotherapy, combined with aromatherapy, to cure the severe joint pain of an eighty-three-year-old patient who had previously failed to improve when treated with conventional therapies.

Some arthritis patients find that a hot bath is particularly soothing after exercise. This helps tired muscles recover more quickly, and helps prevent soreness.

I also recommend that some patients use hot compresses, which can be applied directly to joints. A recent innovation that I often recommend is a hot compress that consists of a gel in a plastic bag, which can be heated in a microwave oven.

Two other relatively new forms of heat therapy are ultrasound and diathermy. Both of these methods, which must be performed at a medical clinic or hospital, are excellent for achieving deep penetration of heat.

Another helpful physical therapy for arthritis patients is use of a TENS unit. For details, see chapter 3.

Use of magnetherapy can also help control the pain of arthritis. Therapeutic magnetic devices can be placed directly on painful joints. For details, see chapter 3.

A final physical therapy that can be of significant value is manipulation therapy, which I discussed in chapter 3. Manipulation therapy will not reverse arthritis, but it will correct the structural problems arthritis creates, and may also boost general health.

As you can see, the key to curing arthritis pain—and all other types of chronic pain—is to be *proactive.*

Level Three: Medication

The worst mistake most arthritis patients make is to take too much aspirin, ibuprofen, and acetaminophen.

Nonprescription pain relievers *do* have a place in arthritis treatment. They're excellent for occasional, short-term use, but the manufacturers of these drugs often promote them as the only viable, practical medications for arthritis. This isn't true; other mild drugs can relieve arthritis pain. Furthermore, when patients take high dosages of nonsteroidal anti-inflammatory drugs (NSAIDs) such as aspirin and Advil, these drugs appear to actually *make arthritis worse.* Many researchers believe that NSAIDs inhibit the action of proteoglycans, the important "water tanks" that keep cartilage healthy. This has not yet been definitively proven, but the evidence is mounting. My personal belief is that NSAIDs *do* damage cartilage. Therefore, if you have arthritis, I strongly urge you to be extremely cautious about not taking to many NSAIDs. Besides aspirin and Advil, other common nonprescription NSAIDs are Aleve, Excedrin-IB, and Motrin. There are also a number of prescription NSAIDs, many of which I listed in chapter 4.

In addition to damaging cartilage, NSAIDs can have horrendous side effects. So does acetaminophen, if taken in large doses over a long period. These side effects include damage to the kidneys and liver, ulcers, confusion, depression, skin rash, and insomnia.

Ulcers are an especially troubling side effect, striking up to 4 percent of all people who regularly take high amounts of NSAIDs. Each year people die from internal bleeding caused by overuse of NSAIDs.

For arthritis patients, damage to the liver can exacerbate arthritis, because the liver helps manufacture the substances that make up cartilage.

Another problem with heavy use of nonprescription analgesics is that they can mask symptoms of the disease, while failing to halt its progression. When this happens, it can keep patients from seeking more effective treatments, which might arrest the progression of their arthritis.

A final problem with heavy use of NSAIDs is that they can decrease the body's absorption of vitamin C, which is vitally important in the manufacture of collagen. Collagen, as I mentioned, is a primary component of cartilage. Taking about ten aspirin daily will cause you to absorb less vitamin C, and excrete more.

Thus, as you can see, nonprescription analgesics are *not* a panacea for arthritis—regardless of what thousands of advertisements may imply.

Occasional, limited use of NSAIDs and acetaminophen can certainly be helpful. It's important, though, that you take acetaminophen for osteoarthritis, and NSAIDs for rheumatoid arthritis. As I explained in chapter 4, acetaminophen is not an anti-inflammatory drug, as are NSAIDs. Therefore, because osteoarthritis is not primarily an inflammatory disease, NSAIDs are not appropriate for it. Rheumatoid arthritis is an inflammatory disease, and requires anti-inflammatory medications, such as NSAIDs.

Some conventional physicians prescribe up to 4,000 mg of acetaminophen daily for arthritis. I generally prescribe significantly less than this, and also encourage patients to skip days, when possible. I prescribe less acetaminophen than most doctors for two reasons: first, I am always very cautious about prescribing drugs, particularly when they have numerous side effects; and, second, my patients simply don't need as much acetaminophen, because they achieve pain relief from many other nontoxic medications and techniques. Often my patients require only about 325–650 mg of acetaminophen daily. When their pain increases, they frequently take a higher dosage.

For osteoarthritis, many doctors prescribe about 2,500 mg of aspirin or ibuprofen daily. Again, I generally prescribe far less than that. Often my patients are easily able to control pain with as little as 200–400 mg daily. If they experience occasional breakthrough pain, they temporarily take higher dosages.

One way to use aspirin without causing undue side effects is to apply the medication topically, as a cream. A cream that contains a form of aspirin called methyl salicylate is helpful for some patients. Another topical medication that can be applied directly to joints is capsaicin cream, which is derived from hot peppers. This cream soothes pain with warmth.

Another common approach that I generally do not employ is administration of the steroid hormones known as corticosteroids. These widely used drugs are synthetic forms of the hormones produced by the adrenal glands. The one used most frequently for rheumatoid arthritis and other inflammatory diseases is prednisone. Corticosteroids are very effective at relieving inflammation, but they can have terrible side effects, including suppression of the immune system and emotional agitation. Ironically, they can also cause bones to become very weak and thin.

Many doctors refrain from administering corticosteroids orally, but inject them into joints when symptoms flare. This can temporarily relieve symptoms, but it can also accelerate joint disease. Therefore, this is generally done only two or three times per year.

As an alternative to medications with potentially devastating side effects, I frequently prescribe homeopathic remedies and herbal medications. Both of these include substances that not only stop pain, but also help cure arthritis.

Homeopathy can be especially valuable for arthritis patients, because it provides immediate relief, is very easy to take, is inexpensive, and has no significant side effects.

To find the best possible homeopathic remedies for your own arthritis condition, you should consult with an accredited homeopath, or with a naturopathic physician or an M.D. trained in homeopathy. A trained professional will be able to find the best possible remedy for you. Responses to homeopathic remedies are often highly individualistic; what works for one arthritis patient may not work for another.

Another approach—which may not be as effective as consulting a professional—is to use some of the following homeopathic remedies, which are among the most commonly used by arthritis patients.

- *Dulcamara*. Effective when joints are red and swollen, and feel worse in damp weather.
- *Cimifuga* 30x. Often used for arthritis that flares up during cold weather, or is worse in the morning.
- *Bryonia* 6x. Effective for patients whose pain is heightened by heat and decreased by cold.
- *Calcarea phos.* 6x. Patients whose pain is worse when the weather changes may benefit from this.
- *Ledum* 6x. Helps relieve arthritis in the smaller joints, including the fingers and toes.

- *Apis* 12x. An effective anti-inflammatory agent.
- *Pulsatilla* 6x. Helps patients whose arthritis is exacerbated by heat.

In addition, patients often benefit from several other homeopathic medications that help with pain. These remedies, which I describe in chapter 4, include *Arnica* 6x, *Aconitum* 12x, *Chamomilla* 3x, and *Rhus tox* 6x. Some patients are helped by formulations of various anti-arthritis remedies; these are sold at health-food stores.

Several herbal medications also help many arthritis patients. For the most part, these herbs are analgesics, rather than medicines intended to help reverse arthritis. One exception is capsaicin, the hot-pepper derivative that is sometimes applied topically. When taken orally, capsaicin can help rebuild cartilage. It does this by blocking the action of substance P, which contributes to the deterioration of cartilage, and is one of the substances the body secretes in response to pain. One of the cruel cycles of arthritis is the cycle of: pain → substance P → cartilage deterioration → pain. Capsaicin helps break that cycle, and is available at most health-food stores.

Other herbs that may help relieve arthritis pain are valerian, chaparral, yucca, and comfrey.

A final form of medication that can be helpful for arthritis patients is hormonal replacement therapy. At approximately age fifty, most people begin to experience precipitous declines in their levels of steroidal sex hormones. Some researchers believe that this decline may indirectly contribute to arthritis.

Even if hormonal decline *doesn't* indirectly contribute to arthritis, it still appears as if steroidal sex hormones often help relieve arthritis pain. As I've mentioned, I rarely prescribe steroids, because of their side effects. However, I do often prescribe steroid "precursors"—the substances the body uses to manufacture steroidal sex hormones. Among the most beneficial steroid precursors for arthritis patients is pregnenolone.

In the 1940s, many doctors treated both osteoarthritis and

rheumatoid arthritis with pregnenolone, which, at that time, was considered one of the best treatments. Shortly after the discovery of pregnenolone, though, the corticosteroids were introduced, and quickly became quite popular as an arthritis treatment, because they produced fast, dramatic effects. As a result, pregnenolone was gradually forgotten.

In recent years, though, the corticosteroids have fallen out of favor as an arthritis treatment, because of their side effects. Meanwhile, pregnenolone has regained popularity. As you will know if you have read *Brain Longevity*, I often prescribe pregnenolone for cognitive decline, and have been very pleased with the results. I also now believe that it can be helpful for many arthritis patients. The only drawback to pregnenolone is that it occasionally makes some people feel jittery. A reasonable daily dosage is 50 mg.

In addition to pregnenolone, I also often prescribe a similar hormonal precursor, DHEA. I have found that if patients combine pregnenolone and DHEA, they may be able to gain positive results with lower dosages of each hormone. For example, many patients do well with just 10 mg daily of pregnenolone, when it is combined with 50 mg of DHEA.

Pregnenolone and DHEA appear to be free of significant harmful side effects, but I recommend that you use them, as well as all other medications, under the care of a physician. Patients with prostate cancer, however, should avoid taking these hormones.

Level Four: Mental and Spiritual Pain Control

Emotional suffering does not appear to play a significant role in causing arthritis, but arthritis often causes emotional suffering.

It's been estimated that approximately 20 percent of all people with severe arthritis are clinically depressed. This depression may start as a purely psychological reaction to pain and disability, but as psychological depression lingers, it can trigger the biological characteristics of clinical depression. Changes occur in the levels of various neurotransmitters and hormones, and those changes create the familiar physical signs of clinical depression: insomnia, changes in appetite, lethargy, and decreased libido.

As clinical depression deepens, it can lower the pain threshold, and reduce the brain's ability to launch an effective counterattack against pain. Also, many arthritis patients suffer from heightened anxiety, which also increases pain. Therefore it is extremely important for arthritis patients to actively seek emotional and spiritual peace of mind.

I strongly urge all arthritis patients to review the information on mental and spiritual pain control that is to be found in chapter 5. For many patients, this chapter will provide the pivotal point of recovery.

7

Curing
Headache Pain

Sweet is pleasure after pain.
—JOHN DRYDEN

Please note that although this chapter contains information specifically about headaches, this material does not replace the previous information about my comprehensive pain program. *All* patients should follow the complete pain program described in chapters 2 through 5, as well as the advice in this chapter.

For many years, migraine headaches have been considered largely mysterious. Most people who suffer from them don't know why they occur, and they don't know what to do about them.

But I believe that I have, to a significant extent, clinically solved the mystery of migraines.

I believe this because of the clinical results I have achieved. Many of my migraine patients have responded superbly to my pain program, and no longer suffer any major discomfort from headaches.

The reason my migraine patients have done so well is that my pain program is so comprehensive. Unlike orthodox physicians who treat migraines, I do not wait until headaches begin, and then try to suppress their symptoms with drugs. Nor, like many holistic physicians, do I simply advise patients to avoid certain foods and environmental substances that trigger migraines.

Instead, I help patients *to improve the fundamental biochemistry of their brains.* This addresses the root cause of migraines—and often cures patients completely.

The root cause of most migraines, I now firmly believe, is *disruption of serotonin levels.* When serotonin levels can be normalized, migraines usually cease.

Here's how low levels of serotonin cause migraines.

Migraines, as you may know, start to hurt when blood vessels in the brain expand, leak blood, and irritate nerves. Thus migraines are, in a sense, a form of inflammation.

However, just before the blood vessels begin to expand, they generally tighten up, or constrict. The painful expansion is a reaction against this constriction.

Many things cause blood vessels to constrict. The most common cause is eating a food that contains an abundance of a vessel-constricting amino acid called tyramine. Foods that contain high levels of tyramine include red wine and aged cheese. Another common constrictor of blood vessels is caffeine. Stress also causes constriction. Even substances such as perfume and carbon monoxide can do it.

However, most people who are exposed to these vessel-constricting substances don't get migraines. That's because most people have sufficient quantities of the chemical that regulates blood vessel elasticity. This chemical not only helps stop constriction, but also allows blood vessels to constrict temporarily without then expanding.

This chemical is serotonin.

Serotonin, as you know, is the neurotransmitter that fights pain, but it also has many actions outside the brain. One of those actions is helping blood vessels stay flexible and not get "stuck" in either a state of constriction or a state of expansion.

Here is some strong evidence indicating the role that serotonin plays in migraines:

• The most effective drug for migraines, sumatriptan, works by mimicking the effects of serotonin.

• Almost all migraine patients have limited ability to retain serotonin in their blood platelet membranes.

• Migraines are almost always preceded by a decline in blood levels of serotonin.

• As a rule, low levels of serotonin in the blood accurately predict vulnerability to migraines.

• Disruption of estrogen levels—which markedly decreases serotonin—is a prime trigger of migraines.

I do not claim to have discovered this evidence. Laboratory researchers discovered it, and I merely interpreted it, and applied it in a clinical setting. Clinical results, though, have convinced me that my interpretation of this evidence is correct. When I've helped migraine patients to attain normal, stable levels of serotonin, it has usually cured their headaches.

Normalizing serotonin levels helps cure headaches by doing more than just improving the elasticity of blood vessels. Serotonin, as I've stated previously, does four other important things that help stop pain: (1) it raises the brain's pain threshold; (2) it promotes healthy patterns of sleep; (3) it reduces pain-amplifying anxiety; and (4) it reduces pain-amplifying depression.

Therefore, if you have migraines, the single most important thing to do is to try to normalize your serotonin levels. I discussed how to do this in the four chapters on my comprehensive pain program. It can be done with nutritional therapy, various physical therapies, medication, mind/body exercises, and relaxation. I urge you to review this material, even though I'll briefly mention some of it again in this chapter.

Migraines are pure torture; they hurt far more than most people realize. When you *do* overcome them—and you *will*—you'll have accomplished one of the greatest achievements of your life.

People who have never had a migraine often assume that a migraine is just another kind of headache, but if you've ever suffered from one, you know that a migraine is *not* just a headache. It is, in fact, a serious malfunction of the brain and the body. Here are the most common symptoms:

- Severe, pulsing pain, generally on one side of the head.
- Nausea, vomiting, and loss of appetite.
- Depression, anxiety, and impaired cognitive function.
- Digestive tract disturbances, including diarrhea and constipation.
- Painful reaction to light and noise.
- Excessive urination, or excessive retention of water.
- Congestion of the nasal cavities, with watery discharge, often accompanied by tearing of the eyes.
- Inability to distinguish colors.

Migraine patients have told me that migraines feel much different from common tension headaches. The primary difference is the vastly greater severity of pain. Patients describe the pain as feeling like repeated blows to the head, inflicted by a sharp, heavy object. The other main difference is the occurrence of widespread symptoms throughout the body.

Migraines are so disabling that each year they result in the loss of 157 million workdays for Americans. The cost of this lost productivity is estimated to be about $50 billion per year. In the United States alone, people spend $4 billion each year on nonprescription headache drugs. Headaches are disabling to approximately 11 million people in America, costing them each an average of almost $5,000 per year in lost income and treatment expense.

Migraines, like many other forms of chronic pain, are most common among women.

Women tend to more frequently suffer from all types of chronic pain because, as I explained earlier, fluctuations in female hormones destabilize serotonin levels.

Approximately 17 percent of all women suffer from at least occasional migraines, compared with just 5 percent of all men. However, before puberty, females are no more vulnerable to migraines than males. When menstruation begins, women become far more vulnerable. About 65 percent of all migraines are directly linked to the hormonal fluctuations of premenstrual syndrome. Similarly, after menopause, migraines usually go away. However, when menopausal women undergo hormone replacement therapy, their headaches often remain.

By the same token, using birth control pills greatly increases vulnerability to migraines. In one study, 70 percent of women with migraines stopped having them when they stopped taking birth control pills.

It is believed that the hormonal action in women that contributes to migraines is a rise in estrogen levels, followed by a sharp drop. This appears to be the factor that destabilizes serotonin levels. When serotonin levels are low, migraine patients are especially sensitive to the triggers that cause blood vessel constriction, followed by painful "rebound dilation." The most frequent triggers are these:

• *Foods.* The worst offenders are high-tyramine foods, food additives, caffeine, and citrus fruits. I'll tell you the foods to avoid in the following section, which discusses nutritional therapy.

• *Environmental factors.* These include carbon monoxide from auto exhaust or cigarette smoke; perfumes and other strong odors; changes in the weather (particularly falling barometric pressure, or decreased ionization of the air, caused by heavy winds); very bright incandescent lights; fluorescent lights; cold food or cold drinks; lengthy exposure to computer screens; visual irritation caused by ineffective glasses or contact lenses; changes in altitude; and vigorous, sudden exercise.

• *Stress.* Severe stress can trigger vascular constriction, especially if it occurs at the same time as exposure to a nutritional or environmental trigger.

Like virtually every other form of chronic pain, migraines are made worse by repetition. Each time a migraine occurs, the brain and nerves "learn" the migraine response. After several severe migraines, this process of sensitization causes many migraine patients to be terribly vulnerable to the onset of further headaches.

Another factor that increases vulnerability is genetic predisposition. If one parent is a migraine patient, or *migraineur*, the parent's offspring has a 50 percent chance of developing migraines. If both parents are migraineurs, their children have a 75 percent chance of developing migraines. This strongly supports the theory that migraines are chiefly a physical phenomenon rather than a psychological one. I believe that the primary genetic factor that is passed along is an instability of serotonin levels.

In addition to migraines, there are three other common types of headaches: (1) "tension" headaches, (2) "cluster" headaches, and (3) "organic" headaches (caused by diseases, such as cancer, or sinus infections).

Tension headaches are far more common than migraines. They account for about 90 percent of all headaches. Tension headaches occur when tense muscles in the neck go into spasm. This causes constriction of blood vessels, and pain. Much of this pain is then neurologically shifted, or "referred," to the brain. This referred pain usually feels like a dull ache that encompasses the whole head.

Tension headaches are approximately as common in men as in women, and are usually caused by stress. Sometimes tension headaches and migraines occur at the same time, and exacerbate one another. Some doctors think tension headaches are just mild migraines, but I don't agree, because I believe there are simply too many basic differences between these two types of headache.

Tension headaches usually last only a few hours, but some people suffer from chronic tension headaches that can be present almost every day, with varying degrees of intensity.

Cluster headaches are similar to migraines, because they're caused by vascular constriction followed by rebound dilation, and strike just one side of the head. These headaches, though, tend to occur in groups, or clusters. They are intensely painful, begin suddenly, usually last only about half an hour, but then recur later in the day. As many as four each day may occur during a cluster period.

Interestingly, cluster headaches are 900 percent more common among men than women. Thus, I sometimes think of cluster headaches as "male migraines." I think it's possible that cluster headaches disappear quickly because most males have a biochemical response system, or feedback mechanism, that allows for better control of blood vessel flexibility, once symptoms arise. This feedback mechanism probably involves serotonin, which is generally more stable among males.

Another clue to the cause of cluster headaches, though, is their seasonal occurrence. They're much more common during the summer and winter solstice periods, when the lengths of the daylight hours are rapidly changing. Thus, cluster headaches may be partly related to the body's level of the hormone melatonin, which governs circadian rhythms and sleep cycles. Another piece of evidence implicating melatonin is the fact that cluster headaches often begin about ninety minutes after the onset of sleep, when melatonin levels are high.

Organic headaches, which are caused by disease and infection, occur far less commonly than the other types of headaches. Sinus infection headaches are relatively common, but they generally go away quickly when the infection is controlled.

Some people who have severe headaches fear that they may have an organic headache caused by a brain tumor, because their pain is so agonizing. However, this is extremely rare. Only 2 percent of all headaches are organic headaches, caused by disease, and the disease is usually minor. Furthermore, only about 15 percent of all brain tumors cause pain.

Therefore, the chance that your severe headache is being caused by a brain tumor is almost infinitely small.

Now let's go through the four levels of my pain program, and I'll tell you about techniques specifically designed to cure headaches. Remember, though, that these techniques should be used as just part of my comprehensive pain program.

A Brief History of Headache Treatment

Among the earliest headache treatments were those devised by the ancient Egyptians. These treatments are described in one of the oldest medical books in existence, the *Ebers Papyrus*. This book lists many herbal treatments for migraine, which is referred to as "a sickness of half the head." One herb that is recommended is willow bark, which is rich in salicylates—the active ingredient in aspirin.

One of the earliest surgeries was for headaches. The surgery, called trepanning, consisted of drilling holes in the skull, to allow the exit of "evil spirits." This surgery was performed in many diverse areas, including what is now Peru, Russia, and Algeria.

In Nero's army, a surgeon named Peandus Dioscorides attached electric fish, such as eels, to the heads of soldiers who had severe migraines. This strange approach was actually quite effective. Even now, doctors treating migraines sometimes use a modified version of electrical stimulation—Transcutaneous Electrical Nerve Stimulation, or TENS.

In the Middle Ages, physicians often used leeches to bleed headache victims. They also prescribed substances they considered medicinal, such as beaver testes, peppermint, and cow's brains.

In the nineteenth century, physicians prescribed opium, mercury, and ammonia.

In the twentieth century, Sigmund Freud and his followers treated migraines by psychoanalyzing patients. For many years, headaches were thought to be mostly psychological in origin.

Very few of these specific approaches are still in use, but many have been successfully modified and adapted by modern physicians.

Special Treatments for Headaches

THE THREE BASIC STRATEGIES

In my pain program, I employ three basic strategies for headache treatment:

PREVENTIVE. Stopping headaches before they start.

ABORTIVE. Stopping headaches immediately after they begin, preferably before blood vessels expand.

ANALGESIC. Stopping pain, after headaches have fully developed.

These strategies are enacted by using elements from each of the four levels of my pain program. As I enact these strategies, I help patients achieve the following goals:

PREVENTIVE GOALS:
- Building serotonin levels.
- Stabilizing female hormone levels.
- Avoiding headache triggers (including food triggers, environmental triggers, and stress triggers).
- Improving blood vessel flexibility, not only with serotonin, but also with other nutrients.

ABORTIVE GOALS:
- Correcting blood vessel constriction and dilation immediately after they occur, with nutrients, physical therapies, medication, and mental control techniques.

ANALGESIC GOALS:
- Stopping migraine inflammation with anti-inflammatory nutrients and medicines.

• Stopping pain with medication, physical therapies, mental control techniques, and nutritional therapy.

Now let's go through each of the four levels of my pain program, and I'll give you the specifics on how to achieve these goals.

Level One: Nutritional Therapy

Let's start with the nutritional preventive strategies. The best nutritional preventive strategy is to eat nutrients that increase serotonin levels. I described how to do this in chapter 2. As you may remember, you can increase serotonin by adjusting your diet, and by taking tryptophan tablets. For exact details, review the pertinent sections of that chapter.

The second most important nutritional preventive strategy is to avoid foods that trigger migraines. Most of these foods are foods that constrict blood vessels, and cause rebound dilation. However, some foods—such as nitrites—directly dilate vessels, all by themselves.

As I mentioned, the amino acid tyramine is the worst blood vessel constrictor. But another amino acid, phenylalanine, also constricts blood vessels. Phenylalanine is the active ingredient in the artificial sweetener aspartame, so you may need to eliminate it from your diet. You may also need to stop eating processed or cured meats, such as hot dogs or bacon, because they contain the vessel-dilating additives sodium nitrites and nitrates.

Another additive that often triggers migraines is monosodium glutamate, or MSG, which is often present in Chinese food, and in many packaged, processed foods. Unfortunately, MSG is often not called MSG on food labels, but is instead referred to as "hydrogenated vegetable protein," "natural preservatives," or "seasonings."

Caffeine is also a potent vasoconstrictor. Many nonprescription pain relievers contain caffeine, so check the labels of your analgesics. Chocolate also contains some caffeine, as well as chemicals called theobromides, which sometimes trigger migraines.

It would be wise to carefully monitor your intake of all high-protein foods, which may contain abundant amounts of tyramine and phenylalanine. Meat, milk products, and eggs trigger migraines in many patients.

Citrus fruits contain chemicals that often trigger migraines.

You may be reactive to all of these foods, but it's probable that only some of them will trigger your migraines. To determine which foods you react to, eliminate all the foods that may trigger migraines, then add these foods back into your diet, one by one. If a food causes a migraine, eliminate it permanently. Remember, however, that your vulnerability to migraines may change from time to time, because of fluctuations in your hormone levels, serotonin levels, or stress levels. A food that does not cause a migraine at one time may cause it at another, so you'll probably have to keep experimenting, and fine-tuning your diet.

Another possible nutritional trigger of migraines is any food to which you're allergic. Not all doctors agree that allergenic foods cause migraines, but I believe it's quite possible, because one aspect of the allergic response is constriction of blood vessels. Several of my patients have suffered migraines after eating allergy-causing foods.

One way to help avoid food allergies—and to reduce your vulnerability to other nutritional migraine triggers—is to improve the general health of your digestive system. Try to increase the amount of healthy bacteria in your small intestine by eating foods such as acidophilus yogurt, and by avoiding high amounts of spicy, acidic, and sugary foods.

If you completely eliminate nutritional migraine triggers from your diet, you will probably experience far fewer headaches. In one study, 93 percent of young migraine patients become totally free of headaches when they eliminated all nutritional migraine triggers from their diets.

Foods that Can Trigger Migraines

red wine

caffeinated beverages

hot dogs

sausage

citrus fruits

peanut butter

aspartame

MSG (monosodium glutamate)

chocolate

pickled or marinated foods

ham

yeast, and high-yeast breads

soy sauce

bratwurst

potato chips

gelatin

salami

corned beef

chicken liver

figs

raisins

bananas

cheddar cheese

Swiss cheese

provolone cheese

beer

eggs

sour cream

bacon

corn products

wheat products

sardines

herring

red meat

smoked meats

bologna

pastrami

frozen prepared food
 (including pizza)

relishes

salad dressings

liverwurst

Another wise preventive strategy, particularly for women, is to eat a diet that supports the function of the liver. The liver helps regulate hormones, and can help control the stability of estrogen levels. To help your liver function properly, eat a minimal amount of fat—especially animal fat—and only a small amount of sugar. Both of these food substances—which make up about two-thirds of the average American diet—are very taxing on the liver. Also, limit your intake of highly refined foods, food additives, and alcohol. Take at least 100 mg daily of the entire B complex of vitamins. To restore optimal function of your liver, take the powerful herbal supplement silymarin, which is an extract of milk thistle. This supplement is available at virtually all health-food stores. A reasonable daily dosage is 500 mg. Silymarin has no known side effects.

Many people find that another important nutritional strategy for preventing migraines is to take generous amounts of magnesium. Magnesium serves two critical functions in preventing migraines: first, it dramatically improves flexibility of blood vessels, and, second, it supports the function of serotonin receptors.

Several studies strongly indicate the value of magnesium for migraine patients. In one study, conducted at Case Western University, 80 percent of female migraine patients became headache-free after taking 200 mg of magnesium every day for three weeks. One of the women in the study, who was completely cured of migraines, had suffered a migraine virtually every week for the prior ten years.

In a related study, researchers found that 40 percent of migraine patients had a deficiency of magnesium. Patients with tension headaches also had a magnesium deficiency.

To ensure sufficient intake of magnesium, take a supplement. It's almost impossible to get 200 mg of magnesium daily from diet alone.

Another nutritional preventive agent is vitamin B_2, or riboflavin. It's believed that riboflavin helps prevent headaches by supporting the brain's energy-producing mitochondria. In one study, migraine severity decreased by 70 percent when migraine patients took 400 mg of riboflavin daily.

A final nutritional preventive technique is simply to stabilize your level of blood sugar. Low blood sugar, or hypoglycemia, triggers migraines in some people. If you feel yourself becoming hungry and tired, eat something.

Now let's consider nutritional strategies for *aborting* headaches. These strategies should be enacted at the first sign of a headache, preferably before blood vessels begin to dilate.

About 15 percent of migraineurs experience an "aura" just before their headaches begin, and for these people, that's the right time to try to abort the headache. The aura consists of visual disturbances such as flashing lights or zigzag patterns.

Most migraineurs, though, don't get this early warning, and therefore have less opportunity to abort their headaches.

One of the most effective nutritional abortive techniques is to take the B vitamin niacin, if it can be taken very early in the headache's development, when blood vessels are still constricted. About 500 mg of niacin will cause blood vessels to dilate slightly, and thereby avoid the exaggerated rebound dilation of a migraine.

Another nutritional abortive strategy is to take a fast-acting, quickly absorbed form of magnesium, such as Epsom salts dissolved in water.

Some of my patients have also successfully aborted headaches by taking high amounts of anti-inflammatory nutrients at the first sign of a headache. For example, some patients have been able to abort headaches by taking 500 mg of ginger, or by drinking a strong cup of ginger tea. (It is available in tea bags from the Yogi Tea Company and other manufacturers, and can be found in any health-food store. Or you can make it yourself from either fresh or dried ginger.)

The primary *analgesic* nutritional strategy for stopping migraine pain, once a headache has fully developed, is to use nutrients that control inflammation.

I described how to stop inflammation nutritionally in chapter 2, so please review that material. The best way to stop inflammation nutritionally is to eat a diet that is low in most common fats, but that contains high amounts of the fats EPA, GLA, and ALA. You should also eat other anti-inflammatory nutrients such as turmeric, boswellin, ginger, and protein-digesting enzymes. All these nutrients are described in chapter 2.

You should also follow the other advice in chapter 2: Eat nutrients that boost the health of your brain and nerves; avoid the four classic dietary pain pitfalls; and, of course, eat nutrients that increase your levels of serotonin.

Since 1983 there has been a 60 percent increase in the incidence of migraines. Many researchers believe this rapid upswing has resulted from the continuing deterioration of the American diet. Over approximately this same time period, obesity in America increased by about 30 percent. Americans are simply eating too much animal fat, sugar, processed foods, and junk foods. This indulgence, I believe, is causing great suffering.

If you currently suffer from migraines, I strongly urge you to improve your diet, and end your suffering.

Level Two: Physical Therapies

The best *preventive* physical therapies for migraines are mind/body exercises, and aerobic exercise.

Many of my migraine patients have responded superbly to the mind/body exercises. These are particularly valuable for migraines because they not only have many of the same effects as aerobic exercise, but also powerfully stimulate serotonin production. In addition, they markedly reduce stress, which is often a primary contributor to migraines.

Some of my migraine patients have found that when they regularly do mind/body exercises, their headaches either cease or dramatically decrease in intensity.

For mind/body exercises that are designed specifically for migraine patients, please see Appendix I.

Aerobic exercise is also extremely helpful in that it helps keep blood vessels flexible, thereby helping to prevent blood vessels from getting "stuck" in rebound dilation. In addition, aerobic exercise reduces both anxiety and depression, primarily by stimulating production of the neurotransmitter norepinephrine. When anxiety and depression are reduced, stress becomes a far less potent trigger of migraines. Furthermore, even if headaches do occur, a reduction of depression and anxiety can significantly reduce the perception of pain.

Exercise also stretches and relaxes muscles, and this reduced muscular tension helps prevent headaches. Tension headaches, in particular, can often be prevented with a regular exercise program that stretches and soothes muscles in the neck, head, face, shoulders, and back.

It's also very important to do stretching exercises *after* a tension headache, to prevent a subsequent headache. Tension headaches, which are caused by tense muscles, cause further muscular tension. When the head starts to hurt, the muscles of the neck tighten even more, as the body attempts to immobilize the head and protect it from pain caused by movement. This increased tightening, however, causes the release of lactic acid in muscle tissues. If lactic acid is allowed to remain in the muscles after the headache has subsided, it will continue to irritate the muscles, and can trigger future headaches. Exercise, however, flushes lactic acid out of muscles.

Several studies show that exercise helps prevent headaches. In one study, eleven migraineurs experienced a significant decrease in headache severity after they began a six-week program of cardiovascular exercise. In another study, migraine patients reduced the frequency of their headaches by an average of 50 percent after they participated in a program of regular aerobic exercise.

If you're a migraineur, though, it's very important that you warm up gradually before you begin to exercise. If you begin strenuous exercise suddenly, you may cause your blood vessels to get locked into dilation. This type of migraine, called an "exertional migraine," has caused many migraineurs to avoid exercise. I once had a migraine patient who absolutely refused to exercise because she had experienced several exertional migraines. But when I finally convinced her that lack of exercise was contributing to her headaches, she began a careful exercise program, and responded extremely well.

Another physical therapy that is especially helpful for *tension* headaches is manipulation therapy. Tension headaches are frequently exacerbated by the muscular strain of poor posture, and osteopathic and chiropractic adjustments are often excellent for correcting bad posture. There is also anecdotal evidence that manipulation therapy can help prevent migraines.

Massage is also very effective for relieving muscle tension and thereby preventing tension headaches. Some of my migraine patients have also responded well to massage, probably because muscular tension was contributing to the constriction of their cerebral blood vessels.

Another important factor in preventing migraines is to make sure you are exposed to adequate amounts of light. As I've mentioned, light is extremely important in the production of serotonin. It has been proven that inadequate amounts of light lower serotonin levels. When this happens, people become far more vulnerable to migraines.

Women particularly need adequate amounts of light during the second half of their menstrual cycles, when their serotonin levels may already be low. For more information on this, please review the material on light therapy in chapter 3, and the material on premenstrual syndrome in chapter 10.

Exercise (including mind/body exercise) is also valuable for *aborting* migraines. When a migraine strikes, though, most migraineurs shun exercise. They tend to quickly withdraw to a quiet, dark room, and lie down. I believe this is the wrong strategy for most patients. Several of my patients have had tremendous success aborting headaches by exercising. Exercise is most valuable when it is performed in the *first* stage of a migraine, when blood vessels are still constricted. It coaxes constricted vessels to gently dilate, and can prevent exaggerated rebound dilation.

To abort a migraine with aerobic exercise, start exercising gradually, at the very first sign of a migraine. Your exercise should be aerobic, causing your heartbeat to maintain a steady, elevated rate. At first the exercise may hurt. Be strong, though, and stick with it. It may help to exercise in a dark, quiet room, using a stairstepper or a stationary bicycle.

Exercise can also effectively abort a *tension* headache. For tension headaches, the exercise should focus on stretching tight muscles in the neck, head, shoulders, and back. Aerobic exercise will also help, though, because it will dilate constricted blood vessels in the neck that are contributing to the "referred pain" in the head.

Besides exercise, several other physical therapies can successfully abort headaches. Most of those abortive techniques can also be used as *analgesic* techniques, once headaches have fully developed. Most, however, provide more relief when they are used as abortive techniques instead of analgesic techniques, simply because headaches are easier to treat in their early stages.

Whether used as abortive measures or analgesic measures, the techniques are applied similarly. Following are descriptions of physical therapies that I recommend as both abortive and analgesic modalities.

One abortive and analgesic therapy for both migraines and tension headaches is combing the hair and scalp with a wooden comb. Some patients are reluctant to try this, because their scalps are sensitive, but the technique can be surprisingly effective. Combing the hair and scalp gives the brain a competing source of neurological input. The touch signals from combing "outrun" pain signals in the "race" to the pain gates. The temporary relief this causes can break the cycle of pain, and can induce muscles, blood vessels, and nerves to return to a state of normalcy. Comb your entire scalp for several minutes. You may not feel relief immediately, and may need to repeat the procedure every couple of hours. If you have a tension headache, you should also gently comb the back of your neck, and massage it.

Cold packs can also help relieve both migraine and tension headaches. In a large study at the Diamond Headache Clinic in Chicago—arguably the world's finest headache treatment center—cold packs reduced pain in 80 percent of migraine patients.

For migraines, cold packs should be placed on the painful side of the face and head, against the forehead, eye, and temple. Apply the pack for about fifteen minutes, and repeat the procedure every two hours, to prevent recurrence. For a tension headache, place the pack not just on the head but also on the neck, which is the original source of the pain.

Another effective form of cold therapy is use of a cooling liniment or gel. The advantage of this type of cold therapy is that it can be done anywhere.

Heat therapy can also help. For tension headaches, a hot pack or hot towel can relax muscles in the neck and shoulders, and can help ease constriction of blood vessels.

For migraines, heat therapy can alleviate constriction in the headache's early stage, and can alleviate dilation in the later stage. In the early stage, when vessels are still constricted, apply heat directly to the head and face. In the later stage, when vessels are dilated, apply heat to the hands and feet; this will draw blood to the extremities, away from the head. One easy way to apply heat to the hands and feet is to immerse them fully in hot water.

Another effective form of abortive and analgesic therapy is acupressure. Acupuncture can also be effective, but it is much less convenient than acupressure. Acupressure can be done immediately, at any time or place. To do it, simply press the tip of your finger on the acupressure point, and massage it gently. If the point is sore, it indicates an energy blockage, which acupressure can help resolve. In general, though, acupressure is more effective if it is performed by people other than the patients themselves.

Following are the primary acupressure points for headaches:

• The point where the bones from the big toe and the second toe meet, about two inches behind the tips of these toes. This point is primarily for migraines.

• The middle part of the webbing between the thumb and forefinger, where the muscle begins. This point is usually sore during a tension headache or a migraine.

• On the outside of the forearm, about one and a half inches above the wrist, between the two bones. This point is effective for pain in the temples.

• The hollow beneath the base of the skull, above the neck. To massage this point, tilt your head backwards. This is especially effective for migraines.

• The top middle part of the collarbone, where there is a small notch. This point helps tension headaches.

• Behind the ear, halfway to the spinal column. This is a good point for tension headaches that hurt behind the eyes.

• Just above and slightly forward of the ear, near the hairline. If only one side of your head hurts, press on the painful side.

• Halfway between the eye and ear. This helps pain in the temples.

• Both sides of the bridge of the nose. Squeeze with your thumb and forefinger for sinus headaches.

• Just above the trapezius muscle, halfway between the shoulder and the neck. This helps relieve pain in the back of the head.

A final physical therapy that can be used as an abortive technique or as an analgesic technique is use of a Transcutaneous Electrical Nerve Stimulation (TENS) unit. These devices send mild electric impulses to the brain, which compete with pain signals. The electric impulses can break the cycle of pain and allow muscles, nerves, and blood vessels to reestablish normal function.

Dr. C. Norman Shealy, director of the renowned Shealy Institute, has achieved impressive results with TENS units. In one study, Dr. Shealy used TENS units in the treatment of migraines. This treatment markedly relieved migraine pain and helped prevent further headaches. In another study of TENS therapy, Dr. Shealy noted a 76 percent reduction in frequency of migraines.

As you can see, there are many physical therapies that help in the preventive, abortive, and analgesic treatment of headaches. You should try *all* of these techniques, more than once, to determine which help most.

My bottom-line advice is, Don't just sit and suffer, *do* something. Your headaches are curable. You *don't* have evil spirits in your head, and you're not being punished by God. You have a physical problem that you *can* solve.

Notable Migraine Patients

Kareem Abdul-Jabbar	Sigmund Freud
Julius Caesar	Ulysses S. Grant
John Calvin	Thomas Jefferson
Lewis Carroll	Karl Marx
Miguel de Cervantes	Edgar Allan Poe
Frederic Chopin	George Bernard Shaw
Charles Darwin	Peter Tchaikovsky
Chris Evert	Virginia Woolf

Level Three: Medication

The best way to *prevent* headaches with medication is to use natural, nonprescription medicines. Prescription medications have been shown to prevent headaches in approximately 10 percent of all migraineurs, but prescription medications tend to have many serious side effects.

Among the best natural preventive agents are homeopathic medications. In one study, the frequency, intensity, and duration of migraines were significantly reduced in 79 percent of migraineurs taking homeopathic remedies. The remedies used in this study included *Belladonna, Ignatia amara, Lachesis, Silicea, Gelsemium, Cyclamen, Natrum muriaticum,* and *Sulphur.* They were administered four separate times, over a two-week period. Each patient was treated with only one or two of these remedies, after doctors determined how well each patient responded to each of the substances. The doctors found that patients responded differently to the various remedies. Thus, to benefit fully from homeopathy, you should consult with a doctor trained in this modality, who can help you find the best possible medication for your own unique biochemistry.

Later in this section, I will tell you about analgesic homeopathic remedies that are used to treat fully developed headaches.

These analgesic medications are also suitable for helping to *prevent* headaches, and *abort* them.

Certain herbs are also effective as preventive, abortive, and analgesic medications. The most popular is feverfew, an anti-inflammatory herb that also has analgesic qualities. In addition, feverfew enhances the production and utilization of serotonin, which is probably why it's more effective for headache prevention than other anti-inflammatory substances. Several studies have shown that feverfew can markedly decrease the frequency and severity of migraines. One major study of feverfew included three hundred migraineurs, all of whom had failed to find relief from various nonprescription and prescription medications. Of these patients, 70 percent reported less frequent and less painful headaches after taking small daily dosages of feverfew. In a related study, reported by the *British Medical Journal*, 30 percent of migraineurs stopped having migraines after they began taking feverfew every day. A reasonable daily dosage of feverfew is 150 mg. The herb has no known side effects.

One migraine patient told me that only two substances had ever relieved his headaches. One was a powerful drug with many side effects. The other was feverfew. This man vastly preferred feverfew, because it worked as well as the drug, but without side effects.

Another anti-inflammatory medicine, aspirin, also appears to help prevent migraines. In a large Harvard University study, migraine patients taking one aspirin every other day experienced a 20 percent decrease in incidence of migraines.

Because fluctuations of estrogen are closely linked to the onset of migraines, female migraine patients should try to stabilize their hormone levels with herbal preparations. Health-food stores carry various herbal formulas that help stabilize estrogen levels. One particularly effective herb is the Chinese herb *dong quai.*

Although I prefer natural medications for prevention of headaches, some mild pharmaceutical drugs can also be helpful. Some of my patients have experienced fewer headaches after they began taking tricyclic antidepressants, such as amitriptyline. Antidepressants improve resistance to stress, and help stabilize serotonin levels. Migraine research is just beginning on the effects of the new Prozac-type antidepressants. These newer antidepressants may soon be proven to be valuable against migraines. My own limited clinical experience indicates that drugs such as Prozac are effective preventive agents for some patients.

Some patients also respond well to the drugs called beta-blockers, which reduce the output of vessel-constricting adrenaline. Other patients have benefited from "calcium channel blockers," which also reduce blood vessel constriction.

Another prescription drug that reduces the tendency of blood vessels to constrict is clonidine. This drug seems to be particularly helpful for patients who have a strong reaction to the nutritional migraine trigger tyramine. However, clonidine can cause drowsiness and other side effects, so I recommend you try other approaches.

Similarly, a drug called *methysergide* is a powerful preventive agent, but its side effects can be quite negative. When methysergide is used for six consecutive months, patients must stop taking it for the next two months. Although other doctors frequently prescribe this drug, I prefer not to, because I believe the risks generally outweigh the benefits.

If you do take headache medication, it's important not to overuse it, which can cause "rebound headaches." When pain medications are taken every day for headaches, the body and brain can become reliant upon the medication, and can experience pain when the medication wears off. Rebound headaches can be triggered by as few as four aspirin every day, or by one daily dosage of a prescription headache medication. Up to 2 percent of the population suffers at least mild headache pain every day as a result of daily use of pain relievers. This phenomenon is especially prevalent among people who have tension headaches. If you are currently suffering from rebound headaches, withdraw from your current medication gradually.

Aborting headaches can also be achieved with certain medica-

250 CURING THE PAIN OF SPECIFIC CONDITIONS

tions. I prefer to use natural medications, such as herbs or homeopathic remedies, because they generally have far fewer side effects. Headaches can often be aborted with feverfew and other anti-inflammatory herbs, which I discussed in chapter 5, and with analgesic homeopathic remedies.

Sometimes headaches can be aborted with nonprescription and prescription NSAIDs. Occasionally a relatively strong dosage of aspirin or ibuprofen will abort a migraine, if the migraine has not yet reached the stage of vasodilation. It may help to take the NSAID with caffeine. Caffeine increases the analgesic effects, and also helps stop vasodilation. The most appropriate *prescription* NSAID for aborting migraines is naproxen sodium.

Unfortunately, though, the nausea and vomiting associated with migraines often makes it hard for patients to take NSAIDs. One solution to this is to use an injectable prescription NSAID, such as ketorolac.

Another prescription medication that some doctors use to abort migraines is isometheptene mucate. A dosage of two capsules per hour reportedly aborts headaches in some patients, especially if the drug is taken at the first sign of a migraine. This is a powerful drug, and the dosage should not exceed five capsules every twenty-four hours. Because of its potential side effects, I am cautious about prescribing this drug.

Other powerful drugs that some physicians use to abort migraines are ergot alkaloids, such as ergotamine. These drugs constrict dilated cranial blood vessels. However, they also constrict blood vessels throughout the body, which can be dangerous for people with cardiovascular problems. Furthermore, some patients can become physically dependent upon ergot alkaloids, just as patients can become dependent upon opioids. I have never prescribed these drugs.

A far less dangerous abortive therapy is oxygen inhalation. Patients can use this technique at home, if it is prescribed by a doctor. Oxygen tanks and masks can be leased from medical supply companies. This abortive technique can be quite effective, and is virtually free of side effects and risks, if performed properly.

Oxygen inhalation therapy can even abort cluster headaches, which develop extremely quickly. Because cluster headaches develop within a matter of minutes, they are the most difficult type to abort.

A final abortive method for migraines is to block a nerve in the head with an injection of lidocaine. When this nerve, the sphenopalatine ganglion, is blocked, the developing headache often ceases. This treatment is usually used only when a patient is already in a hospital.

Analgesic treatment of fully developed migraines recently became more practical with the introduction of a drug called sumatriptin. Sumatriptin mimics the effects of serotonin, and controls the dilation of cranial blood vessels. It is the most effective prescription medication for fully developed migraines. About 70 to 90 percent of migraine patients experience marked relief of pain when they receive approximately 6 mg of sumatriptin. The drug can be taken in pill form, or with a self-injection system.

Sumatriptin has several serious drawbacks. It can be dangerous for patients with coronary artery disease, and for those with insufficient blood flow to the head. Its effects don't last long, so another dosage may be needed later the same day, and it's very expensive, costing about thirty-five to sixty-five dollars per dosage.

Sumatriptin can only be used twice weekly, with a maximum dosage of two injections per headache. When the pill form is used, patients generally take 25–100 mg, but they may not take more than 300 mg every twenty-four hours. Unfortunately, approximately 40 percent of migraine patients using sumatriptin injections have another headache within twenty-four hours. Patients who use sumatriptin in pill form generally don't experience a subsequent headache.

Before sumatriptin was introduced, the primary prescription medication for migraines was ergotamine. Ergotamine not only constricts dilated blood vessels, but also stimulates serotonin receptors. Ergotamine can be effective, especially when migraine pain first begins. However, I prescribe it very sparingly, because of its numerous potential side effects. It can cause nausea, vomiting, and muscle cramps, can be habit-forming, and can severely restrict blood flow to the extremities. Possibly the most effective ergotamine is DHE-45, which has a particularly strong effect on serotonin receptors, and does not cause as much blood vessel constriction as other types of ergotamine. About 70 percent of migraine patients respond favorably to DHE-45.

Other powerful prescription medications also generally stop the pain of migraines, but I almost never prescribe them, because of their potential side effects. These medications include narcotic analgesics such as demerol, morphine, and codeine, and "anti-dopaminergic" drugs such as thorazine and compazine.

Milder drugs are more practical, because they don't have such dangerous side effects. These include antihistamines, which sometimes relieve nausea, and also increase the power of pain medications. Muscle relaxants such as Flexeril can also be helpful for tension headaches.

In addition, many of the NSAIDs can help somewhat with migraines, and can help a great deal with tension headaches. NSAIDs often completely block the pain from tension headaches, and can help soothe migraines by reducing inflammation. For both types of headaches, the drugs work best when used early in the headache's development.

A prescription drug treatment that is somewhat effective is administration of nose drops containing lidocaine. Lidocaine numbs nerves, and has long been used as an intravenous drug treatment for migraines. In 1997, headache specialist Lee Kudrow, M.D., demonstrated that lidocaine can be administered as nose drops. This form of administration is inexpensive and fast-acting. In fact, it can be administered so quickly that it can even abort fast-developing cluster headaches. In a study of lidocaine nose drops, about 60 percent of migraine patients experienced at least a 50 percent reduction of pain. However, 42 percent of these patients soon had a subsequent headache, often within an hour. Also, there is some evidence that patients develop a tolerance to lidocaine drops that decreases the drug's effectiveness. There are no known serious side effects associated with this treatment.

Studies indicate that the duration and severity of migraines can be significantly reduced with homeopathic remedies. In one study, administration of homeopathic remedies resulted in an average decrease in severity of about 70 percent, and an average decrease in duration of about 50 percent.

To get the maximum benefit from homeopathy, I urge you to consult with a physician trained in homeopathic medicine, but you may find relief in the following homeopathic medications, which are among the most commonly administered for headaches. Without a physician's help with your individual case, however, you may not ascertain the proper dosage of these remedies, which may render them ineffective.

- *Bryonia*. The remedy most often used for migraines, this is especially valuable for patients who experience symptoms similar to those of motion sickness.
- *Nux vomica*. Used most frequently for tension headaches, this remedy can also relieve headaches caused by alcohol hangover.
- *Aconitum napellus*. This is used primarily for tension headaches, particularly when the patient feels as if there is a tight band around his or her head.
- *Arnica montana*. Probably the most suitable analgesic for tension headaches, or for headaches caused by a mild injury. If a headache caused by an injury lingers, however, you should consult a doctor.
- *Belladonna*. This can be used for tension headaches or for migraines. It is especially effective for throbbing pain, which is caused by vessels pulsing against nerves.
- *Gelsemium*. Most appropriate for tension headaches, this remedy helps relieve pain, and reduces tightness in the muscles of the neck.
- *Iris versicolor*. Administered most often to patients who experience a migraine preceded by an aura.
- *Kali bichromicum*. Often used for sinus headaches, this is

also used for headaches in which pain is located primarily behind the eyes.

- *Sanguinaria canadensis.* Typically used for migraines, especially when there is considerable nausea.

Level Four: Mental and Spiritual Control

Headache patients should be aware that the mind and spirit do play a significant role in the onset of headaches, and can play an important role in ending them.

Many people who suffer from headaches have a "pain personality," characterized by anxiety, depression, anger, compulsiveness, and rigidity. This type of personality contributes to the onset of many chronic pain conditions, including headaches. As I stated in chapter 5, 58 percent of migraineurs suffer from high levels of anxiety, and 19 percent suffer from clinical depression.

To make matters even more difficult, a pain personality not only helps cause chronic pain conditions, but also greatly magnifies the *perception* of pain. In addition, pain itself can cause even an optimistic, carefree person to develop a pain personality. Thus a destructive downward spiral can be created.

Often the characteristics of a pain personality are deeply rooted in migraine patients. In one large study, 23 percent of migraineurs were found to have been abused as children, and researchers theorized that this trauma had rendered them more vulnerable to migraines.

Biochemistry may play a large part in the personality problems of many migraineurs. It is well known that a deficit of serotonin—which afflicts most migraineurs—contributes to anxiety, depression, and compulsive behavior. Therefore, I believe it's quite possible that a deficit of serotonin may contribute to a pain personality.

Many headache patients, though, don't have clinically diagnosable anxiety, depression, or compulsion disorders, but do have so-called Type A personalities. These hard-driving, ambitious people tend to have high-stress lifestyles that predispose them to headaches. Tension headaches, in particular, are more common among people with Type A personalities.

Having a Type A personality is very rewarding and enjoyable for many people, but it does generally make them more likely to suffer from stress. And stress, unfortunately, is a common trigger of migraine, tension, and cluster headaches. The biological stress response, discussed in chapter 5, contributes to tension headaches mostly by tightening neck muscles. It contributes to migraines and cluster headaches mostly by constricting blood vessels. In addition, the stress response causes the release of various neurotransmitters and hormones that contribute to headaches.

In my practice, my headache patients have generally responded extremely well to the mental and spiritual pain-control techniques that I described in chapter 5. These techniques helped them to react to fewer situations with the stress response. It also helped them to better control their tendencies to be depressed, anxious, or compulsive.

My patients have responded especially well to mind/body exercises, particularly when they are performed early in the morning, as part of the "Wake Up to Wellness" routine. Doing this routine is almost like putting on a "shield" against stress.

Furthermore, the spiritual searching done by many of my headache patients helped them to put their suffering in perspective, and to realize that some degree of pain can *enrich* life, if the person feeling the pain is willing to work for that enrichment.

I urge you to review chapter 5. In it you will find ways to make your pain stop—and to make the best part of your life start.

8

Curing
Back Pain

Pain is deeper than all thought; laughter is higher than all pain.
— ELBERT HUBBARD

Please note that although this chapter contains information specifically about back pain, this material does not replace the previous information about my pain program. Back-pain patients should follow the complete pain program described in chapters 2 through 5, as well as the advice in this chapter.

Back pain *demands* a comprehensive program of integrative medicine, because the symptom-suppression, single-modality approaches are generally not effective. In fact, even most conventional doctors who treat back pain now use a wide variety of holistic techniques, rather than relying on just surgery and drugs, as most doctors did in the past.

Unfortunately, though, many patients still insist on a quick fix for their back problems, and many doctors still try to provide this, with invasive surgeries and powerful drugs. Usually the quick fix doesn't work, and the patient's pain often becomes even worse. Americans have more surgeries and take more drugs than any other people in the industrialized world, but statistics prove that this approach is notably ineffective for back pain.

Consider these facts:

• According to the U.S. Department of Health and Human Services, surgery is helpful in only *one out of every one hundred cases* of back pain.

• Back surgery *itself* creates back pain so frequently that there is a common medical condition called "failed back surgery syndrome."

• The leading cause of back surgery—"slipped discs"—can almost always be treated more effectively *without* surgery.

• It's almost impossible to cure back pain surgically without first having a clear diagnosis, but the cause of 80 percent of all back pain is impossible to diagnose.

• Five years after back surgery, the large majority of patients require further treatment. Second surgeries, however, are even less effective, and more dangerous, than initial surgeries.

• The common conventional treatment of extended bed rest is extremely harmful, creating significant losses of muscle and bone, and increasing pain.

• The pharmaceutical painkillers commonly prescribed for back pain often actually *prolong* symptoms, and further debilitate patients.

Here are the details about why back surgery usually doesn't work:

The most common type of surgery for back pain is the repair or removal of spinal discs that have slipped out of place. These slipped discs often irritate nerves. About 350,000 disc surgeries are performed every year. Their effectiveness is very limited, though, because once a disc has slipped out of place, it can *never* be forced back into its proper position. It can only be trimmed or removed, to keep it from touching nerves.

If a disc is removed, the spine must be partially fused, to immobilize the area that had been occupied by the cushioning disc.

Fusion, however, often creates instability in the spine, which can be repaired only with the insertion of metal plates and screws.

Even if the disc is just trimmed, the surgery often causes scar tissue to form around the spine, and this scar tissue often irritates nerves. Frequently it irritates nerves far more than displaced discs.

Because of these common complications, back surgery—the cost of which averages about $15,000—fails in the majority of cases. In a major study recently reported in the *Journal of Neurosurgery*, only 30 percent of back-surgery patients stated that their surgery had improved their condition, compared with 53 percent who said that their condition was unimproved, and 17 percent who said their condition was "worse" or "much worse."

According to most experts on back pain, back surgery is appropriate only when the patient experiences steadily increasing weakness and numbness, caused by a *clearly identifiable* nerve irritation. Generally, this weakness and numbness will be felt in one of the patient's legs. This happens because the leg's thick sciatic nerve is being pinched.

However, if you don't have weakness or numbness, but simply have pain, back surgery is almost always a poor option. It probably won't help you as much as simple, noninvasive techniques—such as exercise or manipulation therapy—and it might make your pain much worse.

Even most people who *do* have an obvious disc slippage don't need back surgery. In an important 1994 study reported in the *New England Journal of Medicine,* researchers showed that two-thirds of all people with serious structural disorders—including slipped discs—had *no* back pain whatsoever.

For many years, doctors sincerely believed that most back pain was caused by slipped discs, and that the best treatment was surgery. This belief has lost favor only recently, with the advent of new imaging techniques, such as MRI and PET. These imaging techniques prove that many people who have slipped discs don't have pain, and that many people who have pain don't have slipped discs. Nonetheless, many doctors and many patients still cling to the outdated idea that repairing discs is the key to relieving most back pain.

Now I'll tell you what the *real* causes of back pain usually are, and what you can do about them.

Rating Patient Satisfaction with Back Care Practitioners

Percentage of Satisfied Patients	Type of Practitioner
(1) 96% satisfied	Yoga instructors
(2) 86% satisfied	Physiatrists
(3) 65% satisfied	Physical therapists
(4) 36% satisfied	Acupuncturists
(5) 28% satisfied	Chiropractors
(6) 26% satisfied	Orthopedists
(7) 23% satisfied	Neurosurgeons
(8) 20% satisfied	Internists and family practitioners
(9) 4% satisfied	Neurologists

Survey by Arthur C. Klein

The Real Causes of Most Back Pain

To understand why your back hurts, you must first understand how your back is constructed.

Many people think that the human body stands erect and stable because it is built upon the frame of a powerful, weight-carrying spine. But this isn't true. The spine itself is weak and fragile. If the spine were to be stripped of its supporting muscles, tendons, and ligaments, it would be able to support only about five pounds. Without its supporting structures, even just the weight of the head would make the spine crack and crumble. But *with* these supporting structures, the spine can carry hundreds of pounds.

This important anatomical fact reveals the key to curing back pain: To have a healthy back, you must ensure the health of the *entire, interrelated structure* of the back, and not just the spine.

Building the health of the entire structure of the back requires a comprehensive program of exercise, physical therapies, good nutrition, a few natural medications, and relief from stress. A pain-free back *cannot* commonly be achieved with just "magic bullet" drugs and surgeries.

The back, including the spinal column, is an absolute marvel of interrelated structures, each of which supports and protects the other structures. However, the interrelated structures of the back, working together, must accomplish two very different functions: first, they must carry the messages of the brain to the entire body, through a delicate and vulnerable network of nerves; and, second, they must support the body, and give it the strength to do difficult, "backbreaking" tasks.

These two very different functions often conflict. The first function requires an intricate system of nerves and nerve pathways, and the second function requires a brawny system of thick muscles and strong bones. Because of this basic conflict, the back is easily hurt. The delicate structures that protect nerves just don't hold up well against tough physical tasks.

The fragile system that allows nerves to leave the spinal cord includes a series of small openings between the individual back bones, or vertebrae. Between each pair of vertebrae is a spongy cartilaginous disc, and these discs give the nerves enough space to exit the spine. The discs also cushion the vertebrae, and keep them from grinding against each other.

The discs are shaped somewhat like jelly doughnuts, with a tough outer layer enclosing a gelatinous center. The center is about 85 percent water. Sometimes these discs are squeezed out of place, and push against nerves. Occasionally they even rupture, or herniate, and lose all the liquid in the center.

Unfortunately, the liquid in the center of the discs begins to decline gradually during a person's twenties. By age forty, most of us have already lost about 15 percent of the liquid in our discs, and this decline continues as we age. That's why people tend to become somewhat shorter as they get older. Also, this decline in disc height gradually gives nerves less room to exit the spine. That's partly why back pain is more common among older people.

Even the pressure of standing erect during the day temporarily reduces the amount of liquid in the spinal discs. At night, however, when you recline during sleep, this water is reabsorbed into your discs. Therefore, when you first wake up, you are probably slightly taller than you are at the end of the day. Similarly, astronauts who are freed from the earth's gravity often gain up to two inches in height. They quickly lose this added height when they return to earth.

Because of the intense pressure of gravity, it's almost always our *lower* backs that develop pain. The upper part of your back, which carries a far lighter load, doesn't suffer nearly as much strain.

As you probably know, the spine isn't completely straight, but is a beautifully balanced S-curve. The natural curve of the spine allows it to have greater flexibility, but it also makes it somewhat unstable, thus rendering it more vulnerable to structural disruption, and pain.

The spine is able to curve because it's composed of a series of short, separate vertebrae. Each vertebra is connected to the one above it and the one below it by joints near the rear of the spine. Unfortunately, like all the other joints in the body, these spinal "facet joints" are prone to arthritis. Most people eventually suffer some degree of spinal arthritis. If you are forty or older, and feel stiffness in your back every morning when you wake up, you may already have mild spinal arthritis.

Because all of the structures in the back are so dependent upon each other, a problem in one structure can hurt all the others. For example, arthritis in the spinal joints can strain muscles—and chronic muscle strain can contribute to arthritis in the spinal joints. Also, displaced discs can strain muscles—and strained muscles can displace discs.

Thus, to ensure having a healthy, pain-free back, you must maintain the health of each of the three basic components of your back: (1) your muscles, (2) your nerves, and (3) your joints. Each of these three components is crucially important, and each can be the source of pain.

Let's take a look at what can make each of these three components hurt.

MUSCLE PAIN

Very often, severe back pain is nothing more than muscle strain, and can be relieved simply by nurturing sore muscles.

Many back-pain researchers believe that *up to 80 percent* of all chronic lower back pain is caused by strained, overworked muscles. Frequently those muscles are overworked simply because they're not *strong* enough to perform their daily tasks. If they are strengthened by exercise—particularly mind/body exercises—they can usually meet their daily demands.

Because the spinal column itself can carry only about five pounds, most of the work that is done by the back is done by the back *muscles*. Those muscles, however, get a lot of help from tendons, which link one muscle to another, and from ligaments, which link muscles to bones. Unfortunately, tendons and ligaments can also be strained.

When a muscle, ligament, or tendon is strained, it causes a microscopic tear. This creates bleeding, and painful inflammation. If a muscle is badly strained, it will become so inflamed that it will swell and become spongy to the touch.

When muscles are strained, they can cause other muscles to go into a rigid state of spasm, as the other muscles try to protect the injured muscle from further movement, and further damage. Spasms in the back muscles are common. They are very painful, and often completely immobilizing. Sometimes muscles go into *chronic* spasm because of poor posture, or ongoing trauma. For example, an office chair that is too high, and causes a person to hunch over for many hours every day, can cause chronic spasm. Emotional stress also contributes to spasm.

Another result of small muscle tears is the creation of scar tissue. If the tear is repeated several times, or if it is severe, the buildup of scar tissue can weaken the muscle, and irritate nerves.

Weak back muscles can also gradually lead to slipped discs. Muscles hold the spine in proper position, but when *weak* muscles allow the spine to lose its proper position, any sudden twist or trauma can allow a disc to slip out of place. If the sudden trauma is severe, the disc might rupture, and lose its gelatinous center.

Similarly, when weak muscles allow the back to be out of its proper position, it can also stress the *joints*, and contribute to the onset of arthritis.

A common problem among many people with back pain is inactivity. Pain makes people stop using their back muscles, and this just makes the muscles weaker, and the pain worse. This phenomenon, called *chronic disuse atrophy*, can create a vicious cycle of degeneration.

Another common problem caused by lack of exercise is the gradual tightening of muscles. When this happens, tight muscles pull against bones, tendons, and ligaments, and throw the back out of balance. To stay loose, muscles must be regularly stretched by exercise. It's especially important to maintain the flexibility of the powerful hamstring muscle in the back of the leg. When this strong muscle is allowed to tighten, it limits the range of motion of the pelvis, and can strain the lower back. If you are unable to touch your fingers to your toes with your knees locked, your hamstrings are too tight, and may be contributing to your back pain.

Ligaments and tendons also need to be stretched. It's particularly important to do stretching exercises in midlife and beyond, because, as you age, your ligaments tend to shorten. Unless these ligaments are regularly stretched with exercise, they will eventually disrupt the equilibrium in your back.

Another cause of pain in the back muscles is the condition called fibromyalgia, which I will discuss in the following chapter.

Fibromyalgia—a type of chronic muscle pain—can strike any muscle, including the back muscles.

For many years it has been widely believed that weak abdominal muscles often cause back pain. Recently that idea has lost favor among some doctors, but I still agree with it. Your abdominal muscles stretch three-fourths of the way around your back, so they are, in a sense, back muscles. Furthermore, when you need to lift and carry loads, the abdominal muscles do much of the work, and relieve strain on the back muscles. Therefore, I generally include abdominal exercises, such as "stomach crunches," in my exercise routine for back-pain patients.

NERVE PAIN

Like many other doctors, I no longer believe that irritated nerves, pinched by damaged spinal discs, are the primary cause of back pain. However, irritated nerves are still a significant problem. An estimated 5 to 10 percent of all back pain is nerve pain caused by herniated discs, which have lost their gelatinous center. Displaced discs, commonly called slipped discs, usually cause less nerve pain than herniated discs, but they occur more frequently.

Several factors cause discs to become displaced, and herniate: chronically poor posture; weak muscles in the lower back; damage to ligaments; degeneration of the vertebrae; injury; and pregnancy (which places a heavy burden on the back). People are especially vulnerable to these factors in midlife and beyond, because of the loss of water in their spinal discs. By age fifty, most people have suffered some degeneration in approximately 90 percent of their discs.

Nonetheless, most cases of herniated discs occur *before* age fifty. The prime period for herniation is between thirty-five and fifty. In this age group, some degeneration has already occurred, but people are still generally active, and are more likely to attempt difficult physical tasks.

Another condition that causes nerve impingement is a gradual narrowing of the central canal of the spinal column, where the spinal cord lies. By about age fifty, many people begin to suffer from this condition, which is called *spinal stenosis*. It is caused by the degeneration of the vertebrae, and by arthritic deposits called "bone spurs." Back surgery can also contribute to spinal stenosis. People with this condition generally experience numbness or burning in both legs. However, about 20 percent of all patients with this condition will not have any symptoms.

Arthritis can also cause nerve irritation. Arthritic bone spurs often touch nerves. The nerves that are most commonly pinched by a herniated disc are the thick sciatic nerves, which travel from the spine to each leg. Because the sciatic nerves are the thickest nerves in the body, they are the most vulnerable to impingement.

Sciatic pain, however, is not as common as most people think. Many people who have pain in their lower backs, buttocks, or upper legs believe that they have sciatica, but they don't. Sciatica is characterized not just by pain, but also by ever-increasing *numbness and weakness*.

To test for sciatica, I generally have patients lie on their backs, and raise one leg. If they begin to feel a sharp pain in their leg when it's raised to a 30- to 60-degree angle, it can indicate sciatica. If this occurs, I generally order an MRI, which is the most definitive diagnostic test for a herniated disc.

Joint Pain

The third common cause of pain in the back is joint pain. Like all other joints in the body, the facet joints in the back—which link together the twenty-six vertebrae—are vulnerable to arthritis, injury, and degeneration. When any of these conditions occur, pain can result.

Arthritis is the most common cause of pain in the spinal joints. By age sixty-five, almost everyone has some degree of arthritis in his or her spine. Even in midlife, spinal arthritis is relatively common. As I mentioned, if you are in midlife, and your back feels stiff every morning before you stretch or take a hot shower, you may have early arthritis.

If you do have symptoms of arthritis in your spine, read chapter 6; the information in that chapter applies to all types of arthritis, including spinal arthritis. Even if you don't currently have any symptoms of spinal arthritis, you should still read that chapter, to learn how to prevent spinal arthritis, or delay its onset.

One prevention tactic that is *not* mentioned in chapter 6—because the tactic is related solely to spinal arthritis—is the correction of displaced vertebrae by manipulation therapy, which is practiced by doctors of chiropractic and osteopathy. When vertebrae move out of their proper positions, the facet joints suffer extra physical stress, and this stress can contribute to arthritis. Manipulation therapy, however, often restores vertebrae to their proper positions.

In addition to arthritis, another factor that causes joint pain is the general deterioration of the spinal facet joints during the aging process. As we age, all of our bones and joints tend to become weaker, thinner, and more brittle. This degeneration, however, can be significantly slowed by a comprehensive program of exercise, mind/body exercises, good nutrition, meditation, and a healthy lifestyle.

The joint that appears to be the most vulnerable to degeneration—because it carries the heaviest load—is the pelvic joint known as the sacroiliac. Your sacroiliac links your pelvis to your spine, and transfers the weight of your upper body to your legs. For many years, doctors thought that *most* pain in the lowest part of the back was sacroiliac pain, but that belief gradually lost popularity. In 1995, though, an important article in the influential journal *Spine* strongly supported this "old-fashioned" idea. The article described a doctor's success in treating low back pain by injecting sacroiliac joints with anti-inflammatory medication. The doctor estimated that 9 to 30 percent of all patients with low back pain suffered from an inflamed sacroiliac joint.

Thus, it's prudent for people with back pain to try to reduce inflammation. Besides sacroiliac pain, other types of back pain—such as muscle strain and arthritis—cause inflammation. In the chapters on my comprehensive pain program, I described many techniques for reducing inflammation. If you have back pain, you should review this information and follow that advice.

Another common cause of joint pain is physical trauma, caused by an accident, or by extreme exertion (known as overuse syndrome). One example of a traumatic joint injury is whiplash, which is generally caused by rear-end auto collisions. Also, people sometimes injure their joints by lifting heavy objects.

A final cause of joint pain is a genetic condition called scoliosis, which causes the spine to curve sideways. This condition is far more prevalent than most people realize. It's present in an estimated 12 percent of the population, but it rarely requires treatment. Only about 2 percent of all people with scoliosis need treatment.

The ability of the back to adjust to scoliosis underscores the amazing adaptability of the interrelated structures of the back. In fact, about 20 percent of all people have some form of structural abnormality in their backs. Many people have missing vertebrae, and some people actually have openings in the rear portions of their spines. In most cases, though, these conditions cause no pain, because the surrounding structures compensate for the abnormalities. Unfortunately, some overzealous surgeons occasionally cite these abnormalities as justifications for surgery.

PREVENTING AND ARRESTING OSTEOPOROSIS

If you're in midlife, you probably already have some degree of osteoporosis, which can cause back pain.

Osteo is a Latin prefix meaning "bone." *Porosis* means "porous." Thus, *osteoporosis* means "porous bones." If you're forty or older, your bones are probably more porous than they once were. In almost all people, the bones become weaker during the aging process, just as do the eyes and muscles.

You have the power to drastically retard the degeneration of your bones, and to make sure that your osteoporosis never becomes any more troubling than it is now.

Unfortunately, about 25 million Americans have already neglected the health of their bones for so long that they now suffer from clinically diagnosable osteoporosis. These people will endure about 1.5 million broken bones this year. Many of this group will be in chronic pain, and many will be disfigured by skeletal degeneration.

People often neglect the health of their bones because they think of bones as dead, fossilized structures. That's a dangerous misconception. Your bones are dynamic, growing organisms that are changing just as much as your heart, skin, and muscles.

Preventing osteoporosis should be one of your primary anti-pain strategies, because the same things you do to prevent osteoporosis will also keep your spinal bones healthy, strong, and youthful. By preventing osteoporosis, you will also help prevent spinal arthritis and degeneration.

Osteoporosis occurs when the bones lose the minerals that compose them. The primary mineral that composes bone is calcium. Regardless of what certain advertisements may imply, your bones won't stay healthy just from taking calcium tablets alone. In the next section, which covers nutrition, I'll tell you about all the various nutrients your bones need to thrive, and to stay free of osteoporosis.

Besides nutrients, your bones also need a consistent program of physical exercise to avoid osteoporosis. The exercise that works best for bones is weight-bearing exercise, rather than cardiovascular exercise. The most popular weight-bearing exercise for the upper body is weightlifting, and the most popular weight-bearing exercises for the lower body are walking, jogging, and lower-body weight training.

Exercise for the bones can be started at virtually any age, and even a small amount of exercise can be very beneficial. In one recent study, a group of women in their mid-eighties began a program of weight-bearing exercise. Half the group exercised just thirty minutes a week, and the other half didn't exercise at all. After three years, the group that had been exercising had retained about 50 percent more bone minerals than the group that had not exercised.

One form of exercise that can be particularly beneficial for back pain is t'ai chi. T'ai chi is a very nearly perfect exercise for the prevention of osteoporosis. It's both weight-bearing and non-jarring, and it accumulates and mobilizes ch'i. Since one of its principles is proper alignment of the spine, it is also highly therapeutic in many problems involving the spine.

Another factor that helps preserve the minerals in your bones is sunlight, which the body converts to vitamin D. Vitamin D is needed by the body for the absorption of calcium, and also for calcium metabolism within the bones. Interestingly, geographic areas that are notably short of sunshine, such as northern Scotland, tend to have higher rates of osteoporosis. Even in the sunny Middle East, women who wear traditional body-concealing clothing suffer high rates of osteoporosis.

To help prevent osteoporosis, your body needs about fifteen minutes of exposure to the sun each day. If it's difficult for you to get this much exposure, you can substitute for the sun with full-spectrum lights. If you use lights, however, you may need up to an hour of exposure every day. Another alternative is to take approximately 500 to 800 mg of supplemental vitamin D each day.

It's also vitally important for women to maintain adequate levels of female hormones. About 80 percent of all osteoporosis victims are women, and most researchers think this is a result of hormonal deficits. Many doctors advise postmenopausal women to take estrogen for the prevention of osteoporosis. The latest research, though, indicates that the hormone progesterone may be even more effective than estrogen. Furthermore, progesterone is probably safer than estrogen, which has been linked to the onset of some forms of cancer.

These are the primary risk factors for osteoporosis:

- Low calcium intake
- Low intake of the key nutrients
- Hormonal deficits
- Smoking
- Regular use of steroidal medications
- Chronic stress
- Excessive alcohol or coffee consumption
- A sedentary lifestyle—especially confinement to bed

I've already explained why most of these risk factors contribute to osteoporosis; here are explanations of the factors I haven't mentioned: Smoking narrows blood vessels, and blocks delivery of nutrients and oxygen to bones; steroids increase bone demineralization; stress tightens muscles, and also interferes with hormonal balance; alcohol flushes magnesium and calcium from the body; and three or more cups of regular (non-decaffeinated) coffee per day increase demineralization of bones.

If several of these risk factors apply to you, you should be alert for the early warning signs of osteoporosis. One of the first signs of the disease is a slight shrinkage of the jawbone, which is among the first bones to show loss of mineralization. A gradually shrinking jawbone may cause the teeth to become loose, and may cause the gums to recede and expose more of each tooth. In fact, the phrase "long in the tooth" originated from people noticing the increased exposure of teeth in older people with osteoporosis.

Two other early warning signs are increasing transparency in the skin on the backs of the hands and prematurely graying hair. Low-back pain is also a frequent warning sign of osteoporosis, and so is the onset of joint pain.

If you are in midlife and suffer from any of these warning signs, see your doctor. Your doctor may want you to undergo a bone scan, or a nuclear magnetic resonance test. Another helpful test is a blood test that checks for extra calcium in the blood. Your doctor may also order X rays, but osteoporosis generally isn't visible on X rays until the disease is so far advanced that 30 percent of the bone is gone. If you're wise, you'll try to *prevent* osteoporosis before *any* of its warning signs appear.

In the next four sections, I'll show you how each of the four levels of my comprehensive pain program can help prevent osteoporosis and the other conditions that cause back pain. I'll also tell you about the best treatments for back pain, after pain has already developed.

The Terrible Problem of Back Pain

- One-third of all people over forty-five years of age have chronic back pain.
- Back pain is the leading cause of disability in people under forty.
- If back pain occurs once, it's four times as likely to occur again.
- The average annual cost of a back injury is $4,500 in lost earnings, and $1,600 in treatment expense.
- Eighty percent of all people experience back pain at some point in their lives.
- Twenty-two percent of all work injuries are back injuries.
- In America, 7 million new cases of serious back pain occur every year.

Level One: Nutritional Therapy for Back Pain

If you have back pain, you should follow the nutritional therapy program I described in chapter 2. My comprehensive anti-pain nutritional program should end much of your discomfort. You should *also* follow the nutritional advice in chapter 6, even if you don't currently have arthritis. Almost everyone eventually develops some degree of spinal arthritis, and people with *existing* back pain are especially vulnerable to the onset of spinal arthritis.

Following the advice in these two chapters will help you achieve the following:

- You will reduce your painful inflammation.
- You will build your levels of pain-blocking serotonin.
- You will improve the health of your brain and nerves. This will boost your pain threshold, and help your brain and nerves launch a strong counterattack against pain.

- If you are now overweight, you will probably reduce your weight, and relieve strain on your back.
- You will help stabilize your hormonal levels, and prevent hormonal deficits from destroying your bones.
- You will help prevent arthritis, and delay its progression.
- You will give your bones, ligaments, tendons, muscles, and nerves the nutrients they need to regenerate, and stay healthy and youthful.

In addition to following the advice in these two chapters, it would also be prudent for you to engage in the following program of super-nutrition for your bones, nerves, joints, and muscles. The following nutritional guidelines are specifically designed to meet the special nutritional needs of back-pain patients.

SUPER-NUTRITION FOR BACK PAIN

All back-pain patients should regularly ingest the following nutrients (after consulting a doctor in order to tailor a program to their specific needs):

- *Calcium.* Ninety-nine percent of the calcium in your body is in your bones and teeth. The density of calcium in your bones peaked during your twenties. Besides building bones, calcium stops nerve excitation, and thereby helps control pain. Take 1,000–2,500 mg daily.
- *Vitamin C* helps bones metabolize calcium, and is the primary nutritional building block of collagen, the gluey substance that helps hold your bones together. Collagen is also a vitally important component of ligaments and tendons. Take 1,000–2,000 mg of a time-release tablet three times daily.
- *Vitamin D* helps your bones absorb calcium. Without enough vitamin D, the calcium in your bones can decrease by more than half. The sun provides vitamin D, but if you can't get at least fifteen minutes of sunshine each day, take a 500–800-mg vitamin D supplement every day.

- *Boron* prevents the excretion of calcium in the urine. It also appears to help stabilize estrogen levels. Take 3–6 mg daily.

- *Zinc* helps vitamin D to metabolize calcium. Some researchers believe that a zinc deficiency contributes significantly to osteoporosis. Take 50 mg daily.

- *Vitamin K* helps bones to assimilate calcium. It also prevents excretion of calcium. Take 100 mcg daily.

- *Copper.* A deficiency of this mineral increases the demineralization of bones. Take 2–3 mg daily, but do *not* exceed this dosage, because excessive copper can be toxic.

- *Magnesium* activates vitamin K, and thereby aids the absorption of calcium. It also helps make muscles, tendons, and ligaments more supple, and helps the brain fight stress. An estimated 72 percent of all Americans ingest less than the government's recommended daily allowance of magnesium. Take 1,000–2,000 mg daily. Take approximately as much magnesium as calcium.

- *Silica* is essential in the formation of connective tissue, including cartilage, and is used by bones for metabolizing calcium. Take 100 mcg daily.

- *Manganese* is used in the body's production of cartilage and bone. In one study, women with osteoporosis had 75 percent less manganese in their blood than women who didn't have osteoporosis. Take 5 mg daily.

These minerals may be taken individually, or in the form of multiple mineral tablets.

Level Two: Physical Therapy for Back Pain

For fast, enduring results, various physical therapies are superb for back pain. The most effective physical therapies, in my opinion, are the mind/body exercises. Other valuable therapies are exercise therapy, acupuncture, and manipulation therapy. Other helpful physical therapies are massage, heat and cold, TENS, ultrasound, and correction of posture. Here are details about the value of each of these therapies.

EXERCISE THERAPY

According to my own clinical experience, as well as the best recent research, the most valuable exercises for back pain are not the traditional *stretching* exercises, but those that *strengthen* the back muscles. These strengthening exercises include anaerobic floor exercises, yogic exercises, and certain weight-resistance exercises.

Although I believe that stretching is less important than building strength, I still believe it can be valuable for most patients. Therefore, most of the strength-building exercises that I commonly recommend are exercises that also stretch muscles.

Your strength-building and stretching exercises should be performed virtually every day. When you do them, your movements should be slow, gentle, and graceful, rather than fast and forceful. It's acceptable to feel a mild degree of discomfort while performing the exercises, but you should not feel pain. If an exercise hurts, modify it until it no longer causes pain. After you become adept at these exercises, most of them should feel pleasurable.

Occasionally, you may feel and hear a slight popping sound, as displaced joints—including displaced vertebral joints—are pulled back into proper alignment.

1. RECLINING TRUNK ROTATOR. Lie flat on your back, with your knees raised and your feet together. Place a rolled-up bath towel under your neck to support the normal curve of your spine. Keeping your knees together, swing both of your upraised knees down to the floor to one side, while turning your head in the opposite direction. Then swing your knees to the other side, while again turning your head in the opposite direction. Repeat 20–50 times.

2. LOW-BACK TONER. Lie on your back and slowly pull your knees toward your chest. Grasp your knees with your hands, and pull your knees as close to your chest as you comfortably can. Hold the position for approximately 30 seconds to one minute.

3. TORSION TWIST. Lie on your back with your knees raised and your feet flat on the floor. Hold your arms out to your sides for stability. Place one of your ankles on an upraised knee. Gently push your upraised knee toward the floor, with your ankle still resting on it. Push until you stretch the muscles in your hips. Hold the position for about 30 seconds to one minute. Then do the same movement with your other leg.

4. STANDING TRUNK ROTATOR. Stand with your feet spread, and your arms held out to your sides. Gently swing your trunk in a semicircle, using the leverage of your swinging arms to increase your rotation. As you swing, turn your head in the same direction you're swinging. Swing 10–25 times in each direction.

5. PELVIC TILT. Lie on your back with your knees raised and your feet flat on the floor. Lift your buttocks as far off the floor as you comfortably can, and then bring them back down. Repeat 10–20 times.

6. CAT ARCH. Get on your hands and knees, and arch your back toward the ceiling, as cats often do when they stretch. Then lower your back until your stomach sags downward. Repeat 10–20 times.

7. HIP TONER. Sit on the floor with your knees upraised, and your feet on the floor. Bring one foot up and cross it over your upraised knee. As you sit, put your arms behind you, on the floor, for support. Hold the position for about 30 seconds to one minute. Repeat the movement with the other leg.

8. HAMSTRING TONER. Stand with one foot about ten inches directly in front of the other. Raise the toes of your front foot, and bend your knees slightly. Lean forward at the waist, until you feel your calf muscle and the back of your thigh begin to stretch. Do this 10–15 times. Repeat with the other foot.

9. ABDOMINAL CRUNCH. Lie on your back with your knees upraised and your feet flat on the floor. Lift your shoulders about 10 inches off the floor. Repeat 20–100 times.

10. LOW-BACK STRENGTHENER. Lie on your stomach with your arms and legs spread, and your knees and elbows locked. Simultaneously lift one arm and the opposite leg about 10 inches off the floor. Hold the position for a moment, then lift the other leg and arm. Repeat 10–15 times.

WEIGHT-RESISTANCE EXERCISES

In addition to the ten floor exercises described above, you should also do a moderate amount of weight-resistance exercise. As I mentioned, weight-resistance exercises are the best possible exercises for the bones.

Walking is an excellent weight-resistance exercise for the lower body. Jogging is also valuable, but jogging often has a jarring effect on the spine, ankles, and knees, and is often harmful for people with back problems. Remember: If it hurts, don't do it. If you do jog, warm up well, wear shock-absorbing running shoes, and try not to jog on hard surfaces.

For your upper body, you should lift weights. As recently as five years ago, most doctors didn't approve of back patients lifting weights. Now, however, that attitude has begun to change. I have been recommending weightlifting for many years, and my back-pain patients have benefited greatly from it.

To relieve back pain, don't try to lift heavy weights, but focus on high repetitions of light weights. Lifting heavy weights can easily strain the muscles that you need to nurture.

Your weight workout should focus primarily on the muscles of your back, hips, and abdomen, including the latissimus dorsi, the spinae erectors, the gluteus medius, the obliques, the abdominals, the trapezius, and the rhomboideus.

As you can see by the following illustration, all of the muscles in the body are ultimately connected by bones, tendons, and ligaments. Therefore, your back will feel best, and will be most perfectly aligned, if you maintain adequate strength *throughout* your body.

Here are some of the best weight-resistance exercises for strengthening the back. Some can be done with free weights, and some require a weight machine. The exercises that require a weight machine are not essential if you perform all of the free-weight exercises.

PULLDOWN. On a weight machine, grasp the bar above your head with an overhand grip. Pull the bar down to approximately the level of your chest, then slowly return it. Repeat the movement until your upper back muscles begin to tire. This strengthens the latissimus dorsi.

ABDOMINAL TONER. As you sit on the floor, hold a bar with light free weights behind your neck. Lean forward as far as you comfortably can. Straighten to the sitting position. Repeat until you begin to tire.

HORIZONTAL ROWING. Sit on the floor, facing a weight machine, and hold the machine's lower bar with a wide grip. Pull it toward your stomach. Repeat the motion until you begin to tire.

UPRIGHT PULL. Standing erect, raise the lower bar of a weight machine, or the bar of a free weight, from the level of your hips to just under your chin. Lower the bar gradually, and repeat until you begin to tire.

STRAIGHT-ARM LIFT. Using a light free weight, stand erect with the weight bar at the level of your hips. With your elbows locked,

Your Major Muscle Groups

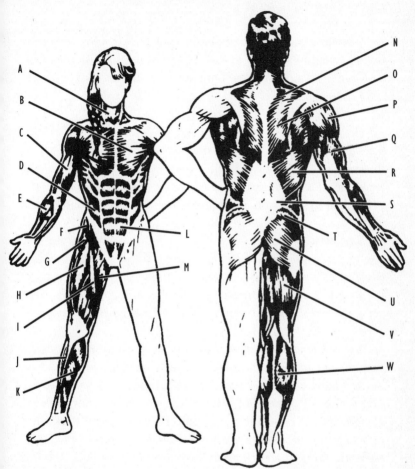

A. Sternomastoid (neck)
B. Pectoralis Major (chest)
C. Biceps (front of arm)
D. Obliques (waist)
E. Brachioradials (forearm)
F. Hip Flexors (upper thigh)
G. Abductor (outer thigh)
H. Quadriceps (front of thigh)

I. Sartorius (front of thigh)
J. Tibialis Anterior (front of calf)
K. Soleus (front of calf)
L. Rectus Abdominus (stomach)
M. Adductor (inner thigh)
N. Trapezius (upper back)
O. Rhomboideus (upper back)
P. Deltoid (shoulder)

Q. Triceps (back of arm)
R. Latissimus Dorsi (mid-back)
S. Spinae Erectors (lower back)
T. Gluteus Medius (hip)
U. Gluteus Maximus (buttocks)
V. Hamstring (back of leg)
W. Gastrocnemius (back of calf)

(Illustration courtesy of Robert Gonzalez, ICON Health & Fitness) raise the bar in front of your body until it is level with your chest. Repeat until you begin to tire.

DUMBBELL SIDE LIFT. Stand erect, your arms at your sides and holding a light dumbbell in each hand. With your elbows locked and your arms straight, raise both arms simultaneously. Continue until you begin to tire.

HIP TONER. Place your ankle inside the lower strap of a weight machine, and stand sideways to the machine. While holding on to the machine for support, pull the leg with the weight attached to it away from the machine, then slowly let the weight back down. Repeat the movement until you begin to tire, then use the other leg.

SIDE BEND. Standing sideways to a weight machine, grasp the lower strap with your hand. Bend your torso away from the machine, thus lifting the weight attached to the strap. Slowly return the weight. Repeat the movement until you begin to tire, then grasp the strap with your other hand, and repeat the exercise.

You will receive the most benefit from weight-resistance exercises if you confine each workout to exercises that use just a few isolated muscle groups, such as the back muscles, or leg muscles. This is more effective than trying to tone the entire body in a single workout. In subsequent workouts, shift your focus from one muscle group to another. This will allow you to more effectively build the strength and endurance of each muscle group, without exhausting your energy.

When you focus an entire workout on just one set of muscles, it dramatically increases the blood flow to that muscle group. This creates growth of the muscle tissue, or hypertrophy. It also engorges the muscle with nutrients and oxygen, and carries away toxic debris.

The back-pain patients of mine who have responded best have all been diligent about weight-resistance exercise. Building the strength of the back can have an almost miraculous effect on most forms of back pain.

For more weight-training exercises, see the weight-training addendum at the back of the book.

MIND/BODY EXERCISE

Another excellent way to strengthen the back, and also to stretch it, is with yogic mind/body exercise.

I have studied yoga for approximately twenty years, and have come to believe that the most effective form of yoga is kundalini yoga, an ancient practice that not only strengthens and stretches muscles but also helps the body to generate and circulate the life-energy called prana or kundalini.

The word *yoga* comes from the same root as *yoke*, meaning "to join." Thus, yoga links together the various parts of the body. The very best forms of yoga join together not only the separate parts of the body, but also the body, mind, and spirit. Kundalini yoga is especially valuable for gathering the body, mind, and spirit into a single, harmonious force. Because kundalini exercises can stimulate the mind and the spirit, they are often referred to as mind/body exercises.

For details on mind/body exercises for back pain, please see Appendix I.

SPORTS AND BACK PAIN

Participating in sports can help most back pain patients, but patients must be cautious about their movements.

One sport that can cause harm, if not done properly, is golf. Golf places a great deal of strain on the back, because of the unique twisting movement of the golf swing. If you're a golfer, you should *always* warm up before playing, by stretching your back and hip muscles. Also, you should not bend over too far during your swing, or rotate your trunk excessively. If any part of your golf swing hurts your back, you should modify your swing immediately, until it no longer causes pain. One patient of mine, a sixty-four-year-old man who'd recently retired, was incredibly upset because back pain had forced him to quit playing golf. However, after he'd begun doing the mind/body exercises, and had undergone six acupuncture treatments, he was delighted to be on the course again.

Another popular therapy among many golfers is the use of magnetherapy. As I mentioned in chapter 3, a number of prominent players on the PGA Senior Tour have responded dramatically to magnetherapy. Magnetherapy is appropriate not just for athletes, but also for anyone who has chronic back pain. For more information on it, please review the appropriate material in chapter 3.

Bowling can also badly aggravate back pain. The worst common mistake is to keep one knee only slightly flexed while the other is fully bent. This places extra strain on the back. Another risky movement is to lift your bowling ball too high during your backswing. You should also remember to warm up properly before you bowl.

Tennis and racquetball can be played by most patients with back pain, but these sports should be played with extra caution. Racquet sports require sudden stopping and frequent bending, both of which can strain back muscles.

Bicycling is an excellent sport for most back pain patients, because it places only moderate strain on the back. However, if you have back pain, you should only ride bicycles with elevated handlebars, rather than the dropped, or racing, type. Racing handlebars require a stooped-over posture that's harmful for most people with back pain. Also, you should frequently stop riding and stretch for a few moments, because maintaining any fixed posture for a long period aggravates back pain.

Swimming is one of the best exercises for back-pain patients. However, if you do the crawl stroke, you should modify its movements. The constant neck twisting required for breathing during the crawl can be harmful. Back-pain patients should use a mask and snorkel when doing the crawl.

Probably the best form of exercise for back-pain patients, as well as arthritis patients, is water aerobics. This type of exercise provides strength training and cardiovascular exertion without stressing weight-bearing joints.

If you have *any* degree of back pain, you *must* exercise. No other single element of your pain program can provide as much benefit.

ACUPUNCTURE AND ACUPRESSURE

About eighteen years ago, when my son was very young, I bent over to pick him up, and felt a terrible pain in my back. It felt as if someone had thrown a spear through my back. I underwent the traditional therapies, including bed rest and use of anti-inflammatory medications, but the pain remained. For almost two years my back often hurt quite badly. Then I got my first acupuncture treatment. The results were spectacular. After just one treatment, the pain decreased by 90 percent, and it has never returned to its former intensity. By using the program I am describing in this section—especially the daily practice of mind/body exercises—I have never missed a day of work because of back pain.

If you have chronic back pain, or acute disabling back pain, I urge you to consider seeing a licensed acupuncturist, or a physician acupuncturist who is a member of the American Academy of Medical Acupuncture. The unique approach of acupuncture elicits certain changes that are impossible to duplicate with any other technique.

You may also gain some relief with acupressure, although I don't find its effects to be as dramatic as those of acupuncture. As you probably remember from chapter 3, acupressure is the massage of specific acupuncture points.

My favorite point for treating back pain with acupressure and acupuncture is point B-60, which is on your foot. To find it, place your thumb on the "ankle bump," or malleolus, on the outside of your ankle. Move your thumb into the indentation between your malleolus and your heel, until you feel a tender, sensitive point. Massage the point vigorously, in an up-and-down direction. To increase the effectiveness, use a lubricating oil. The sciatic nerve ends in this area, so massaging this point is often especially helpful for sciatic pain.

Another point that can ease back pain—particularly upper-back pain caused by a whiplash injury—is B-10. To find it, place your index finger on the thick trapezius muscle that runs from your shoulder to your neck. B-10 is on the inside of the muscle (the side closer to your spine), at the level of the first vertebra of your neck.

Another point that also helps some back-pain patients is GV-26, which is located about halfway between the base of the nose and the top of the lip. This point is often helpful for lower-back pain.

MANIPULATION THERAPY

Until the past few years, many medical doctors were skeptical of the value of manipulation therapies, such as osteopathic manipulation, or chiropractic. In 1992, however, a large study by the Rand Corporation clearly indicated that chiropractic manipulation relieved back pain better than any other treatment, including surgery or drugs. At about the same time the Rand study was released, the *British Journal of Medicine* published a major study on chiropractic that showed it to be superior to conventional medicine in the treatment of back pain.

These days, most medical doctors concede that manipulation therapy can be extremely helpful for people with back pain. If the doctor you are now seeing for your back pain is still skeptical about manipulation therapy, he or she may be out of touch with current medical trends.

If you've never been to a manipulation therapist, you may find that a visit is a pleasant experience. Virtually all manipulation therapy is painless, and often provides immediate relief. Your appointment will probably last about half an hour, and may include an X ray. When you first begin treatment, you may need to visit the therapist every week for several weeks. Soon, though, treatment will probably be necessary only during an occasional flare-up of your back pain.

OTHER PHYSICAL THERAPIES FOR BACK PAIN

Probably the most important of the remaining physical therapies is *postural training*. Poor posture contributes to the onset of spinal degeneration, spinal arthritis, and muscle strain, and badly aggravates existing abnormalities, including chronic pain.

In chapter 3, I described an excellent technique for improving posture, the Trager Approach. If you have chronic back pain and poor posture, you should consider contacting a practitioner of this approach.

If you don't consult with a posture specialist, you should still make an effort to improve your posture. When you stand, your head should be aligned directly over your pelvic area, instead of slumped forward or slouched backward. When you sit for extended periods, the small of your back should touch your chair, and your feet should rest flat on the floor, with your knees bent at ninety-degree angles. When you sleep, you should lie on a firm mattress, and sleep on your side as much as you comfortably can.

You should also, of course, be very careful about lifting. Lift with your legs instead of your back, and squarely face anything you're lifting.

Avoid wearing any shoe with a heel that's higher than two inches. If you do wear high heels, avoid standing or walking in them as much as you reasonably can. If one of your legs is significantly longer than the other, which is a relatively common condition, try using shoe lifts. If the difference in your leg lengths is less than two centimeters, it's unlikely that a shoe lift will decrease your back pain.

Bed rest can be helpful for severe, acute back pain, but should not exceed three to four days. It can help relax muscles that are in spasm, and can sometimes relieve severe leg pain, caused by a pinched sciatic nerve. *Prolonged* bed rest is harmful for virtually all back-pain patients, however. Each day you stay in bed, your muscles atrophy up to about 1.5 percent. Every ten days you stay in bed, you lose about 15 percent of your cardiopulmonary fitness. Every two weeks that you stay in bed, you lose about 7 percent of the density of your bones. Extended bed rest also often causes biological depression. There is no evidence that extended bed rest helps patients recover. Even if you are in significant pain, you should still try to get out of bed, and be as active as possible.

Traction can help some patients, but its benefits are generally quite limited. This form of therapy, which involves stretching muscles by attaching weights to the body, was once very popular among physicians treating back pain. Recent research, though, indicates that traction is helpful only for patients who have pinched nerves, and that even those patients rarely derive lasting relief from it. Long-term traction has the same risks as extended bed rest, and can also contribute to the formation of blood clots in the legs. Also, traction can be very uncomfortable. I almost never recommend it.

Massage can be very beneficial for back pain, especially if it is performed by a licensed professional. In chapter 3, I describe several of the most effective forms of massage. Massage relaxes muscles that are in spasm, speeds the exit of irritating toxins from muscle tissue, improves circulation, and helps stop the cycle of pain.

Heat and cold therapies also have a beneficial effect on back pain. Cold therapy, or cryotherapy, reduces inflammation, can help relieve muscle spasm, and intervenes in the cycle of pain. Heat therapy, or thermotherapy, relaxes muscle fibers, accelerates metabolism in muscles, and also intervenes in the cycle of pain.

Cold therapy is usually done with ice packs or cooling liniments, and heat therapy is generally applied with heating pads and hot water. Many of my patients find that the two therapies work best when they are alternated.

Ultrasound is a relatively new therapy for back pain that is helpful for some patients. In this therapy, a device that emits high-frequency sound vibrations is placed against a patient's back. The signals from the device penetrate up to two inches, and appear to reduce inflammation and increase circulation. This approach, however, has not yet been proven effective by extensive research.

TENS therapy, or transcutaneous electrical nerve stimulation, is somewhat similar to ultrasound, but uses mild electrical currents instead of sound waves. This therapy hasn't yet been proven effective by extensive research, but the anecdotal reports about it tend to be quite favorable. Several of my patients rely upon it. The therapy is relatively safe and comfortable, and can have an instantaneous effect.

The use of *braces*, or back-support belts, can help *prevent* back injuries, but is not effective for treating existing back pain. Nonetheless, it's important for patients to prevent further injuries. Often, back pain becomes severe only when the back suffers a series of injuries.

This concludes the section on physical therapies for back pain, which is one of the longest single sections in the book. This amplifies the important point that physical therapy is generally the most effective single approach for back pain, and is an absolutely indispensable component of any effective back-pain program.

Level Three: Medication for Back Pain

Medication can help many patients reduce their back pain, but it must be used wisely and cautiously. For years, many doctors have prescribed the wrong medications for back pain, and have also kept patients on medications for far too long. This uninformed, careless use of medication has contributed to untold suffering.

The primary mistake doctors and patients make is to expect too much from drugs. Too often, drugs constitute the only therapy that is used, and the results of this narrow approach are often disastrous.

A far more intelligent approach is to use powerful prescription medications *only* for short-term, acute back pain, and for severe flare-ups of chronic back pain. I strongly believe that powerful prescription drugs should *not* be used on a regular, ongoing basis for the most common type of back pain—chronic back pain of moderate intensity.

Chronic, moderate-intensity back pain can, however, be effectively treated year after year with the careful administration of mild pharmaceutical drugs, such as aspirin, and with natural medications, such as herbs and homeopathic remedies. Many of my patients have benefited greatly from this cautious use of medication.

First let's look at the powerful prescription drugs, most of which you should avoid.

Prescription Medications

Opioids can be helpful for some forms of chronic pain, but in my opinion they have no place in the treatment of chronic back pain, even though some doctors still prescribe them. In a medical crisis of acute back pain, opioids can sometimes help. But even in those situations I generally use the mildest possible opioid, such as acetaminophen with codeine. Evidence indicates that opioids are not only dangerous, but are no more effective than nonsteroidal anti-inflammatory drugs, such as ibuprofen.

Steroids are sometimes prescribed to reduce the inflammation from a pinched nerve, but I generally do not recommend use of steroids, even in this situation. Steroids have many dangerous side effects, and I believe they are just not effective enough to warrant the risk.

Muscle relaxants are popular among many doctors, but I rarely prescribe them. For one thing, they don't relax your muscles—they relax your mind, and then your mind relaxes your muscles. If you can relax your mind with a safer method, such as meditation, you'll ultimately be healthier. Muscle relaxants such as Flexeril and Valium can be habit-forming, and have numerous side effects. In my opinion, the only appropriate use of these drugs is on a very short-term basis, for acute back pain.

Antidepressants can sometimes help stop pain, as I mentioned in chapter 4. They can build the levels of pain-blocking serotonin, can help overcome insomnia, and can help with depression (which lowers the pain threshold). However, they have no *direct* benefit for the back.

Analgesic injections can be useful in relieving severe pain from a pinched nerve. The most effective type of injection, in my opinion, is an injection of an analgesic medication directly into the epidural space, the space adjacent to the spinal cord. This can help relieve the pain from a pinched nerve. In my clinical experience, epidural injections are most effective when they are administered in a series of three, over a three-week period. This procedure should be done no more than once a year, however.

Another injection method that occasionally relieves back pain is to inject sore points in muscles with a local anesthetic. These points, which are called "trigger points," can trigger pain elsewhere in the body. For example, a trigger point in the buttocks might cause pain to radiate down the leg, and thus mimic the symptoms of sciatica. Trigger points can also often be eliminated with massage, however. For more information on trigger points, review the information on myotherapy in chapter 3.

NONPRESCRIPTION MEDICATIONS

The best pharmaceutical nonprescription medications for back pain are the nonsteroidal anti-inflammatory drugs, or NSAIDS, such as ibuprofen.

I discussed NSAIDs thoroughly in chapter 4, so you should review that material.

The primary value of NSAIDs, as you may recall, is that they not only block pain, but also fight inflammation. They're of special benefit to back-pain patients, who often have inflammation of muscles, nerves, and joints.

The NSAID that is most commonly used for back pain is aspirin. Its effects are short-term, though, so the dosage usually must be repeated every four hours. Some patients find this inconvenient. Also, aspirin causes more stomach irritation than most other NSAIDs.

Ibuprofen causes less stomach upset than aspirin does, and is also very popular among many back-pain patients. Like virtually all other medications, it works best when it is augmented with other healing modalities. When my own back pain flares up, I take two 400-mg ibuprofen tablets, warm my back muscles with a hot shower, and do mind/body exercises.

An NSAID that has longer-lasting effects than aspirin and ibuprofen is ketoprofen. A convenient medication for back-pain patients, one tablet per day is usually all that is needed. There are other NSAIDs that also require only one dosage per day, but they are harder to flush from the body than ketoprofen, and can cause toxic accumulation.

Another popular NSAID for back pain is naproxen sodium, which is sold over the counter as Aleve. This NSAID is most often taken twice daily, and is considered to be one of the safer types.

Although NSAIDs can be extremely helpful for back pain, you must be very cautious about not taking excessively high dosages, or taking them too often. As I explained in chapter 4, overuse of NSAIDs is very common and often has disastrous results. I urge you to review the material that describes the many dangerous side effects of NSAIDs.

HOMEOPATHIC REMEDIES

Much safer than NSAIDs, in my opinion, and often just as effective, are homeopathic remedies, which I described in chapter 4. These have a much wider range of benefits than NSAIDs. Like NSAIDs, various homeopathic remedies can block pain and reduce inflammation, but homeopathic medications can also reduce muscle tension, improve circulation, optimize the metabolism of muscles, and speed the healing of injuries.

Some of my patients have felt much better after substituting homeopathic remedies for NSAIDs. For example, I had one patient who had developed a bleeding ulcer from taking NSAIDs for his spinal arthritis. After I urged him to rely on homeopathic medications instead of NSAIDs, he did much better. The homeopathic remedies controlled his pain just as effectively as the NSAIDs had, and his ulcer soon disappeared.

Here are the homeopathic remedies I most often prescribe to back-pain patients:

- *Rhus toxicodendron,* often abbreviated as *Rhus tox,* soothes pain originating in muscles, joints, and tendons. It can be taken orally, or used as a topical ointment.
- *Pulsatilla* soothes pain in muscles and joints, and seems to be particularly effective for active, Type A people, who seem to be particularly vulnerable to muscle-pain conditions, including chronic lower back pain and fibromyalgia. My patients use it for back pain and arthritis pain. *Pulsatilla* is also a popular remedy for premenstrual pain.
- *Arnica montana* is the most commonly used homeopathic pain remedy. It is excellent for muscle pain, and can be used orally as well as topically. The effective topical medication Traumeel contains arnica.
- *Arsenicum album* is sometimes effective for sciatic pain, and for arthritic pain. Many pains that are improved by gentle exercise and stretching respond to this remedy.
- *Bryonia* can help back pain that is aggravated by cold weather.
- *Dulcamara.* Some patients who feel worse after exertion respond favorably to dulcamara.
- *Kali carbonicum* often soothes sciatic pain, and other pain that radiates down the legs.

Another wise approach to using homeopathics is to buy specialized formulas. Several companies make formulas that are specifically designed to treat back pain. You can find them in most health-food stores.

Homeopathic medications can also be injected. One of my patients, a fellow physician who had a ruptured disc, responded very favorably when a homeopathic remedy was injected into the epidural space of his spine. When his condition first occurred, it appeared as if he would need an operation. However, after the homeopathic injections, which were accompanied by a course of acupuncture, he no longer required the surgery. Despite his herniated disc, his back caused him no significant further pain.

HERBAL MEDICATION FOR BACK PAIN

A final type of medication for back pain is herbal medicine. For thousands of years, herbal practitioners have helped relieve back pain in patients, while rarely causing any serious side effects.

In the Western herbal tradition, the most commonly used herbs for back pain are black cohosh, cramp bark, willow bark, and horse chestnut.

Black cohosh, which was used by Native Americans, relaxes smooth muscle tissue, and has long been used to treat arthritis and low-back pain. Available in most health-food stores, it is ingested as a tea. Steep one teaspoon in a cup of boiling water, and drink one cup of tea three times daily.

Cramp bark, as its name implies, helps stop muscle cramps and muscle spasm. The herb comes from the bark of the viburnum tree, and is used by many patients with back pain. Available in health-food stores, it is prepared as a tea.

Willow bark is an organic source of salicylate, which is the active ingredient in aspirin. Willow bark is less irritating to the gastrointestinal tract than aspirin, and is therefore a valuable substitute for aspirin. Available at health-food stores, it is brewed as a tea. The tea can also be used as a topical analgesic.

Horse chestnut reduces inflammation, and soothes strained back muscles. It's available at health-food stores.

In the Chinese herbal tradition, practitioners use *radix duhuo,* and also frankincense. *Radix duhuo* is appropriate for back pain that is exacerbated by cold and soothed by warmth. Frankincense is a mild anti-inflammatory agent that reduces swelling.

There are also several Chinese herbal formulations that have been designed especially for back pain. These may be purchased from an herb store, or through a licensed health-care professional, such as an acupuncturist.

Level Four: Mental and Spiritual Pain Control

From recent studies, and from my own clinical experience, I have come to believe that the mind and spirit play an extremely significant role in back pain.

Of all types of chronic pain, back pain may be the one that is most influenced by the mind and spirit. This is primarily because muscle tension plays an important role in back pain. Muscle tension is greatly exacerbated by mental and spiritual discord.

Recent government studies clearly show that mental factors are the best predictors of future back pain. Even more than physical factors—such as obesity, or hard physical labor—mental factors accurately assess vulnerability to back pain.

One of the most important mental factors in predicting the onset of back pain is a person's sense of satisfaction with his or her job. When people hate their work, they are far more likely to eventually suffer from back pain. If they love their work, they are unlikely ever to suffer chronic, disabling back pain, even if their jobs are physically stressful.

In addition, according to the U.S. Department of Health and Human Services, mental factors were the most important elements in predicting response to treatment. People with positive, relaxed personalities tended to respond well to treatment, while people who were negative, tense, and unhappy tended to respond poorly.

When people are tense and unhappy, they almost always tighten the muscles in their necks, shoulders, and backs. Often this tightening is an unconscious reaction. This muscular constriction can exhaust muscles, and cause them to go into spasm. It can also pull vertebrae out of proper alignment, and can contribute to the onset of spinal arthritis. In addition, constriction decreases circulation to muscle tissues, which can cause pain, and further tightening. This stress/pain/stress cycle can proceed endlessly.

To intervene in this cycle, a patient must make a strong effort to relax, and to feel mentally and spiritually at peace. In some cases this is not possible until a person actually changes his or her life—by quitting a nerve-racking job, by ending an unsatisfying relationship, or by moving to a less stressful area. More often, however, people can greatly diminish their stress by engaging in one or more of the stress-reduction techniques, such as meditation, that I described in chapter 5. I urge you to review that chapter, and to take to heart the advice it contains. If you do, it will, in all likelihood, significantly reduce your back pain.

In one large study of meditation and back pain, patients who meditated reduced their pain dramatically over a ten-week period. Half of all patients reduced their pain by at least 50 percent, and another 15 percent of patients reduced their pain by at least 33 percent. In another study, back-pain patients who used simple relaxation techniques cut their number of doctor visits by one-half.

As with other forms of chronic pain, there is no special mental or spiritual technique that is uniquely appropriate for back pain. *All* of the techniques I described in chapter 5 are appropriate for back-pain patients.

If you actively employ these techniques, you are almost certain to notice improvement soon. You must, however, be as proactive as possible. An analogy I sometimes offer patients is that if you go fishing, your likelihood of catching a fish will depend on how long you have your hook in the stream. The same holds true for your back pain: The longer you work on curing it, the more likely a cure will be. The more you relax, the more relaxed you will become. The more time you spend wading in the stream of consciousness, the greater opportunity you will have to enter into the realm of universal healing energy. The more time you spend in the sacred healing space of the meditative mind, the better your health will be, the happier your life will be, and the more attuned you will become to your own true identity, that of *your spiritual self.*

Thus you will discover that life need not be a painful struggle—and that your frustration and your pain can become things of the past.

9

Curing
Fibromyalgia Pain

Death I understand very well; it is suffering I cannot understand.
—ISAAC BASHEVIS SINGER

Please note that although this chapter contains information specifically about fibromyalgia, this material does not replace the previous information about my pain program. *All* patients should follow the complete pain program described in chapters 2 through 5. Fibromyalgia patients should *also* follow the advice in this chapter.

Fibromyalgia has long been one of medicine's most troubling puzzles. Most doctors do not understand it, and are unable to treat it effectively.

However, the pieces of this puzzle seem finally to be fitting together. For the first time, there is now true cause for hope.

The key piece of the puzzle for most patients now appears to be *low levels of serotonin*. When I correct this deficit in my own patients, I often achieve remarkable results. Other doctors have recently begun to achieve similarly positive results with this approach.

As I've noted previously, raising the level of the neurotransmitter serotonin is very important in overcoming virtually all forms of chronic pain. For fibromyalgia patients, boosting serotonin is especially important. I now believe that the terrible pain of fibromyalgia *cannot* be cured in most patients unless serotonin levels are restored to normal, or near normal.

Fibromyalgia, which causes widespread muscle pain, was first reported in the medical literature more than 150 years ago, but the condition was largely ignored by the research community until the late 1980s. For more than a century, almost no research on it was done, and its cause was considered a mystery. Some doctors were even skeptical of its existence, considering it just a neurotic complaint of hysterical patients, most of whom were women. When I was a medical student in the 1970s, fibromyalgia was never mentioned. Prior to 1985, no medical school in America taught physicians how to diagnose it correctly, and the condition was not even properly named. It was commonly called "fibrositis," which implies *inflammation* of the muscles. In fibromyalgia, however, inflammation does not appear to be a significant factor.

Despite the lack of understanding that has long surrounded this syndrome, it is an appallingly common disorder, afflicting up to 3 to 4 percent of the American population, or 7 to 10 million people. A form of muscular rheumatism, it accounts for as many as 30 percent of all cases of rheumatism—more than any other single rheumatic disorder.

Fibromyalgia is a very serious condition. About 20 percent of all fibromyalgia patients are disabled by it, and another 30 percent find it necessary to quit their jobs and find a less strenuous line of work.

The vast majority of fibromyalgia patients are women. Some experts say that the female-to-male ratio is three to one, but others say it is as high as fifty to one. A common figure that is cited is ten to one. In my own practice, all of my fibromyalgia patients except one have been women.

Fibromyalgia usually starts between the ages of twenty and fifty. One particularly common time for women to contract it is during menopause, or shortly before. An increasing number of teenagers have begun to suffer from it, though; about 28 percent of all patients are first diagnosed during childhood.

Technically, fibromyalgia is not a disease, because its exact cause is not certain, and because its existence cannot be confirmed by lab tests. Instead, it is referred to as a syndrome.

The pain of fibromyalgia usually starts in just one part of the body, and then spreads. The quality and degree of pain differ from patient to patient. In some patients the pain is a dull ache, but in others it is an excruciating series of stabbing, searing sensations. The pain is usually more severe than the pain of osteoarthritis or rheumatoid arthritis. The degree of pain waxes and wanes, and patients sometimes go into remissions that last from days to years.

The word *fibromyalgia* is derived from the Latin *fibra,* meaning "fibrous," the Greek *mys,* meaning "muscle," and the Greek *algos,* meaning "pain." Thus, the term refers to pain that originates in muscle fibers and is generally not caused by external trauma, such as a sprain or a bruise.

The three criteria of fibromyalgia are that (1) there must be muscle pain on both sides of the body, above and below the waist; (2) the pain must be present for at least three months; and (3) there must be pain in at least eleven of eighteen localized "tender points," which are indicated in the following diagram. This pain is usually accompanied by stiffness. Generally, the pain is most noticeable when the tender points are touched, or the muscles surrounding them are stretched.

Before these three diagnostic criteria were established by the American College of Rheumatology in 1990, fibromyalgia was notoriously misdiagnosed. In a 1984 study, a rheumatologist who was well versed in fibromyalgia discovered that 94 percent of his fibromyalgia patients had been previously misdiagnosed. Twelve percent had undergone unnecessary spinal surgery, 33 percent had been treated for low-back pain, and 12 percent had been hospitalized for neck pain.

The Fibromyalgia "Tender Points"

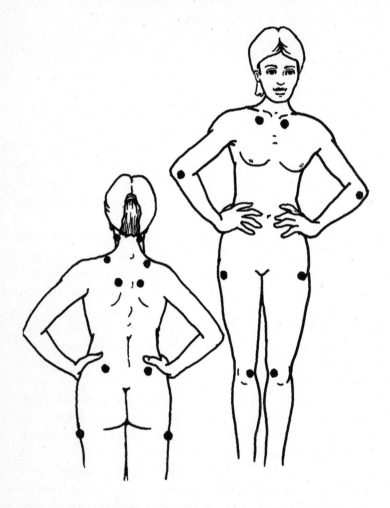

If you have some of the symptoms of fibromyalgia, you should undergo routine lab testing, even though those tests can't confirm a diagnosis of fibromyalgia. The tests *will* help rule out the presence of other disorders. Two dangerous conditions that often mimic fibromyalgia are lupus and hypothyroidism. Both conditions are very serious, and require specific treatments.

In addition to the three primary classic symptoms, there are several other symptoms that are extremely common among fibromyalgia patients. After I tell you about these symptoms, you'll begin to understand why I think that a deficit of serotonin is probably a primary cause of fibromyalgia. As you'll see, most of these common symptoms are *also* related to the low levels of serotonin.

Associated Symptoms of Fibromyalgia

- *Insomnia.* Almost 100 percent of fibromyalgia patients don't get enough deep sleep. This insomnia almost always causes a relentless fatigue.
- *Headaches.* About 50 percent of all fibromyalgia patients have chronic headaches.
- *Irritable bowel syndrome.* About 33 percent of all fibromyalgia patients suffer from the symptoms of constipation, diarrhea, and digestive tract disorder that characterize irritable bowel syndrome.
- *Painful menstruation.* Up to 40 percent of all females with fibromyalgia experience severe cramping and unusually painful menses.
- *Poor circulation in the extremities.* Many fibromyalgia patients have cold hands and feet, caused by the spasming of blood vessels in their extremities. Often this condition is so severe that it is classified as Raynaud's phenomenon, a disease that can cause the hands and feet to turn blue from lack of circulation.
- *TMJ pain.* About 25 percent of all fibromyalgia patients experience chronic tightness and pain in the temporomandibular joints of their jaws.
- *Restless leg syndrome.* Many fibromyalgia patients complain of an inability to keep their legs still, particularly at night, when they are trying to sleep.
- *Irritable bladder syndrome.* About 25 percent of all fibromyal-

gia patients experience frequent urination, or painful urination. The symptoms are similar to those of a bacterial infection of the bladder, but there is usually no evidence of infection in fibromyalgia patients. This problem is more common among women.

• *Cognitive difficulties.* It is very common for fibromyalgia patients to have problems with short-term memory and with concentration. Many of them feel as if they are "in a fog."

• *A feeling of swelling and tingling.* About 50 percent of all fibromyalgia patients report feeling that their hands and feet are swollen. Frequently they experience significant discomfort from this feeling, even when tests indicate that their swelling is actually very limited. This symptom most often occurs shortly after patients wake up in the morning. Many patients also report tingling, or paresthesia, in their hands, arms, and legs.

• *Anxiety and depression.* An estimated 25 percent of all fibromyalgia patients suffer from symptoms similar to those of clinical depression, and many others have pronounced feelings of anxiety. Often, this emotional unrest is a direct result of the suffering caused by chronic pain. In many patients, though, anxiety and depression appear to exist *independently* of the pain, and do not go away when the pain is relieved. Furthermore, fibromyalgia tends to strike highly motivated, Type A people more than others.

• *Dryness of the eyes and mouth.* About 25 percent of patients experience a lack of normal lubrication and saliva in their mouths and eyes.

• *Lack of muscle strength.* Most fibromyalgia patients are in poor physical condition, lacking muscle strength. In many patients, this lack of muscle tone occurs because pain stops them from exercising. Frequently, however, patients have poor muscle tone *before* they develop frank symptoms of fibromyalgia.

Did you notice how many of these symptoms are frequently linked to a lack of serotonin? *Most* of them are, including insomnia, chronic headaches, irritable bowel syndrome, painful menstruation, poor circulation to the extremities, tension in the jaw, restless leg syndrome, cognitive difficulties, lack of muscle strength, anxiety, and depression.

Some researchers believe that several of these symptoms—such as anxiety and poor muscle strength—actually *cause* fibromyalgia. I believe, however, that while some of these symptoms may contribute indirectly to the onset of fibromyalgia, most of them occur independently of fibromyalgia, and are caused by the same root problem that causes fibromyalgia: a serotonin deficit.

Despite this controversy about causation, though, most researchers and clinicians do agree that the best treatments for fibromyalgia are those that *boost serotonin levels*.

Now I'll tell you how I think fibromyalgia is caused. This is currently just a theory; it hasn't thus far been proven by extensive clinical studies. However, because of my own clinical results, and because of the findings of other researchers, I believe that the following theory has considerable merit, and might help you cure your own fibromyalgia.

A Theory on Fibromyalgia Causation

I believe that a deficit of serotonin causes a chain reaction of biochemical processes that can result in fibromyalgia.

As you probably know, the calming neurotransmitter serotonin *must* be abundantly present to ensure both physical and mental health. Serotonin has several vitally important actions in the brain: it helps raise the pain threshold, and helps the brain to launch its counterattack against pain; it improves mood, and is necessary for optimal memory and concentration. Serotonin also has several important physical actions that are not related to the mind. For example, it helps regulate the elasticity of blood vessels. As I mentioned in chapter 7, a lack of serotonin can cause the blood vessels in the brain to contract and expand uncontrollably, and cause migraines.

It's very common for people to have low levels of serotonin.

One indication of this is the popularity of drugs that boost serotonin, such as Prozac.

For fibromyalgia patients, probably the most important actions of serotonin are those related to sleep. Serotonin helps people sleep well. If serotonin levels are disturbed, insomnia often results. Thus, one of the most common medications for insomnia is the serotonin-boosting tricyclic antidepressant called amitriptyline. When serotonin-boosting antidepressants are given in low dosages—much lower than when they are prescribed for depression—the drugs generally help people to sleep peacefully throughout the night.

Without *any* serotonin, it's absolutely impossible to sleep. Researchers have learned that when animals are completely deprived of serotonin, they develop "total insomnia," and soon die.

The serotonin in your brain is especially valuable for helping you achieve the deep, restful sleep that makes you feel energetic and refreshed. This type of deep sleep is called "delta sleep." About one-fourth of your total sleep is delta sleep, and you get most of it relatively early in your night's sleep.

Deep delta sleep is different from rapid-eye-movement sleep, or REM sleep, which occurs when you dream. REM sleep is valuable, but it's quite possible to sleep all night long, have many dreams, and still wake up feeling tired. People commonly describe this type of delta-deprived sleep as "fitful sleep."

One way that serotonin enables you to reach delta sleep is by helping you "turn off" your thoughts and worries. This allows you to sink easily into deep, restorative, delta sleep. When this happens, your brain waves slow down and are dominated by long, "slow" delta waves. These slow delta waves are the opposite of the fast, frenetic alpha waves that you experience while you're awake, and are thinking hard.

Unfortunately, though, some people—particularly those with serotonin deficits—have a hard time turning off their thoughts and worries, even when they're asleep. When they try to slip into deep delta sleep, their brain waves often accelerate into alpha waves. These alpha waves intrude on the delta sleep and ruin its restorative quality. People with this problem can sleep all night long, but wake up feeling tired, irritable, and unrefreshed. Many people with fibromyalgia experience this destructive lack of delta sleep. For some, this occurs practically every night. Sometimes fibromyalgia patients go years without getting a single night of good, deep sleep.

This lack of delta sleep has a terribly negative impact on the ability of patients to withstand pain. It lowers the pain threshold, and makes the patient much less able to launch a strong counterattack against pain.

However, lack of delta sleep also has another very specific, physical effect: *It destroys the health of muscles.* Here's why: One of the important biological functions that occurs during delta sleep is the *repair of muscles.*

You probably weren't aware of it, but every single day you tear and injure your muscles, just by performing your normal, daily activities. The vast majority of these muscle tears are microscopic, and cause virtually no pain. However, these injuries are very real, and can have a cumulative effect if they do not properly heal.

Most people have a wonderfully powerful natural ability to heal these microscopic muscle tears, before the tears cause any noticeable damage, or pain. This repair literally happens overnight.

At night, when you drift into deep delta sleep, you begin to secrete an extremely important hormone called *growth hormone.* Growth hormone is the hormone that enabled you to grow during your childhood—and it is also the hormone that *repairs muscle tissue.* Growth hormone helps muscle tissue to heal the microscopic muscle tears that occur every day. Without sufficient growth hormone, many of these muscle tears do not properly heal.

In addition, growth hormone helps remove the toxic substances from muscles that accumulate during exertion. One of those substances is lactic acid, the chemical that contributes to the soreness in your muscles that you often feel after a hard workout.

Another important function of growth hormone is to help muscles respond favorably to exercise. Growth hormone enables muscles to become toned, and gain strength from exercise. Without a normal supply of growth hormone, muscles grow weak and lax, and exercise tends to just strain and irritate them.

The vast majority of all growth hormone is secreted during delta sleep. If you don't get enough delta sleep, due to a lack of serotonin, you will fail to produce an adequate supply of growth hormone. If this happens to you, you will definitely begin to *feel pain in your muscles.*

In probably the most revealing experiment ever conducted on fibromyalgia, researchers deprived a group of people from reaching delta sleep for three nights in a row. One hundred percent of the group began to suffer from muscle pain symptoms exactly like those of fibromyalgia. When the subjects were again allowed to reach delta sleep, their fibromyalgia symptoms vanished almost immediately.

Similarly, people who have the condition called sleep apnea, a breathing disorder that limits delta sleep, often report symptoms very much like those of fibromyalgia.

Another important study on fibromyalgia showed that patients' pain correlated *directly* to the degree of their sleep impairment.

A number of fibromyalgia patients have tried taking growth hormone injections, to correct their deficiency of it. The response to this treatment has usually been quite favorable. However, growth hormone is extremely expensive, and is usually not covered by insurance policies. Therefore, taking growth hormone is not a practical treatment for fibromyalgia for most people.

A much more practical, comprehensive approach is to boost the patient's level of serotonin. This helps patients to sleep better, and secrete more growth hormone naturally. In addition, restoring serotonin levels helps stop the *other* terrible symptoms that are often associated with fibromyalgia, such as depression, irritable bowel and bladder syndromes, painful menstruation, TMJ pain, anxiety, and poor circulation to the extremities. For the most part, these conditions are *not* helped by growth hormone, only by serotonin.

There are several ways to boost your serotonin level. The mind/body exercises increase serotonin output, and so do certain medications.

Another way to boost your serotonin level is to increase your body's supply of tryptophan, which is, as you may recall, the nutritional "building block" from which serotonin is made. Increasing tryptophan intake is especially important for fibromyalgia patients, because they tend to metabolize tryptophan very poorly. Laboratory tests have shown that most fibromyalgia patients have very low levels of tryptophan in their blood. Some of the most prominent fibromyalgia researchers, including Dr. Muhammad Yunus—the leading fibromyalgia researcher in America—believe that impaired tryptophan metabolism may ultimately trigger fibromyalgia in many patients.

In the following sections, which discuss the treatment of fibromyalgia, I'll tell you how to improve your tryptophan metabolism, and thereby increase your level of serotonin.

Serotonin, though, does even more than help improve sleep, and thus repair muscle tissue. It also has *other* important actions that help prevent and cure the pain of fibromyalgia.

One important action of serotonin is to blunt the effects of substance P, the chemical that promotes the transmission of pain. Fibromyalgia patients generally do not have *enough* serotonin to effectively dampen the effects of substance P. In a study at the University of Alabama, researchers found that fibromyalgia patients had levels of substance P that were three times higher than average. Thus, it was especially easy for these patients' muscle pains to reach their brains.

Another important function of serotonin is to help regulate the immune system. This seems to be especially important for fibromyalgia patients, because many of them appear to have hyperactive immune systems. A hyperactive immune system is characterized by symptoms somewhat similar to those of the flu—a stuffy nose, slight fever, swollen glands, muscle pain, fatigue, and night sweats. These symptoms can shift rapidly and unpredictably.

The immune system tends to become hyperactive when the body produces too many cytokines—chemicals, such as interferon, that stimulate immunity. Cytokine production is normally held in check by serotonin. But when serotonin levels dip, too many cytokines can be produced.

Sometimes, an *illness* can also cause the immune system to become hyperactive, and then stay that way, long after the illness itself is gone. This, too, produces an excess of cytokines, which can then cause symptoms of fibromyalgia. Some patients begin to suffer from fibromyalgia shortly after a bad case of the flu, and others contract fibromyalgia symptoms after a serious systemic infection, such as Lyme disease.

It's possible, I believe, that people with low serotonin levels are especially vulnerable to immune hyperactivity following an illness, because of their inability to dampen cytokine production.

Extreme emotional stress also seems to contribute to the onset of fibromyalgia in some people. No one is sure why this happens, but it might occur because chronic stress can deplete serotonin.

If a serotonin deficit is indeed the most common cause of fibromyalgia, as I believe it is, it may explain why women contract the disorder far more than men. As I've mentioned, women are much more vulnerable than men to fluctuations in their levels of serotonin, because serotonin levels are often destabilized by shifting levels of female hormones, such as estrogen. This hormonal link to fibromyalgia may also explain why women seem especially vulnerable to the disorder during menopause and during their teens; at those times, their hormonal balances are rapidly shifting.

As you can see, the case implicating low levels of serotonin in the causation of fibromyalgia is a strong one.

I'm sure you also noticed that the chain reaction touched off by a serotonin deficit is complicated, and has many variants.

Nonetheless, despite this complexity, many doctors who treat fibromyalgia by simply restoring serotonin levels are having unparalleled success.

Let's now take a look at the various treatments for fibromyalgia. As you'll soon see, most of the best treatments revolve around boosting and stabilizing serotonin levels.

Level One: Nutritional Therapy for Fibromyalgia

Obviously, the most important nutritional therapy for fibromyalgia is to eat nutrients that raise levels of serotonin. I explained how to do this in chapter 2, on nutritional therapy, so *I strongly advise you to review that material,* and put its advice into practice.

As I explained in that chapter, the simplest and most effective way to boost serotonin nutritionally is to take tryptophan supplements. This is especially important for fibromyalgia patients, because most of them appear to have a problem metabolizing tryptophan. Because of this metabolic defect, fibromyalgia patients may require *more* tryptophan than people who have no metabolic deficiency.

At least one study has been done that indicates that the form of tryptophan called 5-HTP can be effective for fibromyalgia. In this study, reported in the *Journal of Internal Medicine Research,* fifty patients with fibromyalgia were given 100 mg of 5-HTP three times daily. Significant improvements were reported in pain intensity, number of tender points, quality of sleep, and fatigue. Approximately 50 percent of the patients reported a fair-to-good response. Some of the patients experienced mild side effects, including drowsiness and diarrhea, but only one patient dropped out of the study because of the side effects.

As I've mentioned, tryptophan supplements are not readily available in the United States. However, a form of tryptophan called 5-HTP is currently available at many health-food stores and is also available from some mail-order supplement companies. You can also get L-tryptophan by prescription from your doctor.

He or she can order it from a compounding pharmacy, which is a type of pharmacy that makes supplements from raw materials.

You can also get tryptophan by ingesting an abundance of foods that are high in it, such as turkey. However, it will be very difficult for you to achieve a high intake of tryptophan from food-stuffs alone.

If you are a fibromyalgia patient, it's very possible that you have a defect in your tryptophan metabolism. However, there are ways to improve your tryptophan metabolism. Some fibromyalgia patients are able to improve their tryptophan metabolisms by taking digestive enzymes. These enzymes help break down protein and the individual amino acids (such as tryptophan) that compose protein. In one revealing study, researchers found that fibromyalgia patients had not only low levels of tryptophan, but also low levels of six other amino acids. This strongly suggests that these patients had a general inability to adequately digest and metabolize protein.

Enzymes that will help you to digest and metabolize protein include papain, bromelain, and chymotrypsin, all of which are available at health-food stores. In addition, most health-food stores sell formulations of combined enzymes that are specifically designed to aid the digestion of protein. I suggest you take one of these formulations every time you eat protein.

Digestion of protein can also be improved by taking the supplement betaine hydrochloride. Chemically similar to your stomach's hydrochloric acid, this supplement helps break down the foods you eat. Betaine hydrochloride supplementation may be especially important for older people because we tend to produce less stomach acid as we age.

Another aid to the digestion and assimilation of protein is the use of full-spectrum vitamin/mineral tablets. Virtually every vitamin and mineral encourages the digestion and metabolism of other nutrients, including protein.

A vitamin that is especially helpful for serotonin metabolism is B_6, which helps convert tryptophan into serotonin. It is also an excellent vitamin for maintaining the health of nerves. To a somewhat lesser extent, the entire B complex of vitamins also improves the metabolism of tryptophan. Because the B complex helps transform tryptophan into the stress-fighting neurotransmitter serotonin, people who don't get enough B vitamins are often very vulnerable to stress.

A more obscure nutrient that also appears to help metabolize tryptophan, and thereby raise levels of serotonin, is pycnogenol, which is available at most health-food stores. Pycnogenol is derived from pine bark, which has been used for many centuries in Asia and Europe as a folk remedy for rheumatism.

Besides nutrients that increase levels of serotonin, other nutrients can help fibromyalgia patients. For the most part, these are nutrients that improve the health of muscles.

Probably the most important of these is magnesium. As I mentioned in the chapter on nutrition, magnesium is vitally important for keeping muscles flexible and loose. In fact, clinical testing has revealed that almost all fibromyalgia patients have a deficiency of magnesium. Muscle tightness is one of the most common symptoms of fibromyalgia; it's possible that this tightness creates a greater demand for magnesium. It's also possible that an *existing* magnesium deficiency may make people more vulnerable to the onset of fibromyalgia.

In addition to keeping muscles supple, magnesium is vitally important in a biochemical activity known as the Krebs cycle, which supplies energy to muscles.

The most revealing signs of a magnesium deficiency are muscle spasms and muscle irritability. If you have fibromyalgia, you may want to have your blood level of magnesium checked. However, this blood test can be misleading, because most magnesium is stored within cells.

I strongly advise all my fibromyalgia patients to take magnesium supplements. A reasonable daily dosage of magnesium for fibromyalgia patients is 300–500 mg daily. For some people, more than 500 mg daily will cause mild diarrhea. If this occurs, reduce the dosage until the symptom goes away.

An excellent way to quickly raise intramuscular levels of magnesium is to administer a combination of nutrients known as a "Meyer's cocktail." This consists of magnesium, calcium, vitamin B complex, and vitamin C. The nutrients are administered with a "slow push" intravenous infusion. Sometimes I add a liver-detoxifying homeopathic medication to the mixture. The only primary side effect I've seen is an occasional feeling of warmth and tingling at the site of the injection, which can be eliminated by slowing down the rate of the IV.

Some of the best food sources of magnesium are chlorophyll-based "green drinks," such as those made from spirulina and blue-green algae. These foods are also a rich source of many micro-nutrients that are not available in more commonly eaten foods.

In one study, magnesium was administered to fibromyalgia patients in conjunction with the nutrient malic acid. Patients were given up to 600 mg of magnesium daily, and up to 2,400 mg of malic acid, which increases energy production in cells. The results were extremely favorable; 100 percent of the patients reported significant relief from pain within forty-eight hours. Some observers of this study felt that the malic acid was even more valuable than the magnesium. You can obtain malic acid from mail-order supplement companies, or from some health-food stores. A reasonable daily dosage of malic acid for fibromyalgia patients is 1,200–2,400 mg.

Another nutrient that enhances the health of muscle tissue is coenzyme Q-10. This nutrient, available at health-food stores, is used by the muscles to produce energy. An appropriate daily dosage for fibromyalgia patients is 100–200 mg.

Creatine monohydrate is a natural amino acid that improves energy production within muscles. This nutrient, widely used by athletes, may help some people with fibromyalgia. I generally recommend that patients begin creatine supplementation by taking approximately 10–15 grams daily for five days, and then taking a maintenance dosage of 5–10 mg per day.

Vanadyl sulfate may help restore muscle strength in some patients. This nutrient, available at health-food stores, improves protein metabolism and increases the absorption of creatine. The daily dosage should be in the range of 30–70 mg.

The minerals selenium and zinc may also be helpful, because they promote healing and growth of muscles. I recommend 50 mg daily of zinc, and 250 mcg daily of selenium.

In addition to these specific nutrients, fibromyalgia patients should try to eat the nutrient-dense, high-energy diet I described in the chapter on nutrition. The only variation from this diet should be an increased emphasis on eating non-acidic foods, because acidic foods, such as citrus fruits and meat, tend to make muscles tighter.

Level Two: Physical Therapies

In my opinion, one of the best physical therapies for fibromyalgia is one that doctors have traditionally advised against: exercise. Until recently, most doctors thought exercise just made the pain of fibromyalgia worse. Now, however, many have reversed their position, and have endorsed the approach that I use: moderate exercise on a daily basis.

Furthermore, the mind/body exercises appear to be even more valuable than standard aerobic exercise for fibromyalgia patients.

For mind/body exercises designed especially for fibromyalgia patients, see Appendix I.

Exercise is helpful because it increases serotonin output. Mind/body exercises are even better for increasing serotonin. Part of the reason you feel more relaxed after you exercise, or do mind/body exercises, is that exercise increases your level of serotonin. The much-discussed phenomenon of "runner's high"—which is usually ascribed to endorphin release—is actually more a result of the release of serotonin and its fellow "feel-good" neurotransmitter norepinephrine. Endorphins are great for killing pain, but, contrary to conventional wisdom, they really don't have much of a direct effect upon the mind.

In addition to boosting serotonin, exercise also directly increases levels of growth hormone. Besides deep sleep, the best creator of growth hormone is exercise.

Fibromyalgia patients should engage in the basic exercise program I outlined in the chapter on physical therapies. This program stresses all four of the most basic forms of exercise: (1) stretching, (2) cardiovascular exertion, (3) strength building, and (4) linking the mind and body. For fibromyalgia patients, each of these three basic forms of exercise is indispensable. Stretching will help relieve tightness in muscles, and prevent muscles from pulling against painful tender points. Cardiovascular exertion will boost levels of serotonin, growth hormone, and endorphins, and will increase blood circulation to muscles. Increased blood flow will improve the metabolism of muscles, speeding the intake of nutrients and oxygen, and aiding the exit of toxins and metabolic waste. Strength-building exercises will make muscles notably more resistant to the minor muscle tears that appear to cause much of the pain of fibromyalgia. Linking the mind and body (with mind/body exercises) will increase serotonin levels, boost mental energy, induce relaxation, and improve the brain's counterattack against pain.

Although I advise my fibromyalgia patients to engage in the same basic exercise program as other pain patients, most fibromyalgia patients must begin with a very mild program and gradually build intensity. When fibromyalgia patients do too much, too quickly, they can suffer from extreme pain and stiffness.

Fibromyalgia patients should not participate in exercise unless they are also engaging in all of the other three levels of my pain program. Those other levels will help protect them from pain and stiffness, and will enable their bodies to derive maximum benefit from exercise.

Another physical therapy that has helped many of my fibromyalgia patients is acupuncture. Interestingly, most of the eighteen classic tender points correlate closely to acupuncture points that are related to pain. Some fibromyalgia patients derive benefit from applying acupressure to tender points, but most seem to respond much better to acupuncture.

In one study done on the use of acupuncture for fibromyalgia, the overwhelming majority of patients receiving acupuncture reported less morning stiffness, less pain, and better sleep. A control group of patients, who were given sham acupuncture treatments that consisted of shallow needle insertions, showed no improvement.

Light therapy can also be very valuable for many fibromyalgia patients. As I explained in chapter 3, people who are not exposed to enough light often develop low levels of serotonin. Light is necessary to help the body switch from nighttime melatonin production to daytime serotonin production. Women in particular need adequate levels of light, because their levels of serotonin often become depleted by hormonal fluctuations. For more information, please review the material on light therapy in chapter 3.

Another valid physical therapy for fibromyalgia is use of heat and cold treatments. As explained previously, heat and cold sensations "outrun" pain signals in the "race" to the brain, and thereby block the perception of pain. This temporary blockage of pain often breaks the recurring cycle of pain. In addition, temporary pain blockage can allow muscle spasms to relax.

Many fibromyalgia patients use heat and cold therapies before and after exercising. This optimizes the benefits of exercise, and decreases the strain. Sometimes, just before they exercise, patients spray a vapocoolant, such as ethyl chloride, on their tender points. This desensitizes the tender points, and allows greater range of motion.

Occasionally, patients using heat therapy are helped by ultrasound treatment, which effectively applies heat to deep muscles, far beneath the surface of the skin. For details on heat-and-cold therapy, please review the relevant material in chapter 3.

Two other physical therapies that can be valuable for fibromyalgia patients are manipulation therapy and massage. Many of my fibromyalgia patients regularly see chiropractors or osteopaths, and report that the adjustments they receive considerably decrease their degree of pain and stiffness. Similarly, many patients derive much relief from therapeutic massage. If you have fibromyalgia, you should reread the information on manipulation therapy and massage in chapter 3.

Level Three: Medications for Fibromyalgia

The most effective medications for fibromyalgia are those that increase levels of serotonin. This includes tricyclic antidepressants, such as Elavil, and selective serotonin reuptake inhibitors, such as Prozac. Of these two classes of drugs, tricyclic antidepressants have a longer history of use, and are still more commonly used. However, selective serotonin reuptake inhibitors, or SSRIs, may eventually prove to be the most effective medications for fibromyalgia, because they are the most powerful drugs for increasing levels of serotonin.

Studies show that tricyclic antidepressants help approximately 30 to 60 percent of fibromyalgia patients to experience less pain and less depression.

When antidepressants raise serotonin levels, they help patients reach deep sleep by stopping the intrusion of alpha waves into delta sleep. When this occurs, patients produce more growth hormone, which heals muscles. In addition, an enhanced level of serotonin reduces the activity of pain-carrying substance P. It also helps stop immune system hyperactivity. Furthermore, boosting serotonin prevents many of the terrible secondary symptoms of fibromyalgia, such as anxiety, poor circulation to the extremities, headaches, and irritable bowel syndrome.

As I mentioned, the dosage of tricyclic antidepressants is lower for the treatment of fibromyalgia than for depression. Fibromyalgia patients may require only about 10–40 mg daily, compared with a dosage of 150–200 mg daily that is prescribed for depression.

Only a limited amount of research has been done on the use of SSRIs, such as Prozac, for fibromyalgia. However, the early evidence, most of which is anecdotal, indicates that SSRIs may soon become a very common treatment. Patients tend to respond well to SSRIs, without suffering excessive side effects. In one study done on Prozac and fibromyalgia, researchers at the Tufts University School of Medicine found that the majority of fibromyalgia patients taking Prozac experienced significant improvement in symptoms. Furthermore, patients tended to fare even better when they took both Prozac and a tricyclic antidepressant.

If you have fibromyalgia, I recommend that you discuss Prozac, and other SSRI medications, with your doctor, or with a rheumatologist.

It appears that a moderate dosage of Prozac, in the range of 20 mg daily, is appropriate for most fibromyalgia patients. If this dosage has no benefit, discuss the possibility of a higher dosage with your physician.

In the past, many doctors treated fibromyalgia with benzodiazepines, such as Valium or Xanax. Recently, however, this treatment has become markedly less popular. This approach can be moderately helpful for overcoming acute muscle spasms and severe sleep disorders, but benzodiazepines tend to suppress delta sleep. Therefore, many patients have reported that benzodiazepines actually made their fibromyalgia worse. Furthermore, these drugs can be addictive, so I generally prescribe them very sparingly.

Other drugs that are generally inappropriate for fibromyalgia are the nonsteroidal anti-inflammatory drugs, or NSAIDs. NSAIDs are primarily valuable for fighting inflammation, but fibromyalgia produces little inflammation. Also, NSAIDs can be dangerous when they are overused. Furthermore, NSAIDs can disrupt sleep by increasing the proportion of time a person spends in alpha-level sleep. Nonetheless, on occasion, a fibromyalgia patient may gain temporary relief from pain with NSAIDs, because they are analgesic drugs, as well as anti-inflammatory drugs. For analgesia, though, patients often do better with acetaminophen, because it has somewhat fewer side effects.

Similarly, steroidal anti-inflammatory drugs, such as corticosteroids, are also of little value in treating fibromyalgia. These drugs have many serious side effects, and should generally be avoided by fibromyalgia patients.

Narcotic analgesics offer temporary relief from pain, but they are highly addictive, and are therefore not appropriate for long-term treatment of fibromyalgia.

A drug treatment that is sometimes helpful is injection of tender points with a local anesthetic or a homeopathic remedy. This temporary solution can disrupt the cycle of pain very effectively. Therefore, its benefits sometimes last long after the local anesthetic has worn off; sometimes, patients remain free of pain for several months. As a rule, though, the effects last only a few hours or days. The injections can be painful, so this is not a practical treatment for most patients.

Muscle relaxants have shown limited ability to decrease pain and improve sleep, but they tend to have no effect on stiffness. For the most part, I do not prescribe them.

Two hormones can also help fibromyalgia patients. DHEA, taken orally, has helped reduce fibromyalgia symptoms in some patients. It helps regulate immunity, and can enable the body to overcome immune hyperactivity. DHEA can also decrease rheumatic joint pain, which is occasionally associated with fibromyalgia. In addition, DHEA is a general "re-youthing" hormone that helps increase energy, improve mood, and protect the body from gradual degeneration. Unfortunately, DHEA levels decline as we age. To determine your dosage of DHEA, you should have your current level checked. Your doctor can do this with a standard laboratory test. Then you should take enough DHEA in supplement form to restore your DHEA level to the same level as that of a healthy person in his or her twenties—which is when DHEA levels peak. You may find that you'll need to take as little as 25 mg or as much as 200 mg daily. The 200-mg dosage would be the amount needed by an elderly person who was producing almost no DHEA naturally.

DHEA is now readily available in health-food stores and pharmacies, but I advise that you take it only under the care of a physician. Before you begin taking DHEA, you should get a complete biochemical profile, including a test of liver function. Men should also get the prostate screening procedure called the PSA blood test, and have their prostate examined. If the prostate is enlarged, DHEA can exacerbate the problem. If you do happen to have an enlarged prostate, or suffer from any of the symptoms of prostate deterioration—such as frequent nighttime urination—I recommend that you take approximately 160 mg of saw palmetto twice daily. This herb can be extremely valuable for promoting prostate health.

Another hormone that can be very beneficial for fibromyalgia patients is melatonin. As I explained in chapter 4, melatonin is a very effective sleep aid. It is the hormone the body naturally produces to achieve sleep. Because poor sleep appears to trigger fibromyalgia indirectly, anything that can improve sleep may be very valuable for fibromyalgia patients. I usually advise patients to begin melatonin supplementation by taking 1–3 mg each night. However, if a patient has severe insomnia—as do many fibromyalgia patients—a higher dosage may be necessary.

Another effective sleep aid is tryptophan. When tryptophan supplements were readily available as an over-the-counter product, they were primarily used as a sleep aid. Fibromyalgia patients should take most of their daily tryptophan dosage in the evening, to promote sleep.

Several homeopathic remedies are particularly effective for muscle pain. A number of these can help the nervous system resist *any* kind of pain, including muscle pain. I recommend that you review the material on homeopathy, in chapter 4.

My own fibromyalgia patients seem to respond well to the following homeopathic medications:

- *Rhus tox* 6x. Two pills every hour will reduce muscle pain, and help connective tissue to heal. It also decreases morning stiffness.

- *Hypericum* 6x is especially valuable for soothing nerves that have become sensitized by pain.

• *Apis* 12x helps reduce the sensation of swelling that some fibromyalgia patients experience. Other medications that reduce swelling are *Bryonia* and *Ledum.*

• *Arnica* 6x. This powerful analgesic medication is helpful for most types of pain.

• *Symphytum* can help relax deep muscle tissue.

Several herbs can help quell the symptoms of fibromyalgia. One is ginseng, the herb that "tones" the function of the adrenal glands, making the glands more responsive to your shifting needs for quick energy. When the adrenal glands are sluggish, the body often compensates by secreting the strong, stimulating hormone cortisol, which frequently triggers insomnia.

Any of the calming and nerve-soothing herbs that I described in chapter 4 can also help fibromyalgia patients. If you have fibromyalgia, you should review that material.

Level Four: Mental and Spiritual Pain Control for Fibromyalgia

There are no mental or spiritual pain control techniques that apply *only* to fibromyalgia. The best mental and spiritual pain control techniques are effective for *all* forms of chronic pain. Review the material I outlined in chapter 5. The material in that chapter is almost sure to help reduce your pain and restore your sense of control over your life.

If you have fibromyalgia, you should be aware that your mind and spirit have been, in all probability, profoundly affected by your condition. Consider the following statistics:

• Approximately one-third of all fibromyalgia patients have a serious psychological disturbance.

• Approximately one-third of all fibromyalgia patients suffer from chronic pain syndrome.

• An estimated 5 to 6 percent of fibromyalgia patients have symptoms of obsessive-compulsive disorder.

• Approximately 25 percent of fibromyalgia patients experience symptoms similar to those of clinical depression.

For years, many doctors believed that fibromyalgia was caused by mental instability. Some doctors speculated that fibromyalgia was caused by having a rigid, anxious personality. Other doctors tried to classify fibromyalgia pain as a symptom of clinical depression. Recent studies, though, indicate that fibromyalgia is *not* caused by the mind.

A far more sensible explanation, in my opinion, is that the same serotonin deficit that indirectly creates muscle pain also causes depression, anxiety, and obsessive-compulsive disorder in some patients.

Anecdotal evidence, and at least one clinical study, indicates that when serotonin levels are restored to normal, psychological problems and muscle pain *both* improve, but this phenomenon has not yet been proven by extensive clinical studies.

It does appear, though, that fibromyalgia pain is often *aggravated* by stress. It's quite possible that this occurs in part because stress further depletes levels of serotonin. Because of this phenomenon, it's extremely important for fibromyalgia patients to engage in stress-reduction techniques—especially meditation, and the "Wake Up to Wellness" routine.

When stress does occur, it can heighten the pain of fibromyalgia, which then adds even *more* stress. Thus, a destructive spiral of stress/pain/stress can be created.

If you have fibromyalgia, I strongly recommend that you carefully review chapter 5, on the mental and spiritual control of pain.

10

Curing Pain Caused by Other Common Conditions

The best way out is always through.
—ROBERT FROST

Please note that although this chapter contains information about various pain conditions, this material does not replace the previous information about my pain program. Patients with the conditions mentioned in this chapter should follow the complete pain program described in chapters 2–5, as well as the advice in this chapter.

Cancer Pain

The treatment of cancer pain is one of the worst failures of modern medicine. Millions of people suffer terrible pain that could easily be avoided.

Sadly, most doctors—including most cancer specialists—don't know how to properly treat cancer pain. They don't prescribe enough medication, use the right types of medications, or administer medications on an effective schedule. Most doctors who specialize in cancer don't even have an adequate education in pain management.

For the most part, cancer specialists realize that their treatment of cancer pain is often inadequate. In a survey of more than one thousand American cancer specialists, or oncologists, only half the doctors rated their own hospital's or clinic's pain management program as good or very good. In the same survey, only 11 percent of the oncologists recalled having received any training in pain management while in medical school. Almost none of the oncologists used any of the powerful pain-control techniques of integrative medicine, even though 85 percent of those doctors said that they thought cancer pain was generally undermedicated.

Unfortunately, many doctors still cling to myths about the drugs that are used to fight cancer pain, and these myths cause great suffering. Here are the two primary myths that are now causing millions of cancer patients to experience excruciating pain:

MYTH NO. I. Cancer patients face a high risk of addiction to painkillers. This myth exists because many doctors don't fully understand the difference between addiction, dependence, and tolerance.

Addiction is a psychological craving for a drug. This craving becomes the focus of the addict's life. Even after all withdrawal symptoms cease, the addict still craves the drug.

Dependence occurs when a patient's body becomes accustomed to a drug. If the drug is suddenly withdrawn, uncomfortable physical withdrawal symptoms occur. However, physical dependence can almost always be overcome simply by withdrawing drugs gradually.

Tolerance means that larger dosages are needed as time passes. In almost every situation, however, larger dosages can be safely administered.

Virtually every cancer patient who uses the common painkiller morphine develops tolerance and dependence. These two conditions are natural, and are essentially harmless. When the morphine is no longer needed, the tolerance and dependence are virtually always overcome, quickly and safely.

Cancer patients almost never become addicted to morphine. In one review of twelve thousand patients on morphine, almost all the patients developed tolerance and dependence. However, only one-tenth of 1 percent of patients became addicted. The other 99.9 percent had no psychological craving, and never used morphine just to achieve a drug high.

Most pain patients don't even experience a drug high when they take morphine. The same dosage that causes euphoria in drug addicts causes a person in severe pain merely to feel normal and comfortable.

Despite the clear evidence that addiction to painkillers is extremely rare among cancer patients, many doctors and nurses still believe the myth that patients can easily become addicted. In one study, approximately one-third of two thousand registered nurses said they believed that the risk of addiction to morphine was 25 percent or more (instead of one-tenth of 1 percent).

In another study, nurses—who are usually in charge of administering medication—administered an average of only 25 percent of the pain medication that doctors had prescribed. They did this because they believed addiction was a major risk.

MYTH NO. 2. If morphine is used for too long, it will stop working. Most people, including many doctors, think that heavy use of morphine will eventually block the drug's effectiveness.

This phenomenon, known as the "ceiling effect," does apply to some drugs, but it does *not* apply to morphine or to the other opioids that are used to treat cancer pain.

In fact, some patients begin treatment with a dosage of 30 mg of morphine daily, and eventually need several thousand milligrams every day. Even though this is a drastic increase, this high dosage can still be administered easily and safely, with no significant increase in side effects. As patients build tolerance to a drug, they also build tolerance to the drug's ability to create side effects.

Because doctors often believe in the myth of the ceiling effect for opioids, they frequently fail to prescribe enough morphine. Instead they withhold morphine, fearing that if they don't, they won't be able to control pain when it becomes most severe. In one study, 60 percent of doctors refused to prescribe enough morphine to fully stop pain, unless the patient had less than six months to live. This is a tragic and glaring clinical error that results in needless torture.

Most *patients* also believe the myth of the ceiling effect for opioids, so they tend to not take their full dosage of pain medication. It has been estimated that as many as half of all patients with cancer pain don't take the full amount of pain medication that is prescribed to them.

Because of these two myths, most cancer patients do not receive adequate treatment for their pain, even when it becomes horribly severe.

As a result of the poor treatment of cancer pain, an estimated 50 to 80 percent of all cancer patients in America suffer unnecessarily.

Unfortunately, pain is one of the most common symptoms of cancer. Approximately 33 percent of cancer patients in the early stages of the disease are in pain, and about 80 percent of patients in the late stages of cancer are in pain. This pain not only destroys their quality of life, but can even contribute to the destruction of life itself. Medical experiments indicate that tumors grow much faster when pain is present. In short, pain kills.

The good news, however, is that relief from cancer pain is possible in 90 to 99 percent of all cases. All that is required is proper treatment. About 85 percent of all patients require only simple medical treatments, including administration of morphine. Almost all of the remaining 15 percent of patients can also be relieved of pain, with the application of somewhat more complex treatments.

Therefore, if you or someone you love has cancer pain, I strongly urge you to find a doctor who can relieve this pain. It may be necessary for you to consult a pain specialist. However, you should *not* passively accept the idea that suffering is inevitable. You *can* be helped—but you may need to actively *seek* that help.

Dr. Charles Schuster, the former head of the National Institute on Drug Abuse, has stated that "the way we treat cancer pain borders on a national disgrace."

Don't allow yourself to be part of that disgrace.

WHY CANCER HURTS

About 75 percent of all cancer pain is caused by the growth of malignant tumors, and about 25 percent is caused by the therapies used to treat those tumors.

Tumors, by themselves, don't hurt, but cause pain when they invade healthy tissues.

The most common pain caused by the invasion of healthy tissues is pain in bones. Many types of cancer eventually spread to bones, and cause a dull ache.

The second most common pain caused by the invasion of healthy tissues is pain in nerves. As tumors grow, they press against nerves, causing a sharp, tingling, constant pain. This occurs in 20 to 40 percent of all patients.

Pain caused by invading tumors also occurs in blood vessels, in the lymphatic system, and in hollow organs, such as those of the gastrointestinal tract. When tumors block blood vessels, lymph ducts, or the intestines, they can cause intense pressure and pain.

Muscles can also be invaded. When this happens, it can feel like an unending muscle cramp.

The other primary source of cancer pain—cancer therapy itself—is also very common.

Some surgeries, including those of the neck, chest, and breast, can cause lasting pain, even after the surgeries have healed. This pain is most commonly caused by nerves that have been damaged by the surgery. One form of nerve pain is the "phantom limb" pain caused by amputations.

Some forms of chemotherapy also cause nerve pain. The two

most troublesome chemotherapy drugs, for many patients, are vincristine and vinblastine. Often the pain caused by chemotherapy is first noticed in the jaw, or the hands and feet. Chemotherapy also causes painful mouth sores, especially when it is combined with radiation. It's well known that chemotherapy can also cause terrible bouts of nausea.

Radiation can injure the skin and nerves, and can cause bleeding and diarrhea. The spinal cord is particularly vulnerable to radiation, and can cause pain that shoots throughout the lower half of the body. Radiation also commonly causes extreme fatigue.

There are, however, certain cancer therapies that do not cause pain. For the most part, these are immunotherapies—therapies that stimulate the body's own immune system to fight cancer. Some immunotherapies are considered conventional, and some are considered experimental. For example, there are experimental therapies that boost natural immunity with nutritional therapy, supplements, detoxification, and stress management. These therapies are controversial, but some appear to be promising. For information about them, please contact the Cancer Control Society, at the address listed in Appendix III.

The Proper Treatment of Cancer Pain

A proper pain management program for cancer is most commonly centered around medications that escalate in power.

The first level of medication is composed of aspirin, acetaminophen, and nonsteroidal anti-inflammatory drugs, such as ibuprofen. These drugs can stop mild pain, and can often control even severe pain, when taken on a careful schedule. For maximum efficiency they should be taken every four hours, even if no pain is present at the time of administration. Pain from the invasion of bones responds particularly well to these drugs. Furthermore, these drugs can amplify the relief provided by more powerful drugs. They work differently from opioids, so a combination of NSAIDs and mild opioids is often much more powerful than opioids alone.

The next level of medication consists of mild opioids, including codeine, oxycodone (Percodan), and dextropropoxyphene (Darvon). These drugs are usually combined with NSAIDs or acetaminophen. Mild opioids can be effective in the early stages of cancer, but many doctors tend to depend upon them for too long, after the pain has become more severe.

The third and final level of medication consists of morphine and drugs like morphine, such as fentanyl, methadone, and hydromorphone.

Morphine administration may begin at a relatively low dosage, such as 30 mg daily, but should then be steadily increased as tolerance increases, and as pain becomes more severe. It is extremely important that the dosage level be increased regularly, in response to increased need. The biggest mistake most doctors make is simply failing to increase morphine dosages when necessary. Doctors who believe in the two primary myths about morphine are usually reluctant to increase dosages to the proper level. If your doctor subscribes to these myths, I urge you to see a pain specialist, who will consult with your oncologist and make sure you are receiving adequate pain treatment.

It's also vitally important that you do not believe in these two myths yourself, so that you do not subvert your own pain therapy. Take your full dosage of pain medication, and tell your doctor if you are not achieving sufficient relief from pain. Many patients try to be stoic about their pain, as if suffering in and of itself has moral value. It does not.

In addition, you should be careful to take your medication on schedule. Many doctors do not stress the importance of adhering to a proper schedule, and this often results in unnecessary pain. A good pain program should provide around-the-clock relief. To achieve this, the program will probably consist of drugs that have a long-lasting effect, combined with fast-acting drugs that relieve the temporary increases in pain known as "breakthrough pain."

A particularly effective form of treatment for breakthrough

pain, and for pain in general, is "patient-controlled analgesia." In this treatment, the patients themselves decide when to administer preset dosages. When this was introduced in the 1980s, many doctors feared that patients would take too much medication. This rarely occurs; in fact, patients tend to take less medication, probably because they feel more in control of the situation. Therefore, this form of treatment is becoming increasingly popular.

When morphine and similar drugs fail to control pain, more complex treatments can generally help. These include anesthetic injections, nerve blocks, and surgeries that inhibit nerve transmission. For more information on these procedures, review chapters 2 through 5.

In addition to these conventional treatments for cancer pain, most patients can also derive great benefit from many of the procedures I use in my general pain program. Nutritional therapy, stress management, and various physical therapies can have a profound impact upon cancer pain. In most cases, though, such therapies must be combined with a medication program.

Treatments that slow tumor growth can also help relieve pain. Doctors frequently use surgery, chemotherapy, and radiation to shrink tumors—and relieve pain—even when the patient is not expected to recover.

Sometimes, late-stage terminal patients begin to suffer from pain that cannot be readily overcome, even with a very aggressive pain program. When this sad stage arrives, patients often ask for very high dosages of powerful drugs, which may cause the patient to sleep around the clock, until death comes. In some cases this sedation hastens death somewhat. In my opinion, accepting the patient's wishes, and prescribing these drugs, is the only humane course of action. For me, this is a much more acceptable approach than assisting a patient's suicide.

Patients should realize, though, that sudden remissions do sometimes occur, even in what appear to be the most hopeless situations. This seems to happen somewhat more often when patients are using nontoxic, immunologic therapies, such as the experimental therapies I described. The immunologic therapies do not injure the body, and they therefore appear to allow for a greater possibility of spontaneous remission.

Also, the immunologic therapies rely on the body's own power to heal, and sometimes this power has a greater potential for miraculous healing than even the best technological therapies.

In any case, I always encourage patients never to abandon hope. As I've said before, where there is life, there is hope.

Irritable Bowel Syndrome

This pain disorder of the gastrointestinal tract is far more common than most people realize. Up to 10 percent of the American adult population suffers from it, occasionally or chronically. It's been estimated that more than one-third of all patients who visit a gastrointestinal specialty clinic suffer from irritable bowel syndrome, or IBS. However, many people who have IBS rarely speak about it, because of embarrassment about its symptoms.

There are three basic types of IBS. One type is characterized by frequent diarrhea, without pain. Another type is characterized by pain and constipation. The third type combines the characteristics of the other two types.

There is no clear physical cause of IBS. Therefore, the only way it can be diagnosed is by a physician excluding other disorders that have similar symptoms.

IBS was first mentioned in the medical literature in 1817, but no real progress has been made in treating or preventing it. In fact, incidence of the disorder appears to be increasing.

Because it is a disorder of digestion and elimination, most of the treatments for IBS involve modification of the diet. Patients are advised, for example, to avoid certain irritating foods, such as fat, and to increase their intake of fiber.

However, I think it's possible that there may be an underlying biochemical factor that contributes to IBS: a deficit of serotonin.

There are several fascinating links between IBS and other disorders that are associated with a deficit of serotonin.

One serotonin-related disorder that is closely linked to IBS is fibromyalgia. As I mentioned in the chapter on fibromyalgia, the leading theory on the cause of fibromyalgia is that it is triggered by a serotonin deficit. There is a significant crossover between IBS patients and fibromyalgia patients. One study, reported in the *Journal of Rheumatology*, showed that 70 percent of fibromyalgia patients had IBS, and 65 percent of IBS patients had fibromyalgia.

Two other problems that are also associated with a serotonin deficit—depression and anxiety—are also very common among IBS patients. It appears that these mood disorders usually exist independently from IBS, and are usually not a direct result of the suffering caused by IBS.

Furthermore, in most IBS patients, stress is one of the most potent *triggers* of symptoms. Up to 80 percent of all IBS patients suffer from its symptoms when they are under stress.

Premenstrual syndrome, another disorder that is often characterized by a deficit of serotonin, also can contribute to IBS symptoms. IBS symptoms are often much more severe for women during menstruation. Furthermore, in a study of 233 females, 34 percent of women who did *not* have IBS reported that during their menstrual periods they suffered from some of the same bowel symptoms that characterize IBS.

Other problems that are sometimes caused by a serotonin deficit—including headaches, and a craving for sweets—also are frequently experienced by IBS patients.

It's not entirely clear why a serotonin deficit would contribute to IBS, but it is known that a serotonin deficit contributes to stress, and that the organs of digestion and elimination do not function effectively under stress. When a person experiences stress, blood flow is automatically shifted away from the organs of digestion and elimination (which causes the sensation of "butterflies in the stomach"). This aspect of the stress response is helpful for survival—because it shifts blood to the "fight or flight" parts of the body, such as the arms and legs—but it makes the stomach and intestines function far less efficiently.

In addition, muscle tension that occurs during stress—particularly tension of the bowel muscles—also interferes with digestion and elimination.

Therefore, I think it's possible that a serotonin deficit—which *increases* stress, and is also *increased by* stress—indirectly contributes to a malfunction of the organs of digestion and elimination.

When the malfunction occurs, it's much more difficult to digest foods—especially foods that are hard to digest even under favorable conditions, such as fat.

Under favorable conditions, food passes through the stomach and intestines in an orderly and rhythmical fashion. When food reaches the large intestine, or colon, rhythmical contractions of the bowel muscle carry it along. However, when digestion is disturbed, these contractions are disrupted. Instead of contracting rhythmically, the muscles of the bowel spasm and cramp, creating pain, bloating, constipation, gas, and diarrhea. Most people have these symptoms occasionally—especially during times of high stress—but when they happen repeatedly, they indicate IBS.

Because I think that a serotonin deficit may be an indirect contributor to IBS, I advise all IBS patients to try to maintain stable high levels of serotonin. To learn how to do this, review the information on it in the chapters on my comprehensive pain program.

Some IBS patients have been treated with serotonin-boosting therapies, but the results have been inconclusive. Nonetheless, I think this approach is very promising.

The other way to help control the symptoms of IBS is to improve the general digestive process. This can be done by avoiding foods that are hard to digest, by eating certain nutrients that improve digestion, and by avoiding stress.

Many of the foods that should be avoided are foods that trigger food allergies, or food sensitivities. These foods are not properly broken down by the digestive system, and appear to disrupt the natural rhythmical contractions of the bowel, especially during times of stress.

The most frequent food trigger of IBS symptoms is milk, and other dairy products. Many people are allergic to, or sensitive to, the lactose in dairy products. Milk is especially hard for many older people to digest, because as we age, we tend to secrete less of the enzyme that breaks down lactose (lactase). Your doctor can give you a test to determine whether you have a lactose intolerance. If you do, and if you also have symptoms of IBS, you should definitely avoid dairy products.

It's possible, though, that you may have only a mild sensitivity to lactose, which may not show up in a lactose intolerance test. Therefore it's wise for all IBS patients to eliminate dairy products temporarily, to see if this helps control symptoms.

Also, some IBS patients feel better when they take supplements containing the digestive enzyme lactase. You can find this enzyme at health-food stores.

If you do eliminate dairy products from your diet, I recommend that you take at least 1,000 to 1,500 mg of calcium every day.

The second most frequent dietary trigger of IBS symptoms is fat. Animal fat seems to be a worse offender in this regard than vegetable oils. One reason fat contributes to IBS symptoms is that it stimulates the release of a hormone called cholecystokin, which causes contractions of the colon.

Also, fat does not mix well in the intestines with other nonfat, water-soluble foods, simply because oil and water don't readily mix. When foods fail to mix properly in the intestines, they disturb the intestine's rhythmical contractions.

The other most common dietary triggers of IBS symptoms are sugar (particularly fructose, or fruit sugar), citrus fruits, and cruciferous vegetables (such as broccoli and cauliflower). These foods tend to irritate the colon, particularly if they are not broken down well by digestive enzymes. Another common trigger is caffeine, which stimulates contractions of the colon.

However, a wide variety of foods may trigger symptoms in various patients. Therefore, I generally advise IBS patients to go on a brief elimination diet, eating only a small number of bland foods at first, and then adding foods one at a time. When particular foods provoke IBS symptoms, they should be permanently avoided.

It's also wise for IBS patients to eat a diet that's high in fiber, because fiber is extremely helpful for moving foods through the intestines. However, a gross excess of fiber can sometimes make IBS symptoms worse.

In addition to avoiding foods that trigger symptoms, IBS patients should also eat particular nutrients that improve digestion. One of the best dietary aids to digestion is yogurt that contains live lactobacillus cultures. These cultures help break down food in the intestines.

Also, peppermint oil and ginger root promote bowel health, by relaxing the smooth muscles of the bowel. This helps prevent cramps. Both of these natural antispasmodics may be purchased as supplements in health-food stores.

Another supplement that often helps is psyllium seeds, which are sold in capsules. These seeds are an excellent source of fiber.

Digestive enzymes also help some IBS patients. These include chymotrypsin, trypsin, and protease (which breaks down protein), amylase (which breaks down starch), and lipase (which breaks down fat). Supplements containing betaine hydrochloride can also improve digestion. The digestion of beans and cruciferous vegetables can be improved by taking a digestive enzyme with the trade name "Beano." Almost all health-food stores sell digestive enzymes. Many people find it easiest to buy a digestive enzyme formulation that contains a variety of enzymes.

In addition to nutritional therapy, certain medications help many IBS patients.

Probably the most effective medications for IBS patients are antidepressants. These drugs, which increase levels of serotonin, have been shown in studies to improve symptoms in a majority of patients. The most commonly used antidepressants are the tricyclic antidepressants, such as amitryptiline. However, the newer selective serotonin reuptake inhibitors, such as Prozac, may eventually prove to be even more effective than tricyclics, because they tend to have a stronger action.

Occasionally, some patients are helped by antispasmodic drugs, which relax the smooth muscles of the bowel, but these drugs have a number of side effects, and are not effective for many patients.

For severe episodes of diarrhea, patients sometimes use mild opioids, which decrease the contractions of the bowel. Opioids, however, should almost never be used on a regular basis. I rarely recommend them.

Some IBS patients occasionally use anti-anxiety drugs, such as Valium. These drugs do sometimes make patients feel better, and experience less stress, but they have only an indirect effect upon IBS. These drugs can be habit forming, though, so I tend not to prescribe them.

Another group of medications that helps some IBS patients are the bile-acid sequestrants, which are commonly used to treat high cholesterol. These drugs seem to help IBS patients whose primary problem is diarrhea. They also help IBS patients who have had their gallbladders removed; after gallbladder surgery, the digestion of fats can become more difficult.

A final medication that is sometimes helpful is the over-the-counter medicine simethicone. Simethicone can help relieve the pain and bloating caused by gas.

A physical therapy that may help patients with IBS is light therapy, which can significantly boost serotonin levels. For more information on light therapy, see chapter 3.

In addition to these therapies, IBS patients should follow my general pain program. Many of the modalities in the general program, including medical acupuncture, will help relieve pain. For IBS patients, the mental and spiritual pain-control techniques are especially important because they help relieve stress, and this alone often prevents the symptoms of IBS.

Carpal Tunnel Syndrome

The carpal tunnel is a narrow channel in the wrist. Traveling through this channel are the tendons, ligaments, and nerves that service the hand.

When people use their hands too much—especially in a single, repetitive motion—their tendons can swell and press against the major nerve that goes to the hand (the median nerve). When this happens, the nerve hurts. If this happens over a long period, the nerve can deteriorate. At that point, pain can become almost constant, and coordination in the hand can become impaired.

Currently, many people suffer from carpal tunnel syndrome, or CTS, because they must make many job-related repetitive movements, which causes their tendons to swell. For example, an assembly-line worker may make 25,000 repetitive movements each day.

The most damaging types of movements are those that cause the hand to bend most of the way back, or most of the way forward. These movements are harmful because they not only cause the tendons to swell, but also cause the carpal tunnel to be squeezed into a narrower shape.

The first symptoms of CTS are numbness and tingling in the fingers. This is followed by pain, which gradually increases during the middle stages of the disorder. The final symptoms include numbness, almost constant pain, and loss of coordination.

If you think you are developing CTS, you should deal with the problem *immediately*; early treatment is by far the best approach. When the problem is addressed in its early stages, complete recovery is likely, without difficult treatment. If treatment is delayed, CTS can require surgery. If the surgery is not successful, CTS can become irreversible.

Several tests are commonly used to diagnose CTS. One is very simple, and can be performed by patients themselves. This test is called Phalen's test, or the wrist flexion test. To do it, bend both your hands all the way forward, and then put the backs of your fingers together, with your fingers pointing down. Hold your hands together gently for about a minute. If you feel pain, tingling, or numbness, you may have CTS, and should consult a doctor immediately.

Your doctor will probably give you further tests, including Tinel's test. In this test, your doctor will tap your inner wrist, directly over your median nerve. If you feel any pain, numbness, or tingling, it's an indication of possible CTS.

Your doctor may also perform other tests that measure the sensitivity of your fingers. Your doctor may also order an X ray, a CAT scan, or an MRI.

If you do have symptoms of CTS, there are physical therapies, nutritional therapies, and medications that may help. As a last resort, surgery may be necessary.

The most important modalities for CTS are physical therapies, because CTS is primarily a mechanical problem rather than a biochemical one.

One of the best things you can do is to simply stop making the repetitive movements that caused the problem. In many early cases of CTS, this alone will solve the problem. However, this is a difficult option for many people, because it may involve changing jobs. Before you rule out this option, though, consider the serious consequences you face if you allow your CTS to continue. If your decision to stick with your job causes you to ultimately spend the rest of your life in incurable pain, you will undoubtedly regret your decision.

If you cannot readily change jobs, the next best option is to rest your hand from the aggravating movement as much as you possibly can. This will help heal your injured median nerve. If you cannot take a sick leave to heal the injury, you should take frequent breaks from the pain-causing movement. These breaks will reduce the swelling in your tendons.

Another excellent option is to wear a wrist splint that will partly immobilize your wrist, and keep it from flexing all the way backward or forward. Wrist splints can usually be worn at work, and can also be worn at night, during sleep. Wearing them at night is important, because at night your circulation declines, further starving your median nerve of the oxygen and nutrients it needs for healing.

Another simple device that helps relieve pain and pressure on the wrist is a forearm brace, a narrow cuff worn just below the elbow. These are sold in most drugstores.

A physical therapy that often helps in the early stages of the disorder is application of ice on the wrist, for about ten minutes at a time. This will reduce swelling and inflammation, and break the cycle of pain. An alternative to ice is a cooling pain gel.

Massage can also help. Many people who have CTS have tight muscles in their shoulders, necks, and backs, and this contributes to tension in their forearms and wrists. It's extremely important to stretch your tight muscles as much as possible while you're working.

Another important factor in CTS treatment is to make sure that your workstation is as comfortable as possible. If you operate a computer, you should keep the keyboard level—not elevated— and use a wrist rest. You should sit in a firm, comfortable chair, with both feet on the floor, and your knees flexed.

Many patients with CTS gain considerable relief with magnetherapy. Magnetic devices especially designed for CTS can be worn over the wrist virtually all day long. For details on magnetherapy, see chapter 3.

A final physical therapy for CTS is acupuncture. In some patients, the healing of the median nerve has been expedited by acupuncture.

Nutritional therapy for CTS is limited, but can be helpful for some patients. The most important nutrient for treating CTS is vitamin B_6, which strengthens the sheaths around tendons; this helps keep tendons from swelling. B_6 is also a mild diuretic, and reduces swelling caused by water retention.

There is evidence that CTS is significantly more common among people who have a deficiency of B_6. You may have a deficiency of this vitamin if you are taking birth-control pills, because they deplete B_6. I recommend that CTS patients take 300 mg of B_6 daily for approximately three months. After three months the dosage should be reduced to 100 mg daily, because heavy, long-term use of B_6 can harm nerves.

Your B_6 supplementation will be more effective if you combine it with a daily dosage of 100 mg of B_2, 1,000 mcg of B_{12}, and 800 mcg of folic acid. These nutritional co-factors increase the power of B_6.

There are also several medications that may help. Many patients take nonsteroidal anti-inflammatory drugs, such as ibuprofen, to reduce swelling and inflammation. These drugs can be beneficial, but, as I mentioned earlier, they have many side effects. As an alternative to NSAIDs, you should consider some of the natural anti-inflammatory medications that I described in the chapters on my comprehensive pain cure program.

Two homeopathic remedies can also help: *Bryonia* and *Rhus toxicodendron,* which can be purchased at most health-food stores.

Sometimes doctors inject cortisone into the wrists of CTS patients. This is very effective for most patients in the short term, but improvements usually do not last. Furthermore, cortisone has many side effects.

A nontoxic topical medication that has helped many patients is Traumeel. This homeopathic formulation relieves pain and reduces swelling. Other pain gels can also reduce inflammation.

When CTS becomes advanced, surgery is often needed. In CTS surgery, doctors cut one of the ligaments in the wrist, which usually relieves pressure on the irritated median nerve. The procedure is often quite effective, but may not work if nerve damage is severe.

Because the treatment options for advanced CTS are so limited, I strongly urge patients to solve the problem before it reaches this late stage.

TMJ Pain

The multi-modality approach of integrative medicine is *essential* for the effective treatment of pain in the temporomandibular joint, or TMJ. No single, isolated modality has proved to be consistently effective for TMJ disorder, probably because this disorder has a number of contributing causes.

The temporomandibular joint is the point where your lower jaw is attached to your skull. You can feel your TMJ by opening and closing your mouth, while pressing against the joint, which is located just in front of your earlobe.

Problems with this joint, and the muscles surrounding it, are very common, occurring in about half the population. Most people, though, experience only minor discomfort, and never seek treatment for temporomandibular joint disorder. However, about 5 to 10 percent of all people who have TMJ disorder experience significant pain. For some, the pain is so severe that it is disabling.

Although the contributing factors vary from patient to patient, the three most common causes are *malocclusion,* or a poor bite, created by the misalignment of the chewing surfaces of the teeth; *muscular tension* of the jaw, caused by stress; and *trauma,* caused by a blow to the head, or by a whiplash injury.

For many years, most doctors thought that malocclusion was the most frequent cause of TMJ disorder. Now, however, many doctors think that stress is a more common cause. Stress not only directly tightens the muscles of the jaw, but also causes many people to grind their teeth, which can then cause malocclusion.

There are two tests you can do yourself to determine whether you might have TMJ disorder.

For the first test, touch your fingers to your temples, and then clench your jaw. You will be able to feel the muscles in your temples tighten. Then leave your fingers on your temples and relax your jaw. If this causes pain, you may have TMJ disorder, and should discuss it with your physician, manipulation therapist, or dentist.

For the second test, place the tips of your little fingers in your ear canal. Press against the front of your ear canal while you open and close your mouth. If you can feel the top of your jawbone push against your fingers, you may have TMJ disorder, and should mention it to a health professional.

If you do have early symptoms of TMJ disorder, you may be able to relieve your problem without a doctor's treatment. It's important, though, that you do not ignore the problem. If you remedy the problem in its early stages, it may never become a significant source of pain. If you ignore it, though, it may progress in severity, and eventually cause you great pain.

To confirm a diagnosis of TMJ disorder, your doctor may order X rays, a CAT scan, or an MRI. However, these tests may not reveal any structural abnormalities. Nonetheless, if you have chronic TMJ pain, you probably do have TMJ disorder.

Treatment for TMJ disorder consists of relieving the immediate pain, reducing inflammation, reducing muscular tension, improving the alignment of the teeth, and stopping the behaviors that contribute to the clenching of the jaw.

A number of techniques temporarily relieve pain and inflammation in muscles and tendons. I described these techniques in the chapters on my comprehensive pain program, so please review that material. In addition, there are several techniques that are specifically helpful for TMJ disorder. One of these is to apply a hot towel to the jaw area, while massaging the jaw. Another is to do isometric jaw exercises, which strengthen the jaw muscles, and also relieve tension in the jaw. For example, you can push your hand against your chin, while resisting the pressure with your jaw muscles.

You may also be able to improve TMJ disorder symptoms by carefully monitoring the level of physical tension in your jaw, and avoiding the activities and behaviors that increase this tension. You should make a concerted effort to refrain from clenching your jaw when you feel stress.

Another valuable approach is use of mouth guards and bite plates. Mouth guards are soft plastic molds that prevent the clenching of the jaw. Many patients wear these during sleep, when they are unable to consciously avoid clenching their jaws. Bite plates are removable, hard plastic dental appliances that fit over teeth, preventing jaw clenching and teeth grinding. These are typically worn throughout the day, except during meals.

Some dentists make bite plates that are designed to not only prevent jaw clenching, but also to properly align the surfaces of the teeth, and improve malocclusion. Occasionally, dentists will also grind down teeth that are exceptionally high, to improve malocclusion.

In severe cases, surgery is needed. However, surgery is not always effective, and can even make the problem worse. I generally do not advise it.

Sometimes doctors inject a local anesthetic, such as procaine, into the most painful areas, and then massage the jaw muscles while the muscles are still numb.

Some doctors inject inflamed TMJ areas with corticosteroids. I generally do not administer steroids, because of their side effects.

Massage without anesthesia can also be helpful. If you use massage, don't confine the massage to the jaw area. You should also focus on your neck, shoulders, and back, because tension in these areas can contribute to tension in the jaw.

Another very helpful approach is to reduce inflammation with aspirin, ibuprofen, anti-inflammatory herbs, homeopathic remedies, and specific nutrients. For information on reducing inflammation, please review the chapters on my comprehensive pain program.

A well-designed stress-management program can also be extremely beneficial, because stress often causes and aggravates TMJ disorder. For information on this, please review chapter 5.

Premenstrual Pain

Premenstrual pain is not only a serious source of pain in itself, but can also indicate hormonal imbalances that increase *all* types of pain.

The biochemical imbalances that are symptomatic of PMS include low levels of serotonin. As I've shown, low serotonin levels reduce the pain threshold, and make people far more vulnerable to every type of pain. In addition, low levels of serotonin appear to directly trigger several terribly painful conditions, including migraine headaches and fibromyalgia.

Hormonal imbalances—primarily decreases in estrogen levels—disrupt the metabolism of tryptophan, the nutritional precursor of serotonin. When this disruption occurs, serotonin levels can plummet.

When estrogen levels are lowest—during the days prior to menstruation, during the weeks after childbirth, and during menopause—serotonin levels can become notably decreased. When this happens, many of the symptoms associated with low levels of serotonin occur, including depression, anxiety, vulnerability to pain, craving for sweets, and insomnia.

Therefore, eliminating premenstrual syndrome can have two important effects: it can stop the specific symptoms of PMS, and it can stop the hormonal imbalances that make *all* types of pain worse.

There are a number of modalities that can help correct premenstrual syndrome. Millions of women, including many of my own patients, have employed these modalities, and have significantly enhanced the quality of their lives. To control PMS, it's important to use a comprehensive, multi-modality approach. Too often, women use a relatively narrow approach—such as exercising more and avoiding sweets—and fail to correct all of the causes of the problem.

In fact, one of America's leading authorities on PMS, author Linaya Hahn, the director of the PMS Holistic Center of Illinois, believes that up to sixteen different factors can contribute significantly to PMS. Among the factors she addresses, which are often overlooked in most PMS treatments, are thyroid dysfunction, intestinal parasites, and food sensitivities. For the address of the PMS Holistic Center, see Appendix III.

One extremely important method of controlling PMS symptoms is to elevate and stabilize serotonin levels. If this is achieved, it can end many of the most disturbing symptoms of PMS, including depression, anxiety, and vulnerability to pain. It can also help prevent other conditions that are triggered by a serotonin deficit, such as migraine headaches and fibromyalgia.

Please review the chapters on my comprehensive pain program. Those chapters contain details on nutritional therapies, medications, physical therapies, mental techniques, and mind/body exercises that raise serotonin levels. One of the modalities discussed in those chapters is use of selective serotonin reuptake inhibitors, or SSRIs, such as Prozac. SSRIs can be especially effective for controlling the symptoms of PMS. A natural SSRI, the herb St. John's wort, can also help correct PMS symptoms in some women.

It is extremely important to try to correct hormonal imbalances *before* they disrupt serotonin levels. There are a number of ways to do this. One way is to engage in hormonal replacement therapy. When PMS or menopausal symptoms are severe, doctors sometimes recommend that women take supplementary hormones. For some women, estrogen is helpful, and for others, progesterone is necessary. To determine the proper hormone to take, your doctor will probably need to do a survey of your existing hormonal levels, with a simple blood test.

Another approach to hormonal replacement therapy is to take DHEA or pregnenolone, the precursor hormones that the body converts into sex hormones. These two hormones tend to be significantly safer than estrogen, which can contribute to cancer. Still, they should be taken only under a doctor's direction, after the testing of existing hormonal levels. Although DHEA and pregnenolone generally improve PMS symptoms, they can aggravate symptoms in some women, particularly if taken at the wrong dosage level.

An even safer way to adjust hormonal levels is to ingest nutrients known as phytoestrogens, which are plant-derived nutrients chemically similar to estrogen. The primary food source of these nutrients is soy. It's quite possible that the high consumption of soy products in Asia accounts for the fact that Asian women tend to have markedly fewer PMS symptoms and menopausal symptoms than most women in Western countries. Other food sources of phytoestrogens include legumes, whole grains, vegetables, and seaweed. A major benefit of phytoestrogens is that they also appear to help prevent certain cancers of the sex-related organs. In one study, conducted at the University of Hawaii, women who ate a diet rich in phytoestrogens were 54 percent less likely to develop endometrial cancer than women who ate a standard Western diet.

Phytoestrogens are sold as supplements in most health-food stores. They may be labeled as "soy isoflavone" products.

Hormonal levels can also be corrected by supporting the function of the liver, which helps to regulate the levels of hormones. To improve liver function, it's very important to avoid excessive dietary fat. Animal fat, in particular, disturbs liver function, because the liver must produce the bile acids that digest fats. Many women notice that their PMS symptoms are aggravated by high-fat foods.

The other major dietary stressor of the liver is sugar. Unfortunately, though, many women crave sweets when they have PMS symptoms, because sugars temporarily increase serotonin levels. Many women especially crave chocolate, not only because it's sweet, but also because chocolate contains other chemicals that temporarily improve mood chemistry. Unfortunately, though, chocolate consumption usually soon creates a rebound effect, characterized by heightened PMS symptoms.

The other important dietary factor that hurts liver function is consumption of foods that are highly processed, allergenic, or tainted with pesticides or herbicides.

Other nutrients, however, *improve* the function of the liver. The most important single nutrient for the liver is the B complex of vitamins, and particularly B_6. I recommend that women with severe PMS symptoms take a relatively high dosage of the B complex daily, in the range of 100 to 150 mg.

In addition, calcium and magnesium supplements can help relieve menstrual cramps. I recommend approximately 1,000 mg of each daily. Vitamin E also appears to have a therapeutic effect upon cramps.

One of the most effective nutritional therapies for PMS is use of the Chinese herb *dong quai*. For many centuries, Chinese women have used *dong quai*, which means "queen of the herbs," to help control a variety of menstrual symptoms. The standard dosage is approximately 200 mg daily. Many health-food stores carry this herb, and it can also be purchased from mail-order supplement companies.

Nutritional therapies can help cure another common condition, candida overgrowth, that is aggravated by hormonal fluctuations. Candida is a single-cell yeast organism that is present in everyone. Women usually become aware of candida only when they have a vaginal yeast infection, but candida cells are also found in all of the mucous membranes in the body, including the intestines and sinuses. Therefore a mild yeast infection, or candida overgrowth, can occur in virtually any part of the body. Often this is not noticeable.

The hormone progesterone, which is more abundant during the last half of the menstrual cycle, stimulates candida growth. Many women suffer from candida overgrowth during this time. Candida overgrowth causes symptoms as candida cells die and throw off toxins. When this occurs, it creates a number of symptoms, many of which are similar to those of PMS. Those symptoms include fatigue, headaches, cognitive dysfunction, acne, and depression.

One of the best ways to overcome yeast overgrowth is to eat yogurt with *Lactobacillus acidophilus,* a helpful bacteria that kills yeast cells. Acidophilus can also be taken as a supplement.

Two other nutrients that control yeast are garlic and caprylic acid, both of which are available as supplements.

You should avoid foods that contain yeast, or that stimulate the growth of yeast. These include sugar, fermented foods (such as vinegar, catsup, alcohol, mustard, and soy sauce), aged foods (such as cheese), and foods with yeast (such as bread, cake, beer, or pizza).

It's also wise to eliminate as much household mold as possible, by cleaning bathrooms, kitchens, and basements thoroughly using bleach and other antifungal products.

Another method of controlling PMS symptoms is to use homeopathic remedies. Among the most commonly used are *Belladonna, Magnesia phosphorica, Colocynthis, Chamomilla, Pulsatilla, Sepia,* and *Natrum muriaticum.* Many women prefer to buy a homeopathic PMS formulation that contains a balanced variety of homeopathic PMS medications.

Certain physical therapies can also be valuable. The mind/body exercises can be extremely helpful, and so can aerobic exercise. Daily exercise often has a profound effect upon PMS symptoms, because it helps balance hormones, stimulates the production of neurotransmitters that reduce PMS symptoms, and relieves stress.

Other effective physical therapies for PMS are acupuncture and acupressure. To help relieve cramps with acupressure, place two fingers about an inch below your navel, and press in as you exhale. Then release the pressure, and inhale. Do this for approximately one minute.

Because a serotonin deficit is a key component of PMS, light therapy can be very helpful. Many women report that their PMS symptoms are worse during the short daylight hours of winter. This problem can strongly contribute to insomnia, which is often present with PMS.

For more information on light therapy, see chapter 3.

May the longtime sun shine
upon you,
All love surround you,
And the pure light within you
Guide your way on.

We close each mind/body session with this verse. It is a positive affirmation bringing blessings to all.

APPENDIX I

Mind/Body Exercise and Meditation

The mind/body exercises that I recommend to pain patients are derived from kundalini yoga, a form of yoga that originated in India several thousand years ago. According to experts, kundalini yoga is the most advanced and complete system of yoga developed over thousands of years. It was introduced into America by Yogi Bhajan in 1969.

When kundalini yoga successfully unites the body, mind, and spirit, it greatly enhances the power of the life-energy called kundalini, or prana, and awakens the power of the spirit.

According to the precepts of kundalini yoga, kundalini energy is an incredibly powerful storehouse of psychic and physical energy that lies at the base of the spine. This energy is symbolized as a coiled serpent that sleeps at the base of the spinal column. In fact, *kundal* means "curled."

When this energy is awakened and channeled, by means of kundalini yoga exercises (or mind/body exercises), it ascends through the body, up the spine to the brain, and then is consolidated. When this happens, more kundalini energy enters the body, and the circulation begins anew. The better this circulation is, the more energy the person experiences.

Kundalini energy is roughly analogous to the nerve energy that circulates throughout the body. However, according to the Eastern tradition, kundalini energy is not merely physical energy, but is also mental and spiritual energy. Therefore, abundant circulation of kundalini energy is thought to create not just increased physical power, but also increased mental and spiritual power.

Many millions of people have practiced kundalini mind/body exercises over the past several thousand years. During this time, specific exercises were found to exert specific effects. What follows are various exercises that are particularly valuable for controlling different forms of pain.

Each exercise consists of a combination of specific movements, postures (or poses), *mudras* (or hand positions), and breathing styles (such as long, slow breathing, or the fast, hard "breath of fire"). In addition, most people do these exercises while they repeat spiritual phrases, or *mantras*.

Here are some of the mudras, postures, meditations, and breathing styles that are most frequently mentioned in the following exercises:

BREATH OF FIRE. This style of breathing increases blood circulation to the brain, increases production of the brain's alpha waves, and powerfully enhances mental energy. To do it, breathe rapidly through the nose, without pausing between breaths. Inhale by bringing your diaphragm down, rather than up, and keep your chest relaxed. Focus your mental energy on your navel area. With practice this will become natural.

LONG, SLOW BREATHING. This is the most common style of breathing during mind/body exercises. It is especially valuable for pain patients because it calms the nervous system and reduces the perception of pain. To do it, inhale through your nose until your abdomen is filled with air, and then fill your lungs. Hold the breath for a brief moment and then exhale through your nose, emptying the lungs first, and then the abdomen. Near the end of your exhalation, pull your stomach in, to force out as much air as possible.

EASY POSE. This posture is the most common posture in the mind/body exercises. To do it, sit on the floor on a mat, a sheepskin, or a rug. Cross your legs in front of you. You may rest one ankle on top of the other, or you may keep both ankles on the floor. Keep your back straight. If this posture is difficult for you, you may use a pillow or sit in a chair, as long as your back is straight. Keeping your back straight helps kundalini energy rise up your spine.

GIAN MUDRA. This hand position consists of touching the tip of the thumb to the tip of the index finger.

VENUS LOCK. This hand position consists of interlacing the fingers, with the left little finger on top for men, and on the bottom for women.

SAT NAM. This simple mantra has a powerful connotation. *Sat* means truth. *Nam* is your divine essence, which is absolute, eternal, and real. *Sat Nam* combined means "to feel your true identity."

Often, several mind/body exercises are performed in a *kriya*, or set of exercises.

It is best to do your mind/body exercises before breakfast.

To begin any mind/body set, it is important to "tune in" to your healthiest image of yourself. To do so, chant the mantra *"Ong Namo Guru Dev Namo,"* which means "I bow before my highest consciousness."

Sit in a comfortable cross-legged posture on a mat or sheepskin on the floor, or sit on a pillow if you like. You can also sit forward in a comfortable but sturdy chair. Bring your hands up to your chest in a typical prayer position, pressing the knuckles of your thumbs against your breastbone. Chant the mantra one time per breath, for a total of three times.

Then take about one minute to center yourself and your mind. If you like, you can take longer and use this time to set your pain cure goals. Say an affirmation such as "I am healthy, strong, relaxed, and happy," or simply pray for optimal health, healing, and peace.

Then follow with a basic set or one for a specific problem, such as back pain, arthritis, migraine, or fibromyalgia.

The final two meditations are excellent to do in the evening alone or in a group. They are effective for every person with pain.

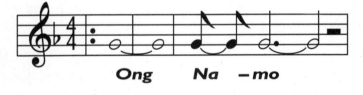

Ong   Na   —mo

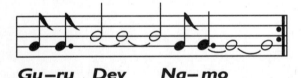

Gu—ru Dev   Na—mo

1. Basic Movement Relaxation and Breath Series for General Pain Control

PART ONE: MOVEMENT

Rhythmic, unforced, graceful, and free movement relaxes your entire body and releases tension. All emotional traumas leave their signature of tension in the body. If these areas of the body are not relaxed, the chronic stress can lead to both physical and mental imbalances. The following simple series is for total relaxation and a cooper ative coordination of mind, body, and spirit to help re- duce pain.

a. Stand straight with the arms completely relaxed. Close the eyes. Feel any tension in each part of the body and consciously let it go. Next, begin to sway and move every part of the body. Dance gracefully, feeling the easy movement of each body area. If there is gentle rhythmic music of a high vibration available, it may be used as a background. Continue for 3 minutes.

a.

b. Immediately stand straight with the eyes still closed. With the hands, begin to lightly feel each part and area of the body without reservation. Every square inch must be touched. Feel sensitively with the palms. Continue for 3 minutes.

c. Lean forward with the arms hanging completely relaxed. All the muscles of the body should relax. Let the breath be normal. Continue for 1 minute.

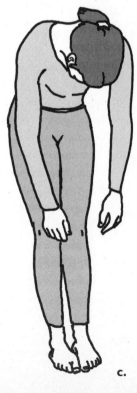

b.

c.

d. Inhale and exhale deeply several times. Next, slowly lean backward with arms hanging loosely down. Breathing is relaxed. Hold for 1 minute. Completely relax.

Feeling the entire body confirms the reality of the relaxation and smooths the area. The remaining exercises strengthen the heart and circulatory system. If this system is weak, then tissues that are tense or are in the extremities of the body and the joints will build up deposits that create pain. True deep relaxation would be difficult.

Please try it, catch the experience, and enjoy enhanced pain relief.

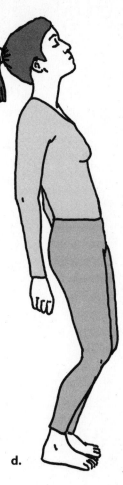

d.

PART TWO: BASIC BREATH SERIES

a. Sit in Easy Pose or in a chair. Cover the right nostril with the thumb of the right hand. Breathe long and deep through the left nostril. Continue for 1 minute.

b. Cover the left nostril with the index finger of the right hand and continue long, deep breathing through the right nostril for 1 minute.

c. Inhale through the left nostril, exhale through the right, using long, deep breaths. Use the right thumb and index finger to close alternate nostrils. Continue for 1 minute.

d. Change hands and repeat exercise c, except inhale through the right nostril and exhale through the left for 1 minute.

e. Sit in Easy Pose with hands on knees, thumbs and forefingers touching, elbows straight. Begin Breath of Fire. Totally center yourself at the brow point. Continue with a regular powerful breath for 2 minutes. Then inhale, circulating the energy. Relax or meditate for 2 minutes, then chant long "Sat Nam" 3 times.

This set, combining movement, breathing, and meditation, is a great way to begin your day. It puts you in a "pain-free" state of mind.

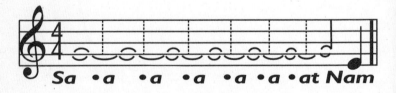

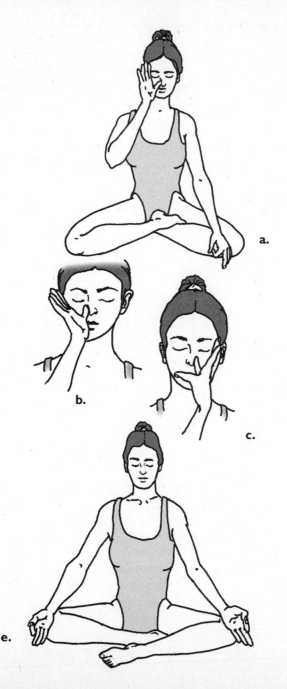

2. A Great Set for Beginners

These two exercises are excellent for relieving stress, and channeling kundalini energy from the body's lower energy centers, or *chakras,* to the highest energy center, in the brain. Both exercises help control pain by building mental energy.

MENTAL ENERGY EXERCISE I

a. Sit in Easy Pose. Place the palms flat together with the fingers pointing up. Put the hands at the center of the chest. Close the eyelids and concentrate through the brow point. Create a positive flow of thought. Focus on your desire to become healthy, happy, and pain-free. Continue 3 minutes.

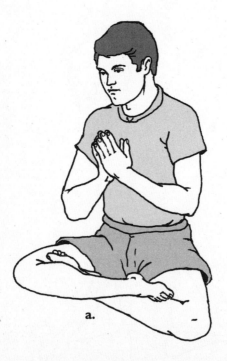

a.

b. Lie down on the back. Point the toes forward. Begin long, deep breaths for 3 minutes. Then relax for 2 minutes.

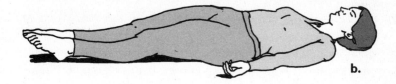

b.

c. Still lying on the back, begin Breath of Fire for 1 minute, then inhale and hold for 15 seconds. Take 8 long, deep, complete breaths. Repeat this entire sequence 3 times.

d. Relax for 2 minutes.

e. Lie on the back. Point the toes forward. Lift both legs 6 inches off the ground, as you inhale deeply. Hold the position for 10 seconds. Lower the legs. Repeat this 5 times.

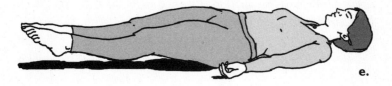

e.

f. Deeply relax the body, part by part, for 10 minutes. Play your favorite relaxing music and let go of all the tension in your body, starting with the toes and proceeding all the way up to your head. Simply say "My toes are relaxed," "My feet are relaxed," and so on.

3. Mind/Body Exercises for General Control of Pain

This is a more advanced exercise, which gives you a definite goal to work toward.

This kriya is named after the energy of the sun. When you have a lot of "sun energy" you do not get cold, and you are energetic, expressive, extroverted, and enthusiastic. It is the energy of purification. It holds the weight down. It aids digestion. It makes the mind clear, analytical, and action-oriented. The exercises systematically stimulate the positive pranic force and the kundalini energy itself. Exercise 1 draws on the "sun" breath and gives you a clear, focused mind. Exercise 2 is for the release of the energy stored at the navel point. Exercise 3 brings the released kundalini energy along the path of the spine and aids its flexibility. Exercise 4 transforms the sexual energy. Exercise 5 stimulates circulation to the head and works on the thyroid and parathyroid glands. Exercise 6 flexes the spine, distributes the energy over the whole body, and balances the magnetic field. Exercise 7 takes you into a deep self-healing meditation. Practice to build the strength of your body, mind, and spirit.

SURYA KRIYA

a. Sit in Easy Pose with a straight spine. Rest the right hand in Gian Mudra on the knee. Block the left nostril with the thumb of the left hand. The other fingers point straight up. Begin long, deep, powerful breaths in and out of the right nostril. Focus on the flow of the breath. Continue for 3 minutes. Inhale and relax.

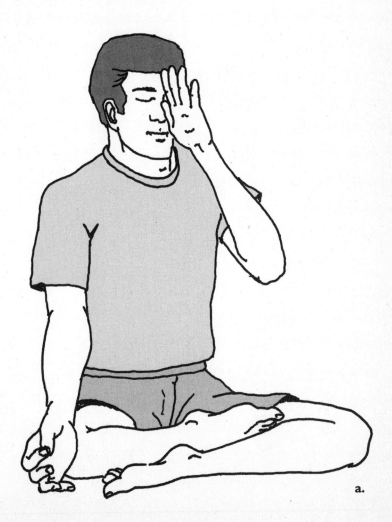

a.

b. Sit on the heels. Raise the arms over the head, elbows straight, palms together. To do Sat Kriya, begin rhythmically chanting "Sat Nam," emphasizing "Sat" as you pull the navel in. Focus at the brow point. Continue for 3 minutes. Then inhale, and hold the breath. Imagine your energy radiating from the navel point and circulating throughout the body. Relax.

b.

c. Sit in Easy Pose. Grasp the shins with both hands. Inhale, and stretch the spine forward and lift the chest. Exhale, and let the spine flex backwards. Keep the head level during the movements. On each inhalation, mentally vibrate the mantra "Sat," on the exhale hear "Nam." Continue rhythmically with deep breaths 26 times. Then inhale, and hold briefly with the spine perfectly straight. Relax.

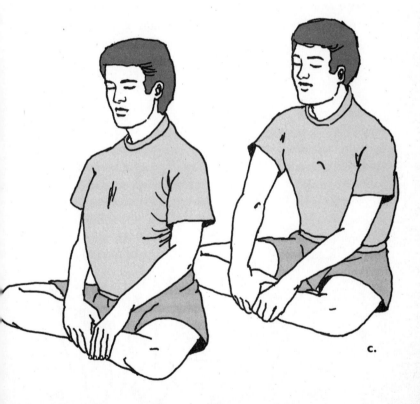

c.

d. Come into the Frog Pose: Toes on the ground with the heels together in the air, place your fingers on the ground between your knees and lift up the head. Inhale, raising the buttocks high while lowering the forehead to the knees and keeping the feet flat on the ground. (Your hands can come up off the ground if needed.) Exhale, coming back to the original squatting position. Go slowly and use your breath. Continue with deep breaths 26 times. Inhale up, then relax down onto the heels.

e. Sitting on the heels, place the hands on the thighs. With the spine very straight, inhale deeply and turn the head to the left. Mentally vibrate "Sat." Exhale completely as you turn the head to the right. Mentally vibrate "Nam." Continue inhaling and exhaling for 3 minutes. Then inhale with the head straight forward. Relax.

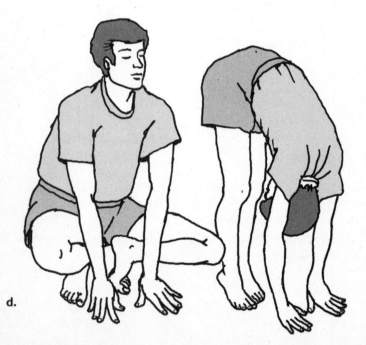

d.

f. Sit in Easy Pose. Put the hands on the shoulders with the fingers in front and the thumbs in the back. The upper arms and elbows are parallel to the ground. Inhale as you bend to the left, exhale and bend to the right. Continue this swaying motion with deep breaths for 1 minute. Then inhale straight. Relax.

f.

g. Sit in Easy Pose with the spine straight. Direct all attention through the brow point. Pull the navel in and hold it. Watch the flow of breath. On the inhale, listen to silent "Sat," on the exhale, listen to silent "Nam." Continue 6 minutes or longer.

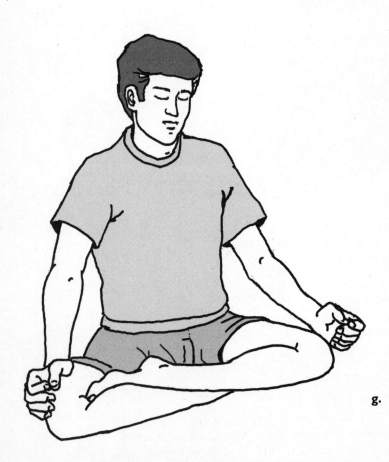

g.

4. Kriya for Back Pain

Do as much as you can without forcing it or overstretching. Take your time and work your way into it. I have used this one myself to help control my back pain over the years.

a. Sit in Easy Pose. Extend the arms up at a 60-degree angle, palms facing forward. Curl the fingertips into the pads of the palms, just below the base of the fingers. Extend the thumbs. Angle the wrists so that the thumbs are pointing straight up and the other fingers are parallel to the ground. Begin Breath of Fire and continue for 1 minute. Then inhale deeply and hold the breath as you bring the thumb tips together above your head. Hold the breath out briefly. Then inhale and relax. *This exercise opens the lungs, and brings the hemispheres of the brain to a state of alertness.*

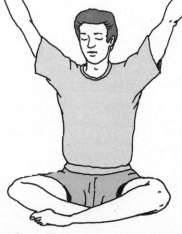

a.

b. Sitting in Easy Pose, grasp the shins with both hands. As you inhale, flex the spine forward. As you exhale, flex the spine back, keeping the shoulders relaxed and the head straight. Continue rhythmically with deep breaths for 1 minute. Then inhale, exhale, and relax. *This exercise stimulates and stretches the lower and mid-spine.*

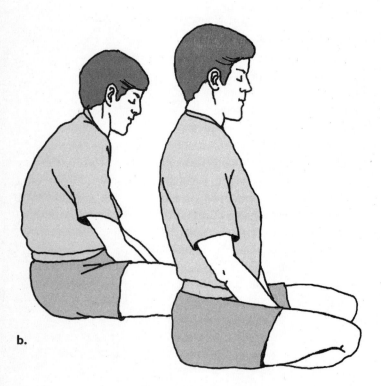

b.

c. In Easy Pose, place the hands on the shoulders, arms parallel to the ground, with the thumbs in back and the fingers in front. Inhale as you twist the head and torso to the left. Exhale as you twist to the right. Continue for 1 minute, then inhale, facing straight forward. Exhale and relax. *This exercise stimulates and stretches the lower and mid-spine.*

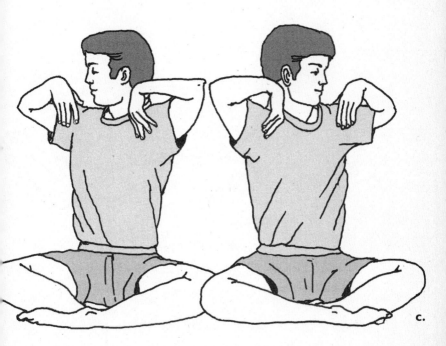

c.

d. Stretch both legs straight out in front. Grasp the big toe of each foot by locking the index finger around the toe and pressing the thumb against the toenail. (If you cannot reach the toes, grab the ankles, calves, or knees.) Inhale and stretch the spine straight, pulling back on the toes and keeping the knees straight. Exhale and bend forward, pulling the elbows to the ground and the head to the knees. Continue with deep, powerful breathing for 1 minute. Inhale, and hold the breath briefly. Exhale completely, holding the breath out briefly. Inhale and relax. *This exercise works on the lower and upper spine.*

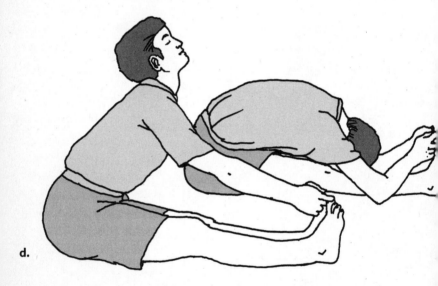

d.

e. Sit on the right heel with the left leg extended forward. (If you cannot sit on the heel, use Easy Pose, with one leg extended. If in a chair, simply straighten your leg.) Grasp the big toe of the left foot with both hands, applying pressure against the toenail. Bring the elbows to the ground and the head to the knee. Begin Breath of Fire. Continue for 1 minute. Inhale. Exhale and stretch the head and torso forward and down. Hold the breath out briefly. Inhale and switch legs. Repeat the exercise, using the opposite side. Relax. *This exercise helps elimination, stretches the sciatic nerve, and brings circulation to the upper torso.*

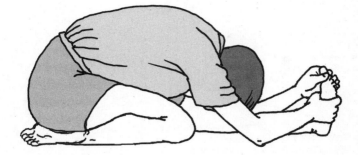

e.

f. Spread the legs wide, and grasp the toes. (If you cannot reach your toes, place your palms on your knees.) Inhale and stretch the spine straight, pulling back on the toes. Exhale. Bending at the waist, bring the head down to the left knee. Inhale, in the center position, and exhale, bringing up the head to the right knee. Continue with powerful breathing for 1 minute. Then inhale in the center position and exhale, bending straight forward from the waist, bringing the forehead toward the floor. Continue this up-and-down motion for 1 minute, then inhale up, stretching the spine straight. Exhale, bringing the forehead down toward the floor. Hold the breath out briefly as you stretch forward and down. Inhale and relax. *This exercise develops flexibility of the lower spine and sacrum.*

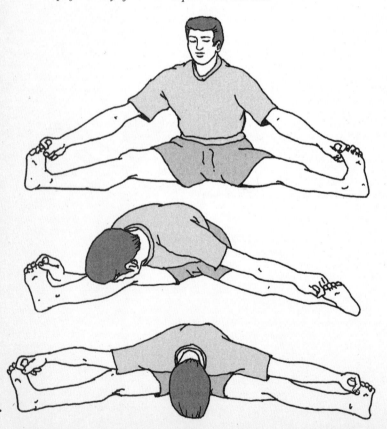

f.

g. Lie on the stomach, with the palms flat on the floor under the shoulders. The heels are together, with the soles of the feet facing up. Inhale, arching the back from the neck to the base of the spine, until the arms are straight, with the elbows locked. (Some chronic pain patients may find it easier to rest the forearms on the ground while stretching.) Begin Breath of Fire. Continue for 30 seconds. Then inhale, arching the spine to the maximum. Exhale and hold the breath out briefly. Inhale. Exhale slowly, lower the arms and relax the spine, from the base of the spine to the top. Relax, lying on the stomach with the chin on the floor and the arms by the sides. *This exercise balances energy, so that the kundalini energy can circulate to the higher centers in the following exercises.*

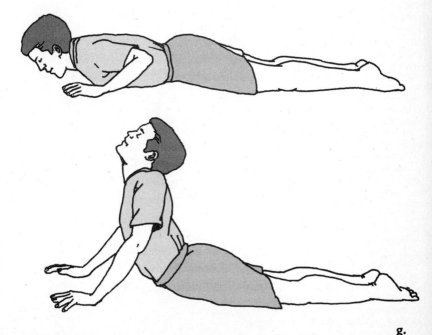

g.

h. Sit in Easy Pose. Place the hands on the knees. Inhale and
shrug the shoulders up toward the ears. Exhale and drop the
shoulders down. Continue rhythmically with powerful breathing for 1 minute. Inhale. Exhale and relax. *This exercise balances
the upper chakras and brings energy to the higher brain centers.*

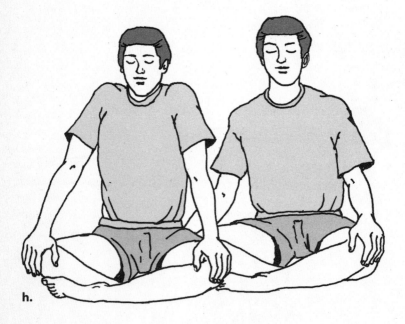

h.

i. Sit in Easy Pose. Begin rolling the neck slowly clockwise in a circular motion. The shoulders remain relaxed and motionless, and the neck should be allowed to gently stretch as the head circles around. Continue for 1 minute, then reverse the direction and continue for 1 minute more. Bring the head to a central position and relax.

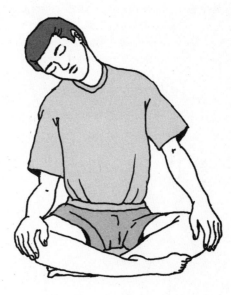

i.

j. Sit on the heels in the position that is pictured. (You may also sit in Easy Pose or in a chair.) Stretch the arms over the head so that the elbows hug the ears. Interlock the fingers, except for the index fingers, which are pressed together and pointed up. Begin to chant "Sat Nam" emphatically, in a constant rhythm, about 8 times per 10 seconds. Chant the sound "Sat" from the navel point and solar plexus, and pull the navel toward the spine. On "Nam," relax the navel. Continue for 1 minute, then inhale and squeeze the muscles tight from the buttocks all the way up the back, past the shoulder. Mentally allow the energy to flow through the top of the skull. Exhale. Inhale deeply. Exhale completely and hold. Inhale and relax. *This exercise circulates the kundalini energy through the cycle of the chakras, and strengthens the nervous system.*

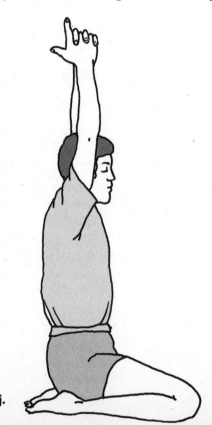

j.

k. Relax in Easy Pose, with the arms at the sides, palms up, in Gian Mudra. *Deep relaxation allows you to enjoy and consciously integrate the mind/body changes which have been brought about during the practice of this kriya. It allows you to sense the extension of the self, and allows the physical body to deeply relax.*

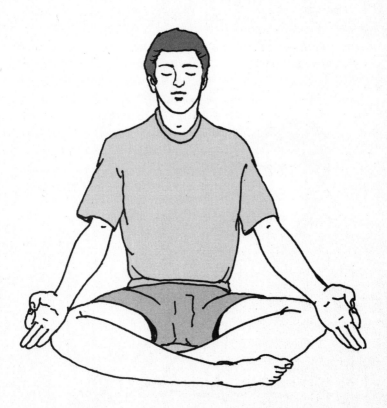

5. Mind/Body Exercises for Arthritis

This kriya, or set of exercises, enhances the function of the endocrine system, and helps build mental energy. It is effective for arthritis because it diminishes the perception of pain signals from all of the body's joints.

BREATH MEDITATION SERIES

a. Sit in Easy Pose. Break your inhale into 4 sniffs. On the first sniff mentally vibrate "Sa," on the second "Ta," on the third "Na," and on the fourth "Ma." When you exhale, break the breath 4 times, again mentally vibrating "Sa, Ta, Na, Ma," as before. With this continuous breathing, pull in the navel point slightly with each sniff. Start with 5 minutes of practice. Then add 1 minute each day, to a maximum of 11 minutes.

a.

b. Lie on the back. Put the arms straight overhead on the ground, with the palms up. Inhale, and raise both legs 6 inches. Exhale, and let the legs down and press the chin to the chest. Continue with long, deep breathing for 3 minutes, then rest for 2 minutes.

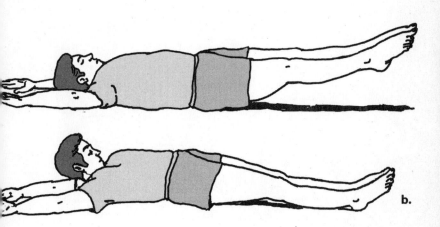

b.

c. Sit in Easy Pose. Grasp your elbows with the arms across the chest. Inhale, and raise to a sitting position. Exhale, and bend forward, gently getting your forehead as close to the ground as possible without tipping over. Take your time. Continue for 1 minute with long, deep breaths.

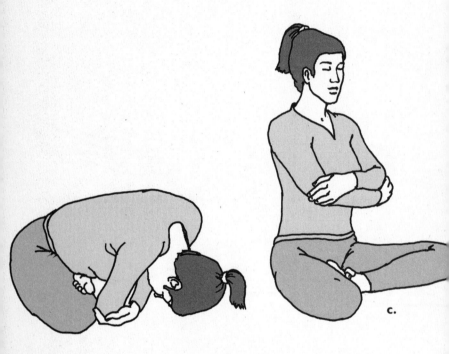

c.

6. Mind/Body Exercises for Headaches

These exercises are effective for tension headaches, and are especially valuable for migraines. They increase blood circulation to the brain, and help stop the vascular contraction that triggers migraines. They also promote release of the neurotransmitter serotonin, which is generally depleted in migraine patients.

HEADACHE EXERCISE I

Sit in Easy Pose, hands in Gian Mudra, arms straight, at a 60-degree angle. Close your eyes and tilt your head slightly backward. Hold the posture with normal breathing for 3 minutes. (You can lower your arms and then bring them back up.) Then relax the hands, rest them on the knees, and chant, in a monotone, "We are the love," for 2 minutes.

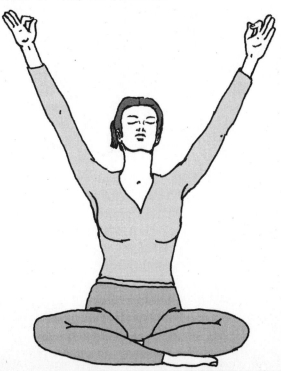

Headache Exercise II

Sit in Easy Pose. Place the hands on the knees. Rotate the shoulders either forward or backward for 3 minutes. Do your best to get maximum rotation—forward, up, back, and down.

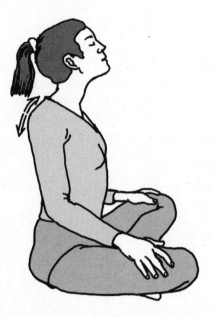

7. Mind/Body Exercises for Fibromyalgia

These two exercises soothe painful muscles by creating deep relaxation, and correcting imbalances of the endocrine system. The exercises also build mental energy, and thus help raise the pain threshold.

FIBROMYALGIA EXERCISE I

Sit in a comfortable meditative posture, spine straight. Place your ring fingers together and interlace all the other fingers, right thumb on the top. Hold your hands several inches out from your diaphragm, with the ring fingers pointed upward at a 60-degree angle.

Close your eyes. Inhale deeply and powerfully. Exhale as you chant out loud the mantra *ONG* ("ooonnnnnnnnnnnnng"), which means "creative healing energy." Keep your mouth open, but let all the air flow through your nose as you chant. The sound is vibrated at the back part of the upper mouth.

Continue for 3 minutes.

The power of this chant, when correctly done, must be experienced to be believed. Only *5 repetitions* are enough to help overcome pain.

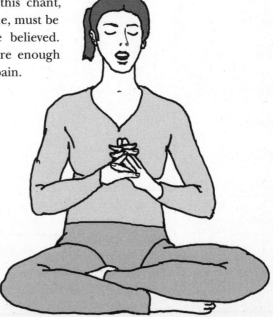

Fibromyalgia Exercise II

Sit in Easy Pose. Arch the arms up over the head, with the palms down. If you are a male, put the right palm on top of the left. Females put the left palm on top of the right. Put the thumbtips together with thumbs pointing back. The arms are bent at the elbows slightly. Keep the eyelids open slightly and look down toward the upper lip.

Chant the mantra "Wahe Guru." Form the sounds with the lips and tongue very precisely. Whisper it so that the "Guru" is almost inaudible. It takes about two and a half seconds per repetition. Continue for 1 to 3 minutes. "Wahe" is an expression of ecstasy, and "Guru" means "divine inner teacher"; taken together, "Wahe Guru" means "from darkness to light."

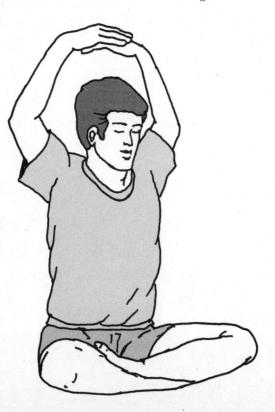

8. Meditations for Relief from Suffering

The following two meditations can be extraordinarily power-ful when they are chanted with conviction and focus.

The first meditation was the primary meditation used by my patient Scott, the supposedly "incurable" polymyositis patient whose story is told in chapter 1.

Scott credited this meditation for much of his healing.

RAA MAA DAA SAA MEDITATION TO HEAL SELF OR OTHERS

Sit in Easy Pose, elbows in snug at your sides, forearms snug against your upper arms, fingers together and pulled down and out so that the palms are parallel with and facing the ceiling.

Close your eyes nine-tenths.

Inhale completely, then exhale completely as you chant the following mantra.

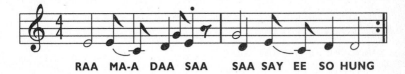

RAA   MA-A   DAA   SAA   SAA SAY   EE   SO HUNG

As you chant "Saa," the navel point is pulled in, so that this syllable is abbreviated. The other syllables are drawn out in a strong, powerful chant that uses all the breath with each repetition of the mantra. Project your voice in a full, conscious sound throughout the meditation.

Continue for 11 minutes. Very gradually, the time may be increased to a maximum of 31 minutes.

Translation: "The healing power of the universe is in every cell of my body." Imagine a glowing green light around yourself as you meditate. If you want to share healing energy with someone else, imagine the same light around them.

This other powerful meditation was used by Tiffany, my patient who had been paralyzed, but who partially regained use of her legs. Tiffany believed that much of her miraculous recovery stemmed from the energy and peace she gained from doing this meditation every day.

This meditation is wonderful, and Yogis believed it to work miracles. It was given by Guru Ram Das, a well-known Indian healer and teacher of the seventeenth century. To this day the Golden Temple in Amritsar, India, which he built, is visited by millions of people of all traditions and faiths who wish to meditate and invoke healing in themselves. Guru Ram Das was a master of Raj Yoga, the Yoga of Kings, as well as the kundalini yoga form I have presented in this book.

Wahe is an expression of ecstasy, and *Guru* means "divine inner teacher."

GURU RAM DAS:
RHYTHMIC HARMONY FOR HAPPINESS AND HEALING

Sit in a peaceful, meditative pose. Keep the eyes one-sixteenth open. Men take the left hand and form Shuni Mudra with the thumb and middle finger. With the right hand, join the thumb to the tip of the ring finger. (Women take the right hand and form Shuni Mudra with the thumb and middle finger. With the left hand, join the thumb to the tip of the ring finger.) Rest the hands on the knees. Chant, in a soft monotone.

GURU GURU WAHE GURU
GURU RAM DAS GURU

Each repetition takes about 8–10 seconds. Continue for 11 minutes in the beginning. You can expand the time to 30 minutes as you progress.

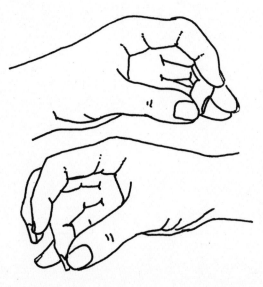

APPENDIX II

Strength Training

Following are illustrations of a weight-training program designed for my pain patients by Nordine Zouareg, M.A., a two-time Mr. Universe bodybuilding champion. Mr. Zouareg, who is my own personal trainer, is extremely skilled at devising strength-training programs that isolate particular muscle groups, without disturbing the delicate structural balance of the overall musculoskeletal system.

I advise patients to focus primarily on only one or two muscle groups during each workout. This allows each muscle group to recover fully before it is exercised again.

For the most part, I recommend that patients use a comfortable weight, and do twelve repetitions. This helps to avoid strain, and still significantly increases muscle mass.

Patients with back pain should also note the exercises found in chapter 8, which also contains an illustration showing the locations of the muscles referred to in this section.

Back

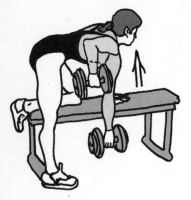

SINGLE-ARM DUMBBELL ROW
MIDDLE LATISSIMUS DORSI MUSCLES ("LATS")

Free arm is used to support the entire upper body, eliminating lower-back strain. Pull the dumbbell up into the midsection and lower until the arm is extended all the way down.

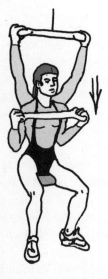

PARALLEL-GRIP PULLDOWN
LAT BELLY

Use a parallel-grip bar, while seated. Pull the bar downward from the arms-straight-overhead position until it is touching the upper chest. Allow the bar to pull back upward, and repeat the movement.

CLOSE-GRIP PULLDOWN
LOWER LATS

Pull the bar down to the front of the chest as shown, tensing your back as you do so. Allow the arms to straighten, and repeat.

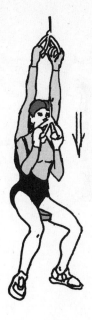

DEADLIFT
LOWER AND OVERALL BACK

Bend over a barbell with your feet apart. Grip the barbell, straighten the back, bend the knees, and pull the bar upward as you straighten to standing position. Keep your head up throughout the exercise.

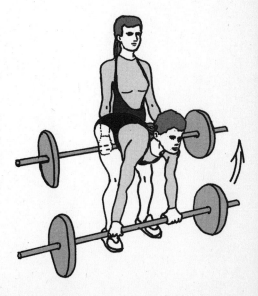

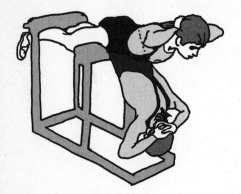

PRONE HYPEREXTENSION
LOWER BACK

This is performed on an exercise unit especially designed for the job. Your upper body will be free to bend upward and downward. Bring the body parallel to the floor.

Legs

SQUAT
ENTIRE THIGH AREA

Hold a barbell behind your neck. Breathe in deeply before squatting. Keep your back flat and your head up throughout the movement. Breathe out forcefully as you raise up.

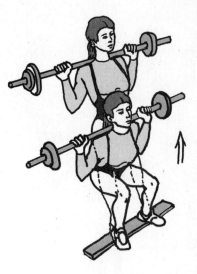

LUNGE
THIGHS, HIPS, BUTTOCKS

Place a barbell across your shoulders. Step forward 2–3 feet with your right leg, keeping your left leg slightly bent. When your right foot touches the floor, bend that leg as fully as possible. Return to original starting position and repeat the action with the left leg.

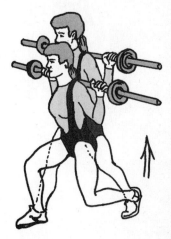

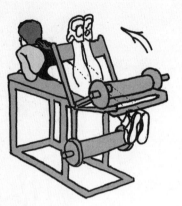

LEG CURL
THIGH BICEPS

Lie on a thigh-curl machine, facedown. Hook your heels under the lift bar and curl your legs upward. Concentrate on feeling the tension in the back of your legs.

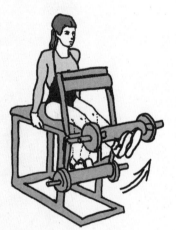

THIGH EXTENSION
LOWER AND MIDDLE THIGH

Sit on the thigh extension machine with the tops of your feet secured under the lift pad. Raise the weight by extending both legs.

Arms

STANDING DUMBBELL PRESS
FRONT AND SIDE SHOULDERS

While in the standing position, hold two dumbbells at the shoulders. Press both dumbbells simultaneously to the overhead position. Lower and repeat, with a steady rhythm.

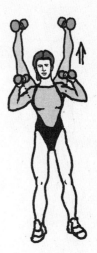

UPRIGHT ROW
SIDE DELTOIDS

Use a grip from narrow to fairly wide. Maintain an upright stance, with feet comfortably apart. Start your pull slowly, and keep your elbows as high as possible, gathering momentum as the weight rises to your chin area. Slowly lower the weight to the straight arm position.

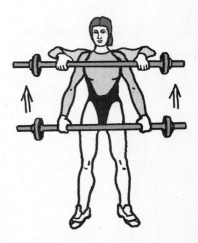

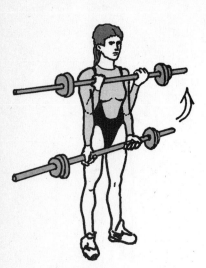

BARBELL CURL
BICEPS BELLY

While in the standing position, hold the bar slightly wider than shoulder width. Keep the elbows close to your body as you curl the weight upward, until it is under your chin.

STANDING TRICEPS STRETCH
LOWER TRICEPS

Hold the weight, as illustrated, behind the head. Keep your elbows pointing skyward as much as possible. Raise and lower the weight rhythmically, without bouncing it at the bottom of the exercise.

SINGLE-ARM LYING TRICEPS STRETCH
OUTSIDE TRICEPS HEAD

Lie on your back on a flat bench, with feet firmly on the floor. Hold a dumbbell in your right hand, at arm's length above your chest. Keeping the upper arm as vertical as possible, bend your elbow to lower the dumbbell to your left shoulder. Raise steadily and repeat. Perform the same movement with the left arm. Do not bounce the weight.

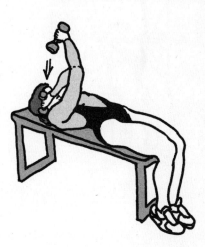

Chest

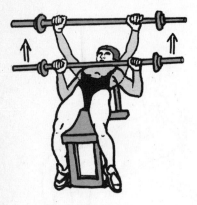

BENCH PRESS
OVERALL PECTORAL AREA

Lie faceup on a bench. Lower the weight from the straight-arm position to the pectorals. Control its descent deliberately. Touch the bar lightly on the chest (no bouncing) and press upward. Keep your elbows under the bar, and don't allow them to come close to the body.

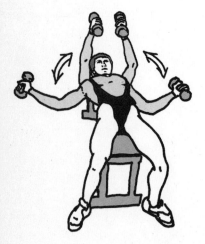

SUPINE FLY
OUTER PECTORALS

Lie faceup on a bench, with your feet planted firmly on the ground. Arms are bent in a fixed position, as though they were in a plaster cast. Lower and raise the dumbbells out to the side.

PEC-DECK FLY
OVERALL CHEST

Hold the "grippers" as indicated, and cross arms over chest by contracting the pectorals. Return to the starting position.

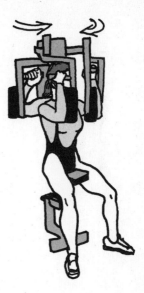

Appendix III

Resources and Referrals

If you would like to inquire about The Pain Cure Seminar Consultation Program please contact:

Dharma Singh Khalsa, M.D.
G.R.D. Center for Medicine and Humanology
P.O. Box 943
Santa Cruz, NM 87567
(800) 326-1322 or (505) 995-2086
Fax: (505) 747-3496
E-mail: healthnow@grdcenter.org

Informational Agencies

For a comprehensive list of certified pain clinics in your area:

American Academy of Pain Management
Richard S. Weiner, Ph.D.
13943 Mono Way, #A
Sonora, CA 95370
(209) 533-9744

For information concerning multidisciplinary pain clinics and academic pain-management programs:

American Academy of Pain Medicine
4700 W. Lake Avenue
Glenview, IL 60025-1485
(847) 375-4731
Fax: (847) 375-4777
E-mail: aapm@amctec.com

For a physician acupuncturist in your area who was trained at UCLA and is certified by the American Academy of Medical Acupuncture:

American Academy of Medical Acupuncture
5820 Wilshire Boulevard, Suite 500
Los Angeles, CA 90036
(213) 937-5514
Fax: (213) 937-0959

For the name of a nearby holistic practitioner who will follow principles similar to those described in this book:

American Holistic Medical Association
6728 Old McLean Village Drive
McLean, VA 22101
(703) 556-9728

A clearinghouse for alternative medical therapies (information available about funding of research):

U.S. Office of Alternative Medicine
National Institutes of Health
9000 Rockville Pike, Bldg. 31, Room 5B-38
Bethesda, MD 20892
(301) 402-2466

For information on mind/body exercises, and for referral to a certified mind/body exercise therapist in your area:

International Kundalini Yoga Teachers Association
Rt. 2, Box 4, Shady Lane
Espanola, NM 87532
(505) 753-0423
Fax: (505) 753-5982
Website: www.yogibhajan.com
E-mail: ikyta@newmexico.com

For information about conferences, and for updated material on anti-aging medicine; also to find a board-certified anti-aging medical practitioner in your area:

American Academy of Anti-Aging Medicine
1341 W. Fullerton, Suite 111
Chicago, IL 60614
(773) 528-4333
Fax: (773) 528-5390

For information about a comprehensive program for PMS:

PMS Holistic Center
Linaya Hahn
942 Twisted Oak Lane
Buffalo Grove, IL 60089
(847) 520-3822
Website: www.pmsholistic.com

For information about new research on myotherapy:

Myotherapy
Bonnie Prudden
7800 E. Speedway Boulevard
Tucson, AZ 85710
(800) 221-4634

For information about the deep, structure-enhancing physical therapy known as rolfing:

The Rolf Institute of Structural Integration
205 Canyon Boulevard
Boulder, CO 00302
(800) 530-8875

For a referral to a chiropractic physician near you, and for research on chiropractic:

American Chiropractic Association
1701 Clarendon Boulevard
Arlington, VA 22209
(703) 276-8800

For information about naturalistic cancer therapies, some of which may be considered controversial:

Cancer Control Society
Lorraine Rosenthal
2043 N. Berendo Street
Los Angeles, CA 90027
(213) 663-7801

For objective, well-documented research on the medical application of herbs:

American Botanical Council
Post Office Box 201660
Austin, TX 78720
(512) 331-8868
Fax: (512) 331-1924

For information on homeopathy:

National Center for Homeopathy
801 N. Fairfax St.
Suite 306
Alexandria, VA 22314
(703) 548-7790

Recommended Reading

Gayle Backstrom, with Dr. Bernard R. Rubin, *When Muscle Pain Won't Go Away* (Dallas: Taylor Publishing Co., 1992).

Roger Cady, M.D., and Kathleen Farmer, Psy.D., *Headache Free* (New York: Bantam Books, 1996).

Ellen Mohr Catalano, M.A., and Kimeron N. Hardin, Ph.D., *The Chronic Pain Control Workbook* (Oakland, Calif.: New Harbinger Publications, 1996).

Margaret A. Caudill, M.D., Ph.D., *Managing Pain Before It Manages You* (New York: The Guilford Press, 1995).

Leon Chaitow, *The Natural Book of Pain Relief* (New York: Harper-Collins, 1993).

Paul Davidson, M.D., *Chronic Muscle Pain Syndrome* (New York: Berkley Books, 1990).

Theresa Digeronimo, *The Natural Way of Healing Chronic Pain* (New York: Dell, 1995).

Larry Dossey, M.D., *Prayer Is Good Medicine* (Harper San Francisco, 1996).

Dr. Joe M. Elrod, *Reversing Fibromyalgia* (Pleasant Grove, Utah: Woodland Publishing, 1997).

Gerard Guillory, M.D., *I.B.S.: A Doctor's Plan for Chronic Digestive Troubles* (Vancouver, B.C.: Hartley & Marks, 1996).

Carol Hart, *Secrets of Serotonin* (New York: St. Martin's Press, 1996).

Dharma Singh Khalsa, M.D., with Cameron Stauth, *Brain Longevity: The Breakthrough Medical Program that Improves Your Mind and Memory* (New York: Warner Books, 1997).

Susan S. Lang and Richard B. Patt, M.D., *You Don't Have to Suffer* (New York: Oxford University Press, 1994). Cancer pain.

Stephen E. Langer, M.D., and James F. Scheer, *Solved: The Riddle of Osteoporosis* (New Canaan, Conn.: Keats Publishing, 1997).

Harris H. McIlwain, M.D., and Debra Fulghum Bruce, *Fibromyalgia Handbook* (New York: Henry Holt, 1996).

Alan Pressman, D.C., and Herbert D. Goodman, M.D., *Treating Arthritis, Carpal Tunnel Syndrome, and Joint Conditions* (New York: Berkley Books, 1997).

Glenn S. Rothfeld, M.D., and Suzanne LeVert, *Natural Medicine for Back Pain* (Emmaus, Pa.: Rodale Press, 1996).

Jason Theodosakis, M.D., Brenda Adderly, and Barry Fox, Ph.D., *The Arthritis Cure* (New York: St. Martin's Press, 1997).

Miryam Ehrlich Williamson, *Fibromyalgia: A Comprehensive Approach* (New York: Walker Company, 1996).

Quality Pain Products

For 5-HTP, anti-inflammatory "green foods," turmeric capsules, anti-arthritis nutrients, and other high-quality nutritional products, available by mail order, contact Smart Basics Inc., (800) 878-6520.

For a natural anti-inflammatory product containing the anti-arthritis nutrients cetyl myristoleate and MSM, contact health-food stores or drugstores for Arthri-Gesic. The product, currently unique in the retail marketplace, is formulated by Quantum, Inc., (800) 448-1448; www.Quantumhealth.com.

To import medications from abroad, for personal use only, contact: Baxamed Medical Center, Hauptstrasse 4, 4102 Binningen, Switzerland, 011-41-61-422-1292 (phone), 011-41-61-422-1286 (fax); or Life Extension Foundation, Box 1097-B, Hollywood, FL 33022, (800) 333-2562, Brain@lef.org (e-mail).

For full-spectrum lights especially designed for bright-light therapy: Light For Health, 942 Twisted Oak Lane, Buffalo Grove, IL 60089; (800) 468-1104; www.lightforhealth.com.

For pain-controlling magnetherapy products, contact: Magnetherapy Inc., (561) 882-0092, or (800) 625-9436.

For quality products to promote natural health and nutrition, get a copy of the Ancient Healing Ways catalog by contacting P.O. Box 130, Espanola, NM 87532; (800) 359-2940.

For high-quality natural pain products and specialty nutrients, contact Life Services Supplements, 3535 Highway 66, Building 2, Dept. R.S., Neptune, NJ 07753, (800) 542-3230.

Index

Tricyclic antidepressants, 144–45,
    248–49, 314, 333–34
Trigger point therapy, 101–102
Tryptophan, 65–68, 236, 305,
    307–308, 309, 317, 342
Tufts University, 98, 315
Turmeric, 57–58, 215, 240
Type A personality, 254–55, 300
Tyramine, 228, 231, 236, 249

Ultrasound for back pain, 286–87
Undereating, 51, 75
U.S. Department of Health and
    Human Services, 105, 258, 293
University of Alabama, 305

Valium, 148, 288, 315, 334
Valproic acid, 146
Vanadyl sulfate, 310–11
Visualization, 162, 179–81
Vitamin A, 60, 71, 213
Vitamin B complex, 71, 76, 78, 213,
    238–39, 239, 240, 308–309, 310,
    337–38, 344
Vitamin C, 60, 71, 73, 213, 214, 273,
    310

NSAIDs and absorption of, 224
Vitamin D, 76, 213, 214, 270, 273, 274
Vitamin E, 71, 213, 214
Vitamin K, 274
Vitamins, 308
    see also specific vitamins
Water aerobics, 283
Weight training, 97–99
    for arthritis, 216
    for back pain, 277–81
    the bones and, 98–99, 269
    for fibromyalgia, 312
Weil, Dr. Andrew, 86
Whiplash, 268
Willow bark, 292
Wintergreen, 138

Xanax, 35, 148, 315

Yeast, 345
Yogurt, 55, 333, 345
Yunus, Dr. Muhammad, 305

Zinc, 213, 274, 311